A Comprehensive Review for the Certification and Recertification Examinations

A Comprehensive Review for the Certification and Recertification Examinations

Published in Collaboration with AAPA and APAP

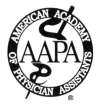 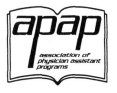

Edited by Sarah F. Zarbock, PA-C

Medical Writer and Editor
Editorial Consultant to the AAPA
Lakeville, Connecticut

Co-edited with Rebecca Lovell Scott

Physician Assistant Program
College of Health Sciences
Roanoke, Virginia

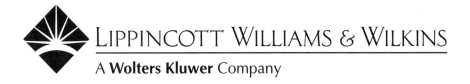
LIPPINCOTT WILLIAMS & WILKINS
A **Wolters Kluwer** Company

Acquisitions Editor: Elizabeth A. Nieginski
Editorial Director of Development: Julie P. Scardiglia
Development Editor: Emilie Linkins
Managing Editor: Darrin Kiessling
Marketing Manager: Debbie Hartman

351 West Camden Street
Baltimore, Maryland 21201-2436 USA

227 East Washington Square
Philadelphia, PA 19106

Printed in the United States of America

Library of Congress Cataloging-in-Publication Data

A comprehensive review for the certification and recertification
    examinations / edited by Sarah F. Zarbock ; co-edited with Rebecca
Lovell Scott. —1st ed.
        p.   cm.
    "Published in collaboration with AAPA and APAP."
    Includes bibliographical references and index.
    ISBN 0-683-30367-8
    1. Physicians' assistants—Examinations, questions, etc.
I. Zarbock, Sarah.   II. Scott, Rebecca Lovell.
III. American Academy of Physician Assistants.   IV. Association of
Physician Assistant Programs.
    [DNLM: 1. Physician Assistants examination questions.   W 18.2
C738 1999]
R697.P45C66   1999
610'.76—dc21
DNLM/DLC
for Library of Congress   98-32027
                                                          CIP

To purchase additional copies of this book, call our customer service department at
(800) 638-3030 or fax orders to **(301) 824-7390**. International customers should call
(301) 714-2324.

99 00 01 02 03
1 2 3 4 5 6 7 8 9 10

Dedication

To Charlotte and Grace—my constant editorial companions

Contributors

Pamela D. Bailey, MHS, PA-C
Clinical Assistant Professor
Department of Physician Assistant Studies
East Carolina University
Greenville, North Carolina

Jo Hanna Friend D'Epiro, PA-C
Staff Physician Assistant, Court Street OB/GYN
Jordan Hospital
Plymouth, Massachusetts

Patricia A. Francis, MS, PA-C
Assistant Professor
Department of Physician Assistant Studies
Medical College of Ohio
Toledo, Ohio

Eunice E. Gunneson, PA-C
Senior Physician Associate
Orthopaedic Surgery
Duke University Medical Center
Durham, North Carolina

Edward D. Huechtker, MPA, AS, PA-C
Chair
Department of Physician Assistant Studies
East Carolina University
Greenville, North Carolina

Susan F. LeLacheur, MPH, PA-C
Assistant Professor
Department of Health Care Sciences
The George Washington University
School of Medicine and Health Sciences
Washington, D.C.

Charles C. Lewis, MPH, PA-C
Clinical Assistant Professor
Department of Physician Assistant Studies
East Carolina University
Greenville, North Carolina

William H. Marquardt, MA, PA-C
Assistant Professor
Department of Health Care Sciences
The George Washington University
School of Medicine and Health Sciences
Washington, D.C.

Robert J. McNellis, MPH, PA-C
Assistant Professor
Department of Health Care Sciences and Department
   of Epidemiology and Biostatistics
The George Washington University
School of Medicine and Health Sciences
Washington, D.C.

Rebecca Lovell Scott, PhD, PA-C
Academic Coordinator and Assistant Professor
Physician Assistant Program
College of Health Sciences
Roanoke, Virginia

Nancy E. Warik, PA-C
Academic Coordinator
Physician Assistant Program
Cuyahoga Community College
Parma, Ohio

Stan Willenbring, PhD
Assistant Professor
Science and Mathematics Department
College of Health Sciences
Roanoke, Virginia

Francis J. Winn, Jr., PhD
Clinical Assistant Professor
Department of Physician Assistant Studies
East Carolina University
Greenville, North Carolina

Contents

Preface

Taking certification and recertification examinations is a fact of life for physician assistants. First, the certification examination is taken upon graduation from an accredited physician assistant program, and the recertification examination is taken every six years thereafter. The National Commission on the Certification of Physician Assistants (NCCPA), using test data from the National Board of Medical Examiners (NBME) and the experience and aptitude of test-question writers, develops the two examinations and refines them on an annual basis to keep current with clinical practice and medical advances.

Test preparation books have traditionally consisted of practice questions and answers. This format provided the opportunity for both new and experienced PAs to improve their test-taking ability by becoming more accustomed to the testing experience; and by reading the answers and explanations provided with each question, the candidate could learn from his or her successes and mistakes.

This book has similar goals, yet goes one very important step further. Again, using data from the NCCPA and NBME, the book's developers and authors have carefully compiled information and created questions that reflect the content and focus of both the certification and recertification examinations. They are based on the objectives, practice settings, and disease lists identified by the NCCPA.

But in addition to the practice questions and answers this book provides, in a condensed outline format, all of the information necessary not only to take and successfully complete either of the tests but also to use on a day-to-day basis in clinical practice. It can be used as a quick and easy-to-read reference. In other words, this book is a practical, "real-time" educational tool for busy practitioners—a handy resource to be used on the front line of patient care.

The chapters are carefully formatted to give general characteristics of diseases (incidence, pathophysiology, prognosis), clinical signs and symptoms, diagnostic and laboratory evaluation, and treatment. These chapters, and the accompanying questions and their explanations, closely mirror the body of knowledge that is tested on the certification examinations and also needed for the realities of clinical practice. For example, more extensive information and questions are provided in cardiology because patients with cardiac problems present very commonly in practice.

The American Academy of Physician Assistants (AAPA) and the Association of Physician Assistant Programs (APAP) have collaborated closely in the development of this book. This partnership—the first for such a review text—serves to enhance the value and credibility of the book, and to ensure that it meets certification and continuing medical education needs of the PA constituency.

We believe that you will find this book helpful in preparing to take either of the NCCPA examinations. But equally important, we hope that you use this book as a quick and valuable reference in clinical practice. We hope you will make the book a permanent addition to your library not only upon graduation and every six years thereafter, but also on a daily basis for the most important use of all—providing care to patients.

Acknowledgments

Many of my colleagues have been immeasurably helpful in the development of this book. At the top of the list is Rebecca Lovell Scott, who helped identify and sign up an impressive group of chapter authors within the PA profession. She provided me with hours of assistance and encouragement as well as pitching in when the repairs needed to be made. Rebecca has the patience I wish I could call my own, the admiration and respect from her fellow PAs, and the ability to steer a straight course in often choppy waters. I am also especially grateful to Greg Thomas, Vice President, Clinical and Scientific Affairs at the American Academy of Physician Assistants. He helped bring this project to my doorstep and took care of all of the behind-the-scenes activities that are involved in a large publishing project such as this. Of course, I appreciate all of the time and hard work of this text's authors. It is no easy task to pull together and condense such a wealth of information, particularly since all of these authors are busily involved in their clinical practices, faculty positions, and myriad of professional activities. I would also like to give special thanks to the Lippincott Williams & Wilkins editors, Melanie Cann and Emilie Linkins, for their input and perseverance. Their close collaboration with the authors and attention to the many details were invaluable. It has been a true pleasure working with both of them—two of the most steadfast and even-tempered editors with whom I have ever had the good fortune to work.

Test-Taking Strategies

Successful completion of the Physician Assistant National Certification Examination (PANCE) or the Physician Assistant National Recertification Examination (PANRE) is dependent not only on how much you know, but also on your ability to handle multiple choice tests. This book is designed to help you, the potential test-taker, to review the knowledge base required for the PANCE or PANRE and to help you practice those important test-taking skills.

PREPARATION

NCCPA Booklet. The process of reviewing for the examination is best begun months, not days (or hours), in advance. The first step should be a thorough review of the information booklet sent out by the National Commission on Certification of Physician Assistants (NCCPA)* with the registration materials for the particular examination you will be taking. Not only does the booklet list the content areas covered on the examination, but it also sets out seven Physician Assistant tasks with fairly detailed objectives to clarify the depth of knowledge expected and tested on the examination. These Physician Assistant tasks include: (1) history-taking and physical examination, (2) diagnostic studies, (3) diagnosis, (4) health maintenance, (5) clinical interventions, (6) clinical therapeutics, and (7) applying basic concepts. Both the booklets for PANCE and for PANRE include a matrix indicating the percentage of questions on the examination allotted to each task within each organ system. For example, the matrices for the 1998 examinations indicate that 16% of the questions on the examination will cover the cardiac system. Of the cardiac questions, 10% will cover history-taking and physical examination, 15% diagnostic studies, 20% diagnosis,

9% health maintenance, 16% clinical interventions, 24% clinical therapeutics, and 6% applying basic concepts. In addition, a small percentage of questions on the examination involve legal or ethical issues. Reviewing this information gives you a reasonable idea of the range and types of materials you need to review.

Diagnostic test. The next step should be taking some kind of a diagnostic test. This will not only help you identify your areas of strength and weakness in various content areas, but will also serve as a point to start reviewing how to take a multiple choice examination. One excellent option is to take the Physician Assistant Clinical Knowledge Rating and Assessment Tool (PACKRAT)**, developed by the Association of Physician Assistant Programs (APAP) as an aid to Physician Assistant students and new graduates in reviewing for the PANCE. PACKRAT takers receive a detailed analysis of their performance within approximately four weeks of submission of the examination. A self-assessment examination for graduate physician assistants (GRADRAT)*** is now available offering a 300-question self-assessment examination. All questions on the examination are classified according to the sixteen clinical areas and seven task categories on the NCCPA's PANRE/Pathway II content blueprint, and were written just for this examination by specially trained educators and clinicians. Although this assessment tool is geared toward first-time certifiers, graduates coming up for recertification may also take the PACKRAT. Sample questions are included in the NCCPA information booklets. Numerous other diagnostic tests are available in book form or on CD-ROM.

It is crucial to remember that none of these practice tests are designed to predict your score on the national examinations. They are only useful in diagnosing your individual areas of strength and weakness in content knowledge and in getting you into the multiple choice mind-set.

Study. The next step is to create a plan for study. To be successful, your strategy should work around your strengths and weaknesses and anticipate pitfalls. Morning people should try to study in the morning; night owls at night! Save the most intricate or difficult materials for the study time when you are brightest and most alert. Scheduling chunks of time in your busy week and treating them as sacred to studying are essential. It is equally important to schedule time for rest, sleep, recreational activities, and physical exercise.

*The National Commission on Certification of Physician Assistants
6849-B2 Peachtree Dunwoody Road
Atlanta, GA 30328
phone (770)399-9971
**American Academy of Physician Assistants/Association of Physician Assistant Programs
950 North Washington Street
Alexandria, VA 22314-1552
phone (703)836-2272; fax (703)684-1924
www.aapa.org and www.apap@aapa.org
***The PACKRAT and GRADRAT examinations can be purchased directly through SpecWorks, 810 South Bond Street, Baltimore, MD 21213, phone (800)708-7581 or fax (410)558-1410.

Where do you study best? Go there to work, and keep the area stocked with books, journal articles, paper, pencils, and practice tests, so you don't waste half of your "study" time trying to locate your materials. Finally, most study skills experts recommend not trying to study with distractions such as TV or music.

Reviewing Content

This review book is designed to present the essential points in different content areas in an easy-to-use format. However, simply trying to memorize the content is not sufficient for passing the examination or, for that matter, mastering any material for use in clinical practice. Learning theorists have demonstrated again and again that interacting with material is essential for mastery. One good way to use this book is to look at a particular topic heading and, before reviewing the outline for that topic, list everything you remember about that topic. Then, compare your list to the outline, noting areas you need to study and review.

Another essential for mastery is reviewing the material multiple times, and the more different ways you review the material, the better. The key is to work to your own learning style in a variety of ways: making and using flash cards, working with another test-taker to quiz each other, underlining, mentally reviewing after each page, reading each section once a week until the examination day, making up sample examination questions, and talking to yourself about the material. Use acronyms and other mnemonics liberally. It doesn't matter why they work; what matters is that these devices really do help you succeed on the test.

For those areas in which you feel weakest, create your own high-yield outline of information from supplemental texts or review articles in journals. Be aware that textbooks are actually a sequence of lists disguised as paragraphs of helpful language. Maximize your ability to master large numbers of lists by minimizing words. Not all words in a sentence are really necessary. You can start by forgetting the adverbs, for example. A brief phrase for subject is all you need, and the predicate will be implied in the phrase.

Make your books and review articles work for you. Retool them if necessary to fit your way of doing things. Use color coding and memory devices. Essential words in a textbook are usually boldfaced or italicized. But during the review, if you find the book's system of highlighting doesn't work for you, try your own underlining. Underline essential words only. You may even develop a fact-sorting system to complement the examination's task-based system. Color codes seem effective for some people, who underline or mark in margins with different-colored pens.

Both the PANCE and PANRE focus on primary care. Your review should cover general medicine and the basics of such subject areas as emergency medicine, dermatology, gynecology, psychiatry, and orthopedics. A certain proportion of the examination will also cover pediatric and geriatric topics, as well as ethics and legal issues.

"THE ONLY THING TO FEAR . . ."

The next challenge is honing your test-taking skills. Take practice tests regularly during your months of review for the examination. Treat the review questions in this volume as a practice test, for example. But don't take the same test over and over; at a certain point, you will be remembering the correct answer without really having to think about the content. Seeking out and taking a variety of tests not only enhances your body of fundamental knowledge, but also sets your mind at ease for the test itself.

The worst part of tests for many people is clutching—fear of failure. Clutching is self-defeating and unnecessary. Start by reminding yourself that the failure rate on certification and recertification tests is low. Most people pass.

In your own mind, create an image of an assembly-line of work, developing a feel for patterns of questions. This is especially important in multiple-choice tests. Develop a pace of from 45 seconds to a minute per question, and finish a sequence of approximately 25 questions before checking for errors and registering answers on the answer sheet. This will be the method you use for taking the actual test.

Even though examination writers try to disguise their methods, they fall into patterns for which you can and will develop a feel. Finding the patterns of questioning both enables you, the test-taker, to intuit the right answer—or to know which will likely be the wrong answers—and to feel some degree of equality with the test makers.

A new wrinkle in certifying and recertifying is a move on the part of NCCPA toward computerized testing. PANCE is on-line starting in 1999 and PANRE is to be on-line by 2000. Seek out on-line practice tests on the Internet or use the increasing number of tests available on CD-ROM. For technophobes, practicing repeatedly in this modality is essential. Pay particular attention to the instructions that come with the NCCPA materials about on-line testing. They should cover how to change an answer, how to mark a question you are unsure of so that you can return to it later, how to submit the examination, and what will happen if the technology fails. Each on-line or computer-based testing system is a little different, but practicing with different systems increases confidence.

Work on your Attitude

Rather than approaching the test with an "I'll-never-pass-this-thing" attitude, assume you *will* pass it—after all, most people do. Positive self-talk helps: "I'm doing what I need to do to pass this examination;" "I may not know everything, but I know enough to pass the examination;" "Every hour I spend studying is helping me pass this examination." Don't sweat the small stuff and remember . . . it's all small stuff. Remember that one small part of your knowledge base you aren't especially sure of does not mean you don't know anything. Be reassured that you know it all, but may be a little weaker in one or two areas, which count only one or two points on an examination with 300+ questions.

Try not to study when you are tired. That will only convince you of a falsehood—that you don't know or can't remember anything. On the other hand, long naps are probably not the solution. There is no better place to snooze productively than sitting at a desk, resting your head on your forearms, under which is a nice wide and firm textbook. That kind of snooze will last for ten or fifteen minutes, which is all you can spare anyway, and will not create a sleep hangover or ruin your regular sleep time.

Arrive Prepared and Cool

Make sure that you rest reasonably well the night before and eat a breakfast that will stick with you (i.e., not sugary doughy stuff). To spare your bladder, have no more than a couple of cups of coffee.

You should already know where the test site is, because several days before, you drove there and scoped out parking. This trip may be doubly useful: If your test center is in a university or school, you will need a visitor's permit, and you should get one in advance, not just before the test. You have allowed enough time to register, and you have adequate identification with a photo, such as a driver's license, as specified in the NCCPA instructions.

If taking the paper-and-pencil PANRE, you have extra number 2 pencils. You are wearing a watch, borrowed, if necessary. (Do not assume there will be a clock. It probably broke yesterday, and nobody called Maintenance.)

TAKING THE TEST

Now comes the hard part. Just kidding, you've already finished the hard part, which was adequate preparation and keeping rested and cool.

But you will need to go the whole route. Ask questions of the examiner before the examination starts (not during), if you are confused about anything in general. After the examination starts, address questions quickly and efficiently, marking those you can't answer immediately for intelligent guessing. It will help to take a break or two—even a minute or two of deep breathing with your eyes closed—during the test, so you don't clutch and you can recompose your mind.

Dealing with the Questions

Do not let the test questions rattle you. Certification tests contain deliberately difficult questions that have baffled legions of test-takers before and will baffle everybody here today. They also contain new questions that are undergoing analysis for effectiveness. That is to say, they may be lousy questions, but they will be equally lousy for everybody. All you can do is pay attention to what you do know or can guess intelligently.

What Kind of Questions?

Most of the questions, as you are aware (having done many practice tests), are multiple-choice, consisting of a "stem" and plausible "answers." The wrong answers are called, with quaint honesty, "distractors." Read each stem carefully, and

underline key words. Mark your question book unless instructed otherwise, and proceed. Some people prefer to transfer answers to an answer sheet as they go along; others prefer to transfer 10–25 answers at a time. Figure out which system works for you. Remember to check periodically, however, to be sure that you are transcribing correctly. You don't want to reach the end of the examination only to discover that you are filling in an answer on answer sheet 301 when you are actually looking at question 300! (This will obviously not be a problem with computerized testing.)

Some test-takers do particularly well by looking at the stem and trying to come up with an answer before looking at the possible answers. You may try to supply an answer in your own words, but don't do that if it cuts into your efficiency. Remember—a minute per question, max.

Look at all answer options and compare. Eliminate systematically. If the answer contains an absolute such as "only," "never," or "always," that is usually a sign to cast it aside. (But not, of course, if you know it is the correct answer. There are deliberately simplistic-sounding answers that may be correct.) Many test questions contain one ridiculous "outlier," which is readily discarded, leaving fewer seemingly plausible answers. Two or three of these options are wrong, containing slightly misleading information. The remaining option contains the correct answer. Which one is it? You know, because you have studied long and systematically.

Lacking certainty of any sort, guess. A good rule of thumb with guessing is to eliminate any options you know are incorrect, then "go with your gut" about the correct answer. You will not be penalized for a wrong answer unless it is of a certain category monitored for actual medical dangerousness or harmfulness. Some of these would be harmful in the act itself (commission), some by omission (negligence).

Guesswork itself is simple. Of five options, the third (c) is the most likely to be correct, because it has been a favored academic "multiple-guess" hiding place since time immemorial. Second option (b) is second best. Over the years, academics have tried to eliminate this tendency, but not with complete success. Neither of these should be chosen if it is a patent absurdity, because (1) you have too much knowledge and self-respect, and (2) because, again, it may be one of the bad guys—in the "harmful" category.

You should look for words or word roots that occur both in the stem and in the answer. Always allowing for trick questions, of course, this may be a clue to the correct answer.

Some choices can be identified as distractors by their very quality. For example, if an item among the choices seems completely odd, unfamiliar, or strange, it is likely to be wrong. There's always the chance you didn't study something both critical and obscure, of course, but probably not, if you did your homework. Conversely, there are choices that seem impossible not to choose, from common sense or fundamental wisdom. They may be right or they may not—but if they are dead wrong, you should be able to screen against being snared by them through the exercise of basic knowledge of medicine.

Again, as in all the above, that's where a well-practiced and well-rested mind will help.

Can you change that well-practiced mind and if so, how often? Change your mind carefully, no matter what. But you may change your mind on an answer, either on the question section or on the answer sheet. If on the latter, be sure to erase completely. The conventional wisdom about changing answers is that it is better to do it sparingly, if at all. Probably the best advice is to change only if you misunderstood or misread the question or if, as the test advanced, you suddenly realized the impossibility of your answer. Often you store up an information level as you go, acquiring a whole lot more usable knowledge than when you started the examination.

That is part of the good news, so to speak. The other is that you won't need to guess or change your answer if you follow the study advice above.

AFTER THE TEST

After the examination, go out and celebrate the completion of an important milestone in whatever manner suits your personal style. Try to avoid those "re-hashers" who spend hours after the test agonizing over questions to try to discover how many they got right (or wrong). You can't do anything about the ones you got right or wrong, so the best tactic is probably to let go of the test and go on to the next important challenge in your life.

1

Ophthalmology and Otolaryngology

Nancy Warik

I. DISORDERS OF THE EYES

A. Disorders of the globe

1. Trauma

a. General characteristics

(1) Traumatic disorders affecting the globe include **blunt** or **penetrating trauma, foreign body intrusion,** and **chemical burns.**

(2) All management **steps should be taken as soon as possible, especially with penetrating trauma and foreign bodies.** The first step of the history is to **find out when and how the accident, trauma, or burn occurred.**

b. Physical examination

(1) After checking when and how the accident occurred, **observe**

(a) **Orbit** (for edema or hematoma)

(b) **Lids** (for laceration, hematomas, edema, and foreign bodies)

(c) **Pupils** (for irregularity—alert suspicion for ruptured globe)

(d) **Extraocular muscles** (for limited movement—likelihood of ocular muscle entrapment)

(e) **Anterior chamber** (for hyphema)

(f) **Interior of eye with funduscope** (for ruptured retinal vessels, which may indicate physical abuse such as shaken baby syndrome)

(2) **Palpate orbital rim** for irregularity, which may indicate a fracture. If **rupture** of the globe is suspected, **do not palpate.**

(3) **Check for intraocular pressure,** carefully using the Schiøtz tonometer.

c. Measurements should be taken.

(1) **Visual acuity** is tested using the Snellen chart. This is important to establish a baseline; any decrease indicates serious trauma.

(2) **Pupillary reactions** should be checked. Unequal reactions might be indicative of severe trauma to the globe.

(3) **Extraocular movements** are tested. A decrease in movement or unequal movement would indicate laceration to the eye muscles.

d. Treatment

(1) Penetrating trauma

(a) The object **should not be removed.**

(b) The patient should be transported to the **emergency room** for **consult** with an **ophthalmologist** and a **computed tomography (CT) scan.**

(2) Foreign body

(a) The eyelids should be **carefully everted, stained with a fluorescein strip** and **observed with a Wood's lamp.**

(b) An attempt to remove the foreign body should be made, **gently using** a **moistened cotton-tipped swab.**

(c) **Patch** the involved eye and **reexamine in 24 hours.**

(d) A **rust ring on the cornea** indicates **metallic foreign bodies.** These may be **removed with a rotating burr** or the patient may be **referred to an ophthalmologist.**

(3) Chemical burns (acid or alkali)

(a) The eye should be **irrigated with water** for at least **30 minutes.** Use sterile water if available. A chemical burn can continue to cause damage even after flushing.

(b) An **eye shield** should be placed on the eye.

(c) Because an **acid or alkali burn is severe,** the patient should be transported to the **emergency room** or **referred to an ophthalmologist.**

2. Retinal injuries

a. Retinal detachment

(1) General characteristics

(a) The underlying pathogenesis is a **tear in the retina flapping in the vitreous humor.**

(b) The tear usually begins at the **superior temporal retinal area.**

(c) The tear can happen **spontaneously,** or can be **secondary to trauma** or **extreme myopia.**

(2) Clinical features

(a) The patient may report the **acute onset of blurred or blackened vision** that occurs over several hours and **progresses to complete** or **partial monocular blindness.**

(b) The symptoms are classically described as **a curtain being drawn over the eye from top to bottom.**

(c) The patient may sense **floaters** or **flashing lights** at the initiation of symptoms.

(3) **Funduscopic examination** will reveal the retinal tear flapping in the vitreous humor.

(4) Treatment

(a) **Emergency ophthalmology consult** regarding possible **laser surgery** or **cryosurgery** is needed.

(b) Patients with retinal detachment should **remain supine** with the **head turned to the side** ipsilateral to the retinal detachment.

b. Macular degeneration

(1) This disorder may be **secondary to the toxic effects of drugs** such as chloroquine or phenothiazine.

(2) It usually has an **insidious onset** and its chief clinical feature **is gradual vision loss.**

(3) There is **no effective treatment.** If detected early, macular degeneration **may respond minimally to laser treatment.**

c. Central retinal artery occlusion

(1) General characteristics

(a) This disorder is considered to be an **ophthalmic emergency.**

(b) **Prognosis is poor,** even with immediate treatment.

(2) Clinical features

(a) It is marked by **sudden, painless,** and **marked unilateral loss of vision.**

(b) The hallmark on physical examination is a **pale retina with a cherry-red–colored fovea.**

(3) Treatment

(a) **Emergency ophthalmologic referral** is necessary.

(b) A **work-up for valvular** and **atrial thrombus** is warranted to prevent further damage.

(c) **Anticoagulation with heparin** is often used.

3. Cataract

   a. General characteristics

      (1) A cataract is **any opacity of the natural lens of the eye.** It may involve a small part of the lens or the entire lens. The degree of opacification is also variable.

      (2) Cataracts may develop secondary to the **natural aging process, trauma, congenital causes,** or **medication use** (e.g., corticosteroids, lovastatin).

   b. Clinical features

      (1) The **insidious onset of decreased vision** is the main clinical feature.

      (2) Usually **far vision acuity is affected** more than near.

      (3) On examination there is a **translucent yellow discoloration in the center of the lens.**

   c. Treatment involves **intracapsular or extracapsular extractions** of the cataract.

4. Glaucoma

   a. General characteristics

      (1) This condition is defined as **increased intraocular pressure that results in loss of vision.**

      (2) Glaucoma may be **acute** or **chronic.** Types include **angle-closure glaucoma** and **primary open-angle glaucoma.**

      (3) Primary open-angle glaucoma affects people **over 40 years of age,** and is more common in **African-Americans,** and in patients with a **family history** of glaucoma.

   b. Clinical features

      (1) **Angle-closure glaucoma** is an **ophthalmic emergency.**

         (a) **Painful eye** and **loss of vision** are important clinical features.

         (b) Physical examination reveals **circumlimbal injection, steamy cornea, mid-dilated pupil,** and **decreased visual acuity.**

         (c) The **anterior chamber is narrowed** and the **globe is hard** to palpation.

      (2) **Primary open-angle glaucoma**

         (a) This is a **chronic, asymptomatic,** and **potentially blinding** disease.

         (b) It is characterized by **increased intraocular pressure,** which can be measured by a Schiøtz tonometer.

         (c) The **peripheral visual field** has **defects.**

         (d) Cup-to-disc ratios are large.

   c. Treatment

      (1) **Angle-closure glaucoma**

         (a) These patients should be **referred immediately** to an ophthalmologist.

         (b) **Mydriatics** may not be administered to these patients.

         (c) Treatment is by **laser or surgical iridotomy.**

      (2) **Primary open-angle glaucoma**

         (a) Patients need to be **referred** to an ophthalmologist.

         (b) Treatment consists of **miotic drops,** such as pilocarpine, **to decrease the pressure.**

5. Orbital cellulitis

   a. General characteristics

      (1) It is **more common in children** than adults.

      (2) Orbital cellulitis has **several possible causes** including **sinusitis** (see III A), **dental infections, facial infections, infection of the globe or eyelids,** and **infections of the lacrimal system.** Less often, it results from **trauma.**

(3) **Causative agents** in children under the age of 4 years include *Haemophilus influenzae* and *Streptococcus pneumoniae*. In **older children and adults** it occurs **secondary to acute or chronic sinusitis** and may have many possible causative agents.

b. Clinical features. Orbital cellulitis presents with **ptosis, eyelid edema, proptosis, purulent discharge, conjunctivitis,** and **decreased range of motion in the eye muscles.**

c. Laboratory studies

(1) Work-up includes **complete blood cell count (CBC), blood cultures,** and **cultures of any drainage.**

(2) **Sinus radiographs** and **CT scans** may help determine etiology.

d. Treatment

(1) It **constitutes a medical emergency** requiring **hospitalization** and **intravenous antibiotics.**

(2) Antibiotics should be broad-spectrum until the causative agent is identified.

B. Disorders of the adnexa

1. Nasal lacrimal duct obstruction

a. This disorder is **common** in the newborn **after the first month of life,** and occurs when the duct does not open.

b. The obstruction usually **resolves by 9 months of age.**

c. **Treatment** includes **warm compresses** and **massage;** and, if no resolution, **surgical probe.**

2. Eyelids

a. Blepharitis

(1) This condition refers to **chronic inflammation** of the **lid margins** of unknown etiology.

(2) Clinical features

(a) **Vision** is **not impaired** in these patients.

(b) **Eyelashes adhere together.**

(c) The **conjunctiva** is **clear** or **slightly erythematous.**

(d) **Mild pruritus** is present.

(3) Treatment

(a) **Lid scrubs** using **diluted baby shampoo** on **cotton-tipped swabs** are helpful.

(b) **Topical antibiotics** should be used if needed.

b. Hordeolum

(1) **General characteristics**

(a) A hordeolum is an **acute development** of a **small abscess within a gland** in the upper or lower **eyelid** of one eye.

(b) **Types**

(i) **Internal hordeola.** These are due to inflammation and **infection of a meibomian gland,** with **abscess formation** in that gland. They are situated **deep from the palpebral margin.**

(ii) **External hordeola** (commonly referred to as a **"sty"**). These are due to the **inflammation** and **infection of the glands of Moll or Zeis,** with **abscess formation** in those glands. They are situated **immediately adjacent** to the **edge** of the **palpebral margin.**

(c) *Staphylococcus aureus* is the gram-positive coccus that is the **pathogen** for either type of hordeola.

(d) Hordeolum is **not contagious.**

(2) **Clinical features**

(a) Hordeolum is characterized by **acute onset** of **pain** and **edema** of the involved eyelid.

(b) **Increased tearing** and **redness** of the involved eye may occur.

(c) There is a **palpable, indurated area** in the **involved eyelid,** which has a **central area** of **purulence** with **surrounding erythema.**

(3) Treatment

(a) **Warm compresses** should be applied for **48 hours.**

(b) **Topical antibiotics** should be used.

(c) **Incision and drainage (I&D)** may be performed if indicated.

c. Chalazion

(1) **General characteristics**

(a) This is a **painless, indurated lesion deep** from the **palpebral margin.**

(b) It is often **secondary** to a **chronic inflammation** of an **internal hordeolum of the meibomian gland.**

(2) **Clinical features**

(a) The chalazion is characterized by **insidious onset** with **minimal irritation.**

(b) It can become **pruritic** and cause **erythema** of the **involved eye** and **lid.**

(3) **Treatment** involves **referral** to an **ophthalmologist** for an **elective excision.**

d. Entropion and ectropion

(1) **Entropion.** The **lid** and **lashes** are **turned in, secondary** to **scar tissue** or a **spasm** of the **orbicularis oculi muscles.**

(2) **Ectropion.** The **edge** of the **eyelid everts** secondary to **old age, trauma, infection,** or the **palsy of the facial nerve.**

(3) **Treatment** involves **correcting the pathology** if possible, and **surgical repair.**

C. Disorders of the conjunctiva

1. Viral conjunctivitis

a. General characteristics

(1) Viral conjunctivitis is **more common in children.**

(2) **Viral infection in the conjunctiva** is usually caused by **adenovirus type 3, 8, or 19.**

(3) Viral conjunctivitis is **highly contagious. Transmission** is by **direct contact,** usually **via the fingers,** to the **contralateral eye** or other persons.

(4) It can be transmitted in **swimming pools** and it is most common in **midsummer to early fall.**

b. Clinical features. Viral conjunctivitis is characterized by the **acute onset of unilateral** or **bilateral erythema** of the conjunctiva, **copious watery discharge,** and **ipsilateral preauricular lymphadenopathy.**

c. Treatment

(1) Specific therapy includes the **application of topical antibiotics.**

(2) Treatment may also include **concurrent systemic antibiotics** such as **erythromycin** or **doxycycline.**

2. Bacterial conjunctivitis

a. General characteristics

(1) Bacterial conjunctivitis is **more common in adults.**

(2) **Bacterial infection in the conjunctiva** may occur with common pathogens or rare pathogens.

(a) **Common** pathogens include *S. pneumoniae, Staphylococcus aureus, Haemophilus aegyptius,* and *Moraxella.*

(i) Transmission is via **direct contact of secretions** or by **autoinoculation,** from one eye to the other, usually via the fingers.

(ii) The **natural history** of an infection caused by these common pathogens is usually **self-limiting** but can develop into a **secondary keratitis.**

(b) **Rare pathogens** include *Chlamydia trachomatis* and *Neisseria gonorrhoeae.*

(i) Transmission is either by **direct contact** of **eye secretions via the fingers** or **via contact of the eyes with water** in nonchlorinated swimming pools. It can also be **transmitted to a neonate** via vaginal delivery.

(ii) The **natural history** of an infection caused by these rare pathogens is a **severe conjunctivitis** and **keratitis** with the development of **permanent visual impairment.**

b. Clinical features

(1) Bacterial conjunctivitis is characterized by **the acute onset** of **copious, purulent discharge** from **both eyes.**

(2) Patients may have a **mild decrease in visual acuity** and **mild discomfort.** The eyes may be **"glued" shut upon awakening.**

c. Laboratory studies

(1) **Common pathogens**—**Gram stain** should show the **presence of polymorphonuclear cells (PMNs)** and a **predominant organism.**

(2) **Rare pathogens**—**Gram stain** and **Giemsa stain** should show PMNs.

(a) When **C. *trachomatis*** is the pathogen, no organisms will be seen.

(b) When **N. *gonorrhoeae*** is the pathogen, **intracellular gram-negative bacilli** will be present.

d. Treatment

(1) Specific therapy includes the **application of topical antibiotics.**

(2) For the **rare pathogens,** treatment may also include **concurrent systemic antibiotics** such as **erythromycin** or **doxycycline.**

D. Optic nerve and visual pathways

1. Papilledema

a. This condition can be defined as **an increase in intracranial pressure.**

b. **Causes** are numerous but may include **malignant hypertension, hemorrhagic strokes, acute subdural hematoma,** and **pseudotumor cerebri.**

c. **The disc appears swollen** and the **margins** are **blurred** with an **obliteration** of the **vessels.**

d. The patient may be **asymptomatic** or may complain of **transient visual alterations** that last for seconds.

e. Treatment consists of **treating the underlying cause.**

2. **Blurred vision** and **decreased visual acuity** may be caused by lesions to the eye.

a. The **location of the lesions** determines the effect on vision.

(1) **Lesions anterior** to the **optic chiasm** will affect **only one eye.**

(2) **Lesions** at the **optic chiasm** will affect **both eyes partially.**

(3) **Lesions posterior** to the **chiasm** will yield corresponding defects in **both visual fields** of the **opposite side.**

b. The **quality of visual loss** helps determine the diagnosis.

(1) **Transient visual loss** may be **secondary** to a **transient ischemic attack (TIA), temporal arteritis,** or **giant cell arteritis. Temporal arteritis** is one of the more common causes and is characterized by a **tender temporal artery, fever, malaise,** and a **strikingly increased erythrocyte sedimentation rate (ESR).**

(2) **Sudden visual loss** may be secondary to **central retinal vein** or **branch vein occlusion, optic neuropathy, papillitis,** and **retrobulbar neuritis.**

(3) **Gradual visual loss** may be secondary to **macular degeneration, tumors, cataracts,** or **glaucoma.**

3. Strabismus

a. Strabismus is a condition in which **binocular fixation** is **not present.**

b. Strabismus may occur **in one eye** or **both.** A **cover test** or **corneal light reflex test** will reveal this abnormality.

c. **It may be corrected with exercise** or, in severe cases, with **surgery.**

4. Amblyopia

a. Amblyopia is **reduced visual acuity not correctable by refractive means.**

b. It may be caused by **strabismus, or drugs** such as **alcohol, tobacco, lead,** and **toxic substances,** or from uremia.

II. DISORDERS OF THE EARS

A. Hearing impairment (hearing loss) **may be of acute or chronic onset**. It results from either **conductive** or **sensorineural** physiologic causes.

1. **Conductive hearing loss** is due to **impaired transmission of sound** along the external canal, across the ossicles, and through the oval window.

    a. There is an **increased threshold for perceived sound intensity.**

    b. Possible causes of conductive hearing loss:

        (1) **Impacted cerumen** may build up and require removal by either irrigation or the use of a wire loop or cerumen spoon.

        (2) **Acute otitis externa** can also cause a conductive hearing loss because of the exudate in the external canal.

        (3) **Otosclerosis**, which is caused by abnormal new bone formation in the oval window, causes conductive hearing loss and is amenable to surgery.

        (4) **Otitis media** may also cause conductive hearing loss.

    c. A **Weber test** and **Rinne test** are used to help establish the diagnosis.

2. **Sensorineural hearing loss** is any **hearing loss secondary to a disruption in the nerves or the mechanics of hearing.** It has many causes (e.g., neural degeneration, decreased cilia, problems in the ossicles).

    a. Presbycusis

        (1) General characteristics

            (a) Presbycusis is the **most common cause** of sensorineural hearing loss.

            (b) It **occurs with age** in most people, with **men affected more often than women.**

            (c) It may be caused by **noise exposure.**

        (2) Clinical features

            (a) It **usually involves the higher frequencies** and may be **associated with tinnitus.**

            (b) The patient or family members may complain that there is **difficulty in discrimination.**

        (3) Treatment. This type of loss **may or may not be helped with hearing aids.**

    b. Meniere's disease

        (1) General characteristics

            (a) This is a **recurrent** and usually **progressive group of symptoms** including acquired chronic hearing loss, tinnitus, and dizziness or vertigo.

            (b) The **etiology** of Meniere's disease **is unknown.**

        (2) Clinical features

            (a) It is accompanied by **vertigo** and **nausea** and **vomiting.** The attacks may last from minutes to hours, but unsteadiness may last longer.

            (b) The **hearing loss** may abate with each attack but **rarely returns to the pre-attack level.**

        (3) Treatment. Most cases can be **managed with diuretics and salt restriction.**

    c. **Acoustic trauma** (e.g., an explosion or shotgun blast) or **chronic noise exposure** can cause hearing loss.

    d. **Acoustic neuroma** is another cause of hearing loss. It is **more predominant in females** and is **usually unilateral.** The patient may present with **hearing loss, tinnitus, vertigo, and facial drooping.** It is **diagnosed with CT or magnetic resonance imaging (MRI) scans** and the **treatment is surgical.**

3. Drug-induced hearing loss

    a. It may be caused by **streptomycin, kanamycin, neomycin, ethacrynic acid, chloramphenicol,** and other drugs.

    b. The **onset is insidious** and **tinnitus may be the first symptom.**

    c. Hearing loss is **usually high frequency.**

    d. It **may or may not be reversible with cessation of the drug.**

4. Infancy and childhood hearing loss

    a. It may be from **congenital causes** such as **asphyxia, erythroblastosis,** and **maternal rubella.**

    b. It may also be from **acquired causes,** including **measles, mumps, pertussis, meningitis, influenza,** and **labyrinthitis.**

    c. Clinical features include **inattentiveness to mother** or **lack of reaction to noise.**

    d. Treatment involves **correction of underlying causes.**

B. Otitis media (infection of the middle ear)

  1. General characteristics

    a. The pathophysiology involves underlying **poor drainage from the eustachian tubes because of age** (i.e., the tubes may be straight in children) **or a congenital deformity** (e.g., Down syndrome, cleft palate, adenoidal hypertrophy).

    b. Otitis media is **most common in children from 4–6 months old to 2 years old,** but can persist into adulthood.

    c. It is **caused by bacteria in 70%–90% of the cases,** with the most common organisms being *S. pneumoniae, Haemophilus influenzae, Moraxella catarrhalis,* β-hemolytic *Streptococcus pyogenes,* and *S. aureus.*

    d. **In recurrent cases,** it can be associated with **food allergies** or **exposure to secondhand smoke.**

  2. Clinical features

    a. The patient may present with **fever, pain,** and **hearing loss.** The pain and fever are both variable components.

    b. The **eardrum will be immobile** and may appear **erythematous** and **bulging.**

  3. Treatment

    a. First line **antibiotics** include **amoxicillin, clavulanic acid/amoxicillin, trimethoprim** and **sulfamethoxazole,** or **ampicillin.** If the patient is allergic to penicillin, erythromycin or clarithromycin is indicated.

    b. **When medication fails** to heal the otitis media, the patient may need **myringotomy, tympanostomy, adenoidectomy,** or a **combination** of these procedures.

C. Otitis externa (swimmer's ear)

  1. General characteristics

    a. Otitis externa, commonly known as swimmer's ear, is **common in the teenage years.**

    b. The cause is a **combination of mechanical obstruction to drainage of bathing water from the external ear canal** and **an infectious agent.**

    c. Certain conditions may predispose one to otitis externa (e.g., eczema, seborrheic dermatitis, psoriasis). The causative organisms include *Pseudomonas,* Enterobacteriaceae, or *Proteus,* and, rarely, fungi.

  2. Clinical features

    a. Physical signs include **pain in the ear** and **tenderness when traction is applied to the tragus or the auricle.**

    b. **Otoscopic examination** reveals a **canal that is edematous** and **obscured with purulent debris.**

  3. Treatment

    a. Use of **otic antibacterial drops** and **keeping the canal dry** are usually effective.

    b. In diabetic or immunocompromised patients, **malignant otitis externa** may develop, which is an **osteomyelitis of the bones of the ear,** and requires **hospitalization** and **parenteral antibiotics.**

D. Vertigo

  1. General characteristics

    a. **True vertigo** is the **sensation of spinning around in space** or a person's sensation of **objects spinning around him or her.**

b. It is caused by **irritation of the labyrinth** or the **central nervous system, brain stem,** or **temporal lobe.**

c. It **may also be caused by labyrinthitis** (vestibular neuronitis) or **Meniere's disease.**

2. Clinical features

a. Vertigo is usually **accelerated with movement.**

b. It may be accompanied by **nystagmus.**

c. The condition may last from **days to weeks.**

3. The **Hallpike maneuver,** quickly turning the patient's head 90° while the patient is in the supine position, is **used to reproduce the vertigo.**

4. Treatment may include administration of **meclizine** or **diphenidol.**

III. DISORDERS OF THE NOSE, SINUS, AND THROAT

A. Sinusitis

1. General characteristics

a. Sinusitis refers to **any inflammation of the sinus cavities.**

b. It usually **follows an upper respiratory tract infection (URI)** [see Chapter 2].

c. The causative agents are the **same as for otitis media** (see II B).

d. Specific **risk factors** for the development of acute sinusitis include a **recent URI, history of trauma or a foreign body,** either of which can obstruct drainage and increase the risk of infection.

2. Clinical features

a. Pain in the face when leaning forward, green purulent drainage, fever, and **malaise.**

b. Physical examination reveals **tenderness to palpation over the sinuses,** or **opacification of the sinus with transillumination.**

3. Laboratory studies

a. A **radiograph** using the Waters view will reveal **opacification, air-fluid levels,** or an **abnormally thick mucosa.**

b. A CT scan is indicated only in the case of **recurrence** or other complications or **if the host is immunocompromised.**

c. Osteomyelitis, cavernous sinus thrombosis, or an **orbital cellulitis** (see I A 5) are among the complications of sinusitis.

4. Treatment

a. Treatment of sinusitis includes **antibiotics, decongestants, antihistamines,** and **hot packs.**

b. Treatment **should last for at least 14 days** and be **carefully monitored** for any signs of complications.

B. Rhinitis

1. General characteristics

a. Rhinitis refers to **any inflammation of the nasal mucosa.**

b. There are three basic types: **allergic rhinitis, vasomotor rhinitis,** and **rhinitis medicamentosa.**

(1) Allergic rhinitis is a **component of the syndrome of hay fever.** It is immunoglobulin E (IgE)-mediated reactivity to airborne antigens. It occurs in people who have other atopic diseases (asthma, eczema, and atopic dermatitis) and with family history.

(2) Vasomotor rhinitis is rhinitis with **rhinorrhea due to increased secretion of mucus from the nasal mucosa.** It may be caused by an allergy or neurovascular imbalance.

(3) Rhinitis medicamentosa is caused by the overzealous use of decongestant drops or sprays. This causes a rebound congestion requiring the increased use of the agent.

2. Clinical features

    a. Allergic rhinitis. Symptoms may be confused with those of a common cold. Signs may include allergic shiners (bluish discolorations below the eyes), scratchy eyes, rhinorrhea, itchy conjunctivitis, and pale boggy mucosa. The discharge is usually clear and watery.

    b. Vasomotor rhinitis. In its purest form, vasomotor rhinitis consists of bogginess of the nasal mucosa associated with a complaint of stuffiness. The symptoms are labile and go quickly. It may be precipitated by odors or perfumes.

    c. Rhinitis medicamentosa

3. Treatment

    a. Allergic rhinitis. Treatment includes the **use of antihistamines, cromolyn sodium and corticosteroids, nasal saline drops,** and **immunotherapy.**

    b. Vasomotor rhinitis. The treatment is **avoidance of the irritant.**

    c. Rhinitis medicamentosa. Treatment is **discontinuance of the irritant.** It may be quite uncomfortable for the patient and sometimes the use of **topical corticosteroids** may be helpful.

C. Pharyngitis (sore throat)

    1. General characteristics. The causes of pharyngitis are bacterial, viral, Epstein-Barr virus (EBV), *Corynebacterium diphtheriae*, or *N. gonorrhoeae.*

    2. Clinical features. The overall manifestations of pharyngitis include sore throat, difficulty swallowing, fever, erythema of the tonsils and posterior pharynx, lymph node enlargement, rhinitis, and cough, all in varying degrees.

    3. Types of pharyngitis and their management

        a. Streptococcal pharyngitis

            (1) Clinical features—acute onset, fever, exudate in posterior pharynx or on tonsils, cervical adenopathy. In children, it may present as abdominal pain secondary to adenopathy in the abdomen. Throat culture should be obtained to confirm the diagnosis.

            (2) Treatment is with penicillin or erythromycin. Complications of improper or incomplete treatment include rheumatic fever, Ludwig's angina, and tonsillar abscess.

        b. Viral pharyngitis

            (1) Clinical features—more insidious onset, often with coryza, usually lacking exudate. Fever is low grade and may or may not have lymphadenopathy. Obtain a throat culture to rule out streptococcal infection.

            (2) Treatment is supportive in nature.

        c. Epstein-Barr virus (mononucleosis)

            (1) Clinical features. There is a **prodromal phase of malaise** and **constitutional symptoms** of at least a week's duration. There is **exudate, pharyngitis,** and **petechiae** on the mucous membranes; **tender widespread adenopathy, possible splenic enlargement,** and **jaundice.** A **monospot test** should be performed.

            (2) Treatment is supportive and a **short course of corticosteroids** may be required to decrease pharyngeal edema. An **antibiotic** may be used to cover concomitant strep infection. Ampicillin should be avoided, as a rash will often ensue.

        d. *Corynebacterium diphtheriae*

            (1) Clinical features—a **rare cause** of pharyngitis. The features of *Corynebacterium diphtheriae* include **severe sore throat, fever,** a **discrete white exudate** that, if removed, bleeds easily on the tonsils or posterior pharynx, and **marked cervical adenopathy.**

            (2) Treatment is with **antitoxin, penicillin,** and **quarantine.**

        e. *N. gonorrhoeae*

            (1) Clinical features—a **rare cause** of pharyngitis, more commonly seen in immunocompromised patients. This form of pharyngitis has **acute onset of severe sore throat; exudate** is present with **multiple ulcer-type lesions** and **tender cervical lymphadenopathy.** May have a **concurrent urethritis** or **cervicitis.**

            (2) Treatment is **ceftriaxone,** or **amoxicillin** and **probenecid.**

D. Epiglottitis

    1. General characteristics

        a. Epiglottitis is a **life-threatening infection** of the epiglottis and surrounding tissues that **leads to obstructive respiratory disease.**

        b. Commonly **caused by** *H. influenzae* **type B, group A streptococcus, pneumococcus, or staphylococci. Is more common in children** but can occur at any age. It has become **more common in adults** because most children have had the vaccination against *H. influenzae*.

    2. Clinical features. Onset is abrupt, with **high fever, difficulty swallowing, sore throat, drooling,** and, in children, **sitting in the tripod position.**

    3. Laboratory studies

        a. **A lateral soft tissue neck radiograph** reveals **a thumb-like projection** (the classic **"thumb" sign**).

        b. **Controlled intubation** should be performed and the patient **should not be left alone** until intubation has occurred.

        c. Examination should be limited **causing no undue distress until airway is maintained.**

    4. Treatment

        a. Patients need **intravenous fluids** and **antibiotics for 24–72 hours.**

        b. All **family members** should be given **prophylaxis with rifampin.**

E. Epistaxis (nosebleed)

    1. The anterior aspect of the nose is the **most common site** of epistaxis, which is termed **Kiesselbach's plexus.**

    2. **Causes** are minor trauma, dry mucosa, nasal trauma, or an acquired or genetic coagulopathy.

    3. Treatment

        a. Begin with the patient sitting or standing **upright** and apply **firm pressure to the nares for 10–15 minutes,** then **identify the bleeding site.** Visualization is aided by using a light source and a nasal speculum.

        b. If a bleeding site can be identified, **cautery with a silver nitrate stick** is preferred. **Five percent cocaine spray** may be used.

        c. **Recauterize with packing** if necessary. **The packing is left in place for 24 hours.**

        d. The patient should be told **to return if bleeding begins.**

        e. **Posterior bleed is uncommon** and significant, requiring emergency evaluation and treatment; it is usually caused from acute trauma and the bleeding is usually arterial. Often, blood is seen in the posterior pharynx.

        f. The bleeding may **compromise the airway** and a **posterior pack** must be placed. This usually **requires an ENT consult.**

        g. The patient is **at risk for toxic shock syndrome,** secondary to retained packing.

F. Polyps

    1. Polyps are **pedunculated tumors found on the nasal mucosa.**

    2. They are often **seen in patients with allergic rhinitis** and often are **easily visualized.**

    3. Patients may have **nasal phonations** and complain of **feeling congested** all the time.

    4. In most cases, **polyps are benign** and **should be removed.**

2

Pulmonology

Patricia A. Francis

I. CHRONIC OBSTRUCTIVE PULMONARY DISEASE (COPD)

A. General characteristics

  1. COPD is a clinical and pathophysiologic **syndrome comprising three diseases: emphysema, chronic bronchitis, and asthma.** These three disorders **have overlapping features,** and because patients often have characteristics of more than one disorder, all three are classified together as COPD.

  a. Emphysema is a condition in which the air spaces are enlarged as a consequence of destruction of alveolar septa.

  b. Chronic bronchitis is a disease characterized by a chronic cough productive of phlegm occurring on most days for 3 months of the year for 2 or more consecutive years, without an otherwise defined acute cause.

  c. Asthma is described in II.

  2. COPD has one major, reversible risk factor— **smoking.**

B. Clinical features

  1. The physical examination of a patient with advanced COPD may reveal **asthenia, dyspnea, pursed lip breathing,** and **grunting expirations.**

  2. A chest examination shows signs of **hyperinflation** with **increase in anteroposterior (AP) dimension.** Percussion yields increased resonance. **Auscultation** reveals decreased breath sounds and early inspiratory crackles. **Wheezing** may not be present at rest, but **can be evoked** with forced expiration. The duration of **expiration is prolonged.**

  3. In patients with chronic bronchitis, **rhonchi reflect secretions** in the airways and **breathing is typically raspy and loud.**

C. Laboratory findings

  1. A chest radiograph shows hyperinflation of the lungs and flat diaphragms. Although suggestive, a chest radiograph is not sensitive or specific enough to serve as a diagnostic or screening tool.

  2. Pulmonary function testing. Airflow obstruction demonstrated on forced expiratory spirometry is suggestive. The ratio of forced expiratory volume in 1 second (FEV_1) to forced vital capacity (FVC) is decreased.

  3. A complete blood cell count (CBC) may show polycythemia caused by chronic hypoxemia.

D. Treatment. In symptomatic patients, the goal of treatment is to **improve functional state** and **relieve symptoms.**

  1. Smoking cessation should be encouraged.

  2. Bronchodilators can reverse airflow obstruction.

  3. Oral antibiotics may be necessary to treat acute lung infections.

  4. Continuous low-flow oxygen is indicated when the partial pressure of oxygen in alveolar gas (PaO_2) is below 55 mm Hg.

5. Diuretics should be administered to control peripheral edema in patients with cor pulmonale.

6. Patients should receive **prophylactic influenza vaccine. Pneumococcal vaccine** may also be of value.

II. ASTHMA

A. General characteristics

1. Asthma is characterized by three components: **obstruction to airflow, bronchial hyperreactivity, and inflammation of the airway.**

2. Many asthma syndromes have been identified: extrinsic allergic, allergic bronchopulmonary aspergillosis, intrinsic asthma, extrinsic nonallergic, aspirin sensitivity, exercise-induced, and asthma associated with COPD.

B. Clinical features

1. Patients have an **intermittent occurrence of cough, chest tightness, breathlessness,** and **wheezing.**

2. Patients undergo **asymptomatic periods** between these attacks.

C. Laboratory findings

1. Pulmonary function is less than 25% of predicted value.

2. Arterial blood gas measurements reveal hypoxemia and hypocarbia as a rule with a partial pressure of oxygen in arterial blood (PaO_2) less than 60 mm Hg and a partial pressure of carbon dioxide (PCO_2) of less than 40 mm Hg.

D. Treatment. The primary goal is to **relieve airway obstruction** and to **maintain adequate oxygenation and ventilation.**

1. β-**Adrenergic agonists** should be administered to induce bronchodilation.

2. Inhaled corticosteroids are the most effective anti-inflammatory medications for asthma management.

3. Daily evaluation of pulmonary function with a peak flow meter or spirometry is an important component of optimal asthma management. This type of monitoring permits medication adjustments.

III. BRONCHIECTASIS

A. General characteristics

1. Bronchiectasis is defined as an **abnormal dilatation of the bronchi** and is categorized as **cylindrical** or **saccular.**

2. Bronchiectasis **results from bronchial injury subsequent to severe infection.**

B. Clinical features

1. Chronic purulent sputum, often foul smelling, and **hemoptysis** are not uncommon.

2. Physical examination may reveal localized **chest crackles** and **digital clubbing.**

C. Laboratory findings

1. Chest computed tomography (CT) scan reveals dilated, tortuous airways.

2. Plain chest radiographs in patients with clinically significant bronchiectasis are abnormal. The degree of abnormality depends on the extent and severity of the disease.

D. Treatment

1. A productive cough should be managed with the **appropriate antibiotic, bronchodilators,** and **chest physiotherapy.**

2. Patients with disabling symptoms or progressive bronchiectasis can be considered for **surgery**; however, surgery has been found to be of little benefit.

IV. ADULT RESPIRATORY DISTRESS SYNDROME (ARDS)

A. General characteristics

1. Three clinical settings account for 75% of cases of ARDS—**sepsis syndrome** (the single most important), **severe multiple trauma,** and **aspiration of gastric contents.**

2. The underlying abnormality in ARDS is **increased permeability of the alveolar capillary membranes,** which leads to the **development of protein-rich pulmonary edema.**

B. Clinical features

1. The physical examination shows **tachypnea, frothy pink or red sputum,** and **diffuse rales.**

2. Many patients are **cyanotic** with **increasingly severe hypoxemia that is refractory to administered oxygen.**

C. Laboratory findings

1. Chest radiograph may at first be normal. Infiltrates tend to be peripheral with air bronchograms.

2. Pulmonary capillary wedge pressure is normal.

D. Treatment

1. The treatment remains **largely supportive** with several primary therapeutic aims.

  a. Oxygen delivery should be maintained.

  b. Excessive breathing workload should be **relieved.**

  c. Electrolyte balance should be established while **preventing further damage** from oxygen toxicity.

2. The **mortality rate** associated with ARDS is **60%–70%.** The high death rate reflects the severity of the predisposing conditions.

3. One third of deaths occur within 3 days of the onset of symptoms. The remaining deaths occur within 2 weeks of diagnosis and are caused by infection and multiple organ failure.

V. PLEURAL DISEASES

A. Pleural effusion

1. General characteristics

  a. Pleural effusions, **the accumulation of significant volumes of pleural fluid,** may result from **inflammation of structures adjacent to the pleural space or lesions within the chest.**

  b. The effusions **may not cause symptoms** and may be first discovered on a routine radiograph.

2. Clinical features

  a. With a small inflammatory effusion, **pleural pain (pleurisy)** is often present, and a **friction rub** may be heard.

  b. Large or bilateral pleural effusions may lead to **dyspnea,** but **orthopnea is uncommon** in the absence of congestive heart failure.

  c. A **dull-to-flat percussion note** over the area of fluid may be heard with **reduced or absent breath sounds.**

  d. The **mediastinum is usually shifted away** from the side of the large effusion.

3. Laboratory findings

  a. Radiographic findings include blunting of the costophrenic angle, loss of sharp demarcation of the diaphragm and heart, and mediastinal shift to the uninvolved side.

  b. CT may be useful if plain films cannot separate parenchymal and pleural densities.

4. Treatment

- **a.** Unless the cause has been clearly established, the presence of fluid is an indication for **thoracentesis.** Removal of fluid via thoracentesis allows fluid examination, radiographic visualization, and relief of symptoms.

- **b. Transudate pleural effusions can resolve when underlying causes are treated** [i.e., congestive heart failure (CHF) treated with diuretics, digitalis, and aferload reduction]. Effusions resolve over days to weeks.

B. Pneumothorax

1. General characteristics

- **a.** Pneumothorax is **the accumulation of air in the pleural space.**

- **b.** Entry can be through **an opening in the visceral pleura** or the **parietal pleura.**

- **c.** The cause may be **spontaneous, traumatic,** or **iatrogenic.**

- **d. Tension pneumothorax** is secondary to a sucking chest wound or pulmonary laceration allowing air to enter the chest with inspiration but not allowing it to leave on expiration.

2. Clinical features

- **a.** Pneumothorax is characterized by the **acute onset of ipsilateral chest pain** and dyspnea. Minimal physical findings occur in mild cases (e.g., unilateral chest expansion, decreased tactile fremitus, hyperresonance, diminished breath sounds).

- **b. Tension pneumothorax** is associated with a **mediastinal shift to the contralateral side** and **impaired ventilation** leading to cardiovascular compromise.

3. Laboratory findings

- **a. Chest radiographs** reveal the presence of pleural air.

- **b. Arterial blood gas analysis** reveals hypoxemia.

4. Treatment depends on the severity.

- **a. Small pneumothoraces resolve spontaneously.**

- **b.** For severely symptomatic or large pneumothoraces, **chest tube placement** is performed. If tension pneumothorax is suspected, a **large-bore needle should be inserted to allow air to move out of the chest.**

C. Pleurisy

1. General characteristics

- **a.** Pleurisy is **chest pain caused by the stimulation of pain fibers in the parietal pleura, as a result of pleural inflammation.**

- **b.** The inflammation associated with pleurisy is usually caused by **viral, bacterial,** or **tuberculous** infection, but may have numerous other causes.

2. Clinical features

- **a.** The pain, located over the lower portion of the chest, is usually **sharp or stabbing.**

- **b. Deep breathing, coughing,** or **sneezing** make the pain much worse.

3. Laboratory findings. **Consideration of the setting in which the pleuritic pain** developed helps to narrow laboratory studies because conditions that cause pleurisy can be associated with a virus, bacteria, fungus, or tuberculosis.

4. Treatment

- **a.** The **underlying disease** must be treated.

- **b. Simple analgesic** and **anti-inflammatory drugs** are helpful for pain relief.

- **c.** If not contraindicated, **codeine** may be used to control cough associated with pleuritic pain.

- **d. Intercostal nerve blocks** are sometimes helpful.

VI. PULMONARY NEOPLASMS

A. Squamous cell carcinoma

  1. General characteristics

   a. Squamous cell carcinoma, in the past, was the **most common variety** of carcinoma, and accounted for 50% of all bronchogenic carcinomas. By the mid-1980s, however, the percentage had decreased to approximately 30%–40%.

   b. Squamous cell carcinoma tends to **originate in the central bronchi** and **metastasize to regional lymph nodes.**

  2. Clinical features

   a. The clinical features **depend on the primary cancer, metastases, systemic effects,** and **coexisting syndromes.**

   b. The initial symptoms include **cough, chest pain, weight loss, dyspnea,** and **hemoptysis.**

  3. Laboratory findings

   a. **Anteroposterior (AP) and lateral (L) chest radiographs** may show hilar masses, peripheral masses, atelectasis, infiltrates, cavitation (10% of patients), and pleural effusions.

   b. **Cytologic examination of sputum** permits definitive diagnosis of a specific cell type if malignant cells are seen in approximately 85%–95% of cases.

   c. **Bronchoscopy, examination of pleural fluid,** and **biopsy** are also used to establish a diagnosis by looking at specific cell types through direct visualization.

  4. Treatment

   a. Options include **surgery, radiation therapy, and chemotherapy.**

   b. **Surgery remains the treatment of choice.** The 5-year survival rate after resection is 35%–40%.

B. Adenocarcinoma

  1. General characteristics

   a. During the past 2 decades, adenocarcinoma has emerged as the most common histologic subtype of all lung cancers. These tumors **usually appear in the periphery of the lung** and are **not amenable to early detection** through sputum examination.

   b. These cancers typically **metastasize to distant organs.**

   c. **Bronchoalveolar cell carcinoma**, a subtype of adenocarcinoma, is a low-grade carcinoma.

  2. Clinical features. Patients may exhibit **lymphadenopathy, hepatomegaly,** and **clubbing.**

  3. Laboratory findings

   a. Usually **carcinoembryonic antigen (CEA) positive** because adenocarcinomas express low-molecular weight cytokeratins and epithelial membrane antigen.

   b. **Small peripheral masses** can usually be seen with **radiography** and often **in relation to focal scars** or regions of interstitial fibrosis.

  4. Treatment

   a. The **interval between the development of the first lung cancer cell and clinical presentation of the disease has been estimated at 5–10 years.** This delay in recognition usually allows ample time for metastasis.

   b. **Symptomatic lung cancer is usually advanced and often not resectable.**

   c. If resectable, **solid tumor with mucin production is associated with poorest prognosis** and bronchoalveolar with the most favorable.

C. Small (oat) cell carcinoma

  1. General characteristics

   a. Small cell carcinomas **account for approximately 20%–25% of lung cancers.**

   b. This is the **most aggressive type of carcinoma**, and tends to metastasize early.

2. Clinical features

    a. **Paraneoplastic syndromes** occur in 15%–20% of lung cancer patients.

    b. There is **little or no atelectasis,** and **early lymphatic** and **hematogenous spread** (i.e., brain, liver, bones, kidney, adrenal glands).

3. Laboratory findings

    a. **Chest radiographs** commonly show a **hilar mass** and **mediastinal widening.**

    b. **Cavitation** is exceedingly **rare.**

    c. The majority of small cell lung cancers are **located centrally, arise in the peribronchial tissues, and infiltrate the bronchial submucosa.**

4. Treatment. **Combination chemotherapy** is the treatment of choice for patients with small cell carcinoma and results in improvement in median survival, although patients rarely live for more than 5 years after the diagnosis is made.

D. Solitary pulmonary nodule

    1. General characteristics

        a. Only **10%** of solitary pulmonary nodules **are metastases from extrathoracic cancer.** Metastases to the lung are usually multiple.

        b. Approximately **25% of cases of bronchogenic carcinoma** present as a solitary pulmonary nodule. The 5-year survival rate detected in this form approaches 50%.

    2. Clinical features

        a. A solitary pulmonary nodule is a **round** or **oval, sharply circumscribed,** pulmonary lesion **(up to 5 cm in diameter)** surrounded by normal lung tissue.

        b. **Central cavitation, calcification,** or **surrounding (satellite) lesions** may occur.

    3. Laboratory findings. In a large study of surgical node evaluation, approximately **60% of solitary pulmonary nodules are benign** and 40% are malignant.

        a. **Benign lesions.** A lesion that has not enlarged in ≥2 years suggests a benign etiology.

        b. **Malignant lesions** are occasionally symptomatic, tend to **occur in patients who are older than 45 years of age,** are usually **larger than 2 centimeters in diameter,** often have **indistinct margins,** and are **rarely calcified.**

    4. Treatment

        a. **Exploratory thoracotomy** or, in some cases, **thoracoscopy** is advised as soon as possible after a solitary pulmonary nodule is detected.

        b. **A conservative approach** may be justified if there are strong indications of a benign diagnosis or contraindications to surgery.

VII. DIFFUSE INTERSTITIAL LUNG DISEASE

A. General characteristics

    1. Interstitial lung diseases comprise a heterogeneous group of chronic disorders characterized by **inflammation** and **fibrosis of the alveolar walls** and **air spaces.** Approximately **1% of disease entities** share the **manifestations** of interstitial lung disease.

    2. **No specific cause can be identified** in most patients. In the remainder, drugs and a variety of inorganic and organic dusts are the predominant causes.

B. Clinical features

    1. **Exertional dyspnea** and **a dry cough of insidious onset** are the usual presenting symptoms.

    2. **Digital clubbing** is common.

    3. **Systemic manifestations** such as fever, fatigue, anorexia, and weight loss predominate in some disorders.

C. Laboratory findings

   1. **Chest radiograph** shows diffuse ground-glass, nodular, reticular, or reticulonodular infiltrates.

   2. **Pulmonary function tests** show a restrictive pattern with FVC and FEV_1 proportionally reduced.

D. **Treatment.** Primary therapy can consist of specific **antimicrobials, removal from exposure, discontinuation of drugs, corticosteroids, cessation of smoking, plasmapheresis, whole lung lavage,** or **chemotherapeutic agents.**

VIII. PNEUMOCONIOSES

A. General characteristics

   1. Pneumoconioses are **chronic fibrotic lung diseases** caused by the **inhalation of coal dust** and various inert, inorganic, or silicate dusts.

   2. Clinically important pneumoconioses include **coal workers' pneumoconiosis, silicosis,** and **asbestosis.**

B. Clinical features

   1. In simple cases, pneumoconioses are **usually asymptomatic.**

   2. In complicated cases, patients have **dyspnea, inspiratory crackles, clubbing,** and **cyanosis.**

C. Laboratory findings

   1. **Pulmonary function tests** show restrictive dysfunction and reduced diffusing capacity.

   2. Chest radiographs

   (a) Coal workers' pneumoconiosis—small opacities are prominent in the upper lung fields.

   (b) Silicosis—small, rounded opacities are seen throughout the lung, and hilar lymph nodes may be calcified.

   (c) Asbestosis—interstitial fibrosis, thickened pleura, and calcified plaques appear on the diaphragms or lateral chest wall.

D. **Treatment** is primarily **supportive.**

   1. **Corticosteroids** may relieve the chronic alveolitis in silicosis.

   2. **Smoking cessation** is especially important for patients with asbestosis because smoking interferes with short asbestos fiber clearance from the lung.

IX. SARCOIDOSIS

A. General characteristics

   1. Sarcoidosis is a **multi-organ disease of unknown cause.** It is characterized by **noncaseating granulomatous inflammation in affected organs** (e.g., lungs, lymph nodes, eyes, skin, liver, spleen, salivary glands, heart, nervous system).

   2. The incidence is highest in North American blacks and northern European whites.

B. Clinical features

   1. Common respiratory symptoms include **cough, dyspnea of insidious onset,** and **chest discomfort.**

   2. Patients may present with **malaise, fever,** and symptoms consistent with **various organ involvement.**

C. Laboratory findings

   1. Serum blood tests may show **leukopenia, eosinophilia, an elevated erythrocyte sedimentation rate (ESR), hypercalcemia,** and **hypercalciuria.**

   2. **Angiotensin-converting enzyme (ACE)** levels are elevated in 40%–80% of patients.

3. Radiographic findings demonstrate **symmetric bilateral hilar** and **right paratracheal adenopathy, and diffuse reticular infiltrates.**

4. **Transbronchial biopsy of the lung** or **needle node biopsy** confirms the diagnosis.

D. **Treatment.** Ninety percent of cases are very responsive to **corticosteroids** and can be controlled with modest maintenance doses.

X. KYPHOSCOLIOSIS

A. General characteristics

1. Kyphoscoliosis is a skeletal abnormality that leads to chronic deterioration in lung function.

2. This condition causes **reduced lung volumes** and **increased stiffness** (reduced compliance) of the chest wall. **Progressive atelectasis also decreases lung compliance.**

B. Clinical features

1. Severe kyphoscoliosis causes **increased work of breathing**, leading to a **fall in minute ventilation** and eventually **chronic hypercapnic respiratory failure.**

2. Patients complain of **dyspnea** and are **noticeably breathless. Use of accessory muscles** is noted on physical examination.

3. **Infection, bronchospasm, or heart failure may precipitate acute respiratory failure.**

C. Laboratory findings. **Blood gas analysis** shows carbon dioxide retention and respiratory acidosis.

D. Treatment. Patients may need **mechanical ventilatory support** if diaphragm dysfunction occurs.

XI. PULMONARY EMBOLISM

A. General characteristics

1. Pulmonary embolism **arises from thrombi** in the venous circulation or the right side of the heart, from **tumors** that have invaded the venous circulation, and from other sources. More than **90%** of pulmonary emboli **originate as clots** in the deep veins of the lower extremities.

2. Approximately 80% of **pulmonary emboli spontaneously resolve.**

B. Clinical features

1. Symptoms include **pleuritic chest pain, dyspnea, apprehension, cough, hemoptysis,** and **diaphoresis.**

2. Signs include **tachycardia, tachypnea, crackles, accentuation of the pulmonary component of the second heart sound,** and a **low-grade fever.**

C. Laboratory findings

1. **Arterial blood gas measurements** show acute respiratory alkalosis.

2. **An electrocardiogram (ECG)** shows tachycardia and nonspecific ST-T wave changes.

3. **On chest radiograph, elevation of a hemidiaphragm** and **pulmonary infiltration** are the most common abnormalities found.

4. A **ventilation–perfusion lung scan** shows perfusion defects. A normal scan rules out clinically significant thromboembolism.

5. **Pulmonary angiography** remains the definitive test for diagnosis.

D. Treatment

    1. **Anticoagulation therapy** is initiated, heparin being the anticoagulant of choice.

    2. Duration of therapy depends on the clinical situation. **A minimum of 3 months** is advised.

XII. INFECTIONS

A. Upper respiratory tract infection

    1. **General characteristics.** Most upper respiratory tract illnesses are caused by viruses and resolve spontaneously.

    2. **Clinical features.** Patients with upper respiratory tract infections can present with coryza, pharyngitis, sinusitis, otitis media, or bronchitis.

    3. **Laboratory findings. Gram stain** and **cultures** may be used to detect upper respiratory illnesses that are caused or complicated by bacterial infections. Common causative agents are anaerobic fusobacteria, *Bacteroides* species, and anaerobic, as well as aerobic streptococci.

    4. Treatment

        a. **Supportive measures** include decongestants, antipyretics, and cough suppressants.

        b. **Antibiotics may be prescribed for complications** (i.e., otitis media or sinusitis).

B. Pharyngitis (see also Chapter 1). Pharyngitis is **primarily caused by a viral infection.** Eighty percent of cases are caused by the **same viruses that cause the common cold.** One must **differentiate streptococcal pharyngitis from acute epiglottitis.**

C. Tracheobronchitis

    1. General characteristics

        a. Most tracheobronchitis is **caused by viruses** and patients **recover spontaneously.**

        b. **Bacterial superinfections** can occur.

    2. **Clinical features.** Patients characteristically have a persistent cough, and may have fever or headache, sore throat, and coryza.

    3. **Laboratory findings.** Patients with chronic lung diseases who develop bacterial superinfections have abnormal findings consistent with the infection.

    4. Treatment

        a. In patients with chronic lung disease, **antibiotics** are warranted.

        b. Viral tracheobronchitis treatment should include **humidity, cough suppressant,** and **reassurance.**

D. Pneumonia

    1. Pneumonia denotes **inflammation in the alveoli or interstitium of the lung caused by microorganisms.**

    2. Pneumonia ranks as the **primary cause of mortality from infectious diseases.**

    3. Classic community-acquired pneumonia

        a. **General characteristics.** "Community-acquired" denotes pneumonia caused by the **inhalation of an organism with relatively high virulence.**

        b. **Clinical features.** Typical presentation is a 1- to 10-day history of increasing cough, yellow sputum, shortness of breath, temperature, tachycardia, and pleuritic chest pain.

        c. Laboratory findings

            (1) **Sputum culture** may reveal *Streptococcus pneumoniae, Haemophilus influenzae, Staphylococcus aureus, Klebsiella pneumoniae,* or gram-negative bacilli.

            (2) **Physical examination** may reveal dullness to percussion and bronchial breath sounds over an area of consolidation.

(3) **Hematologic evaluation** reveals leukocytosis with shift to the left or sometimes leukopenia.

(4) **Chest radiography** shows lobar or segmental infiltrates.

  d. Treatment

(1) The patient who is otherwise healthy and free of respiratory distress or complications may be managed as an outpatient with **oral antibiotics** and **appropriate supportive care.**

(2) The presence of neutropenia, involvement of more than one lobe, or poor host resistance indicates a need for **hospitalization.**

(3) **Bed rest, supplemental oxygen,** and **antibiotics** are the cornerstones of therapy.

4. Atypical community-acquired pneumonia

  a. **General characteristics.** As the term "atypical" implies, this form of pneumonia has a clinical presentation different from that of classic community-acquired pneumonia. ***Mycoplasma pneumoniae*** is the most common cause of atypical pneumonias. Other causes include viruses (influenza type A and B and adenoviruses), *Chlamydia pneumoniae, Legionella,* and *Moraxella.* These organisms, such as mycoplasma, can be detected on culture in selective media.

  b. Clinical features

(1) The typical presentation is a **low fever** with relatively **mild pulmonary symptoms** that are self-limited, occurring in young, **otherwise healthy** adults.

(2) **A nonproductive cough, myalgia,** and **fatigue** are common.

  c. Laboratory findings

(1) Organisms usually are **not detected with conventional stain** or **culture of sputum.**

(2) **The white blood cell count (WBC)** is normal or slightly elevated.

(3) **Radiography** shows segmental unilateral lower lung zone infiltrates.

  d. Treatment

(1) **Antibiotics.** Because serology results can be prolonged, treatment is done **empirically** based on the clinical features. Regimens include **erythromycin** (for M. *pneumoniae* infection and *Legionella* infection) and **tetracycline** (for *Chlamydia*).

(2) **Amantadine** is effective in shortening the duration of symptoms of influenza A.

5. Hospital-acquired pneumonia

  a. General characteristics

(1) Hospital-acquired pneumonia is **caused by organisms that colonize ill patients, staff, and equipment.** After colonization, the organisms are aspirated.

(2) The causative organisms are unique and the mortality rate is high.

  (a) The usual organisms are *S. aureus* and **gram-negative bacilli**, which are easy to recover from respiratory secretions.

  (b) *Pseudomonas aeruginosa* is the most likely pathogen in intensive care units and carries the worst prognosis.

  b. **Laboratory findings.** Diagnosis is with Gram stain and culture of sputum and blood.

  c. **Treatment** is with appropriate antibiotics. Despite therapy, patients may develop bacteremia or ARDS.

E. Tuberculosis

1. General characteristics

  a. *Mycobacterium tuberculosis* infection is acquired by **inhaling organisms within aerosol droplets expelled during coughing** by people who have tuberculosis.

  b. Most exposed people mount an immune response sufficient to **prevent progression** from primary infection to clinical illness, but approximately **5% of exposed people fail to contain the primary infection** and progress to active tuberculosis within 2 years.

Table 2-1.

Treatment of Tuberculosis

Latent infection
  Isoniazid 300 mg every day for 6–12 months (non–HIV- infected)
  Isoniazid 300 mg every day for 12 months (HIV-infected)
Active infection (adults)
  Initial phase (months 1 and 2):
      1. Isoniazid 300 mg/d
      2. Rifampin 600 mg/d
      3. Pyrazinamide 20–30 mg/kg/d not to exceed 2 g*
      4. Ethambutol 15–25 mg/kg/d (until drug susceptibilities are available)
  Continuation phase (months 3 through 6):
      1. Isoniazid 300 mg/d
      2. Rifampin 600 mg/d

---

* If pyrazinamide cannot be tolerated, isoniazid and rifampin should be given for a total of 9 months.

   c. Some **nosocomial outbreaks** have seen the **emergence of organisms resistant** to multiple antituberculous drugs.

2. Clinical features

   a. **Systemic complaints** include fever, chills, night sweats, anorexia, weight loss, and fatigue.

   b. **Cardiopulmonary symptoms** are a chronic productive cough lasting more than 3 weeks, with or without hemoptysis.

3. Laboratory findings

   a. **Radiography** reveals a cavitary infiltrate in a posterior apical segment of an upper lobe or in a superior segment of a lower lobe.

   b. A positive **purified protein derivative (PPD) skin test** indicates tuberculosis.

   c. **Sputum should be examined** in the form of **smears** for acid-fast bacilli, as well as **cultures.**

4. Treatment

   a. **Antituberculous drugs** are the cornerstone of therapy (Table 2-1)**.**

   b. Patients with active disease require **combination chemotherapy** for 6–9 months; patients infected with HIV require therapy for at least 1 year.

   c. **Isoniazid (INH)** for 6–12 months is **indicated for prophylaxis** in patients who have tested negative in the past but who are now positive with known or unknown exposure (converters).

   d. For **biologic prophylaxis,** the **bacille Calmette-Guérin** (BCG) vaccine can be administered to a tuberculin-negative person in cases where there is a high risk for intense, prolonged exposure to untreated or ineffectively treated cases of infectious tuberculosis.

XIII. SLEEP APNEA

  A. General characteristics

   1. Sleep apnea may **result from central suppression of respiration** or **from airway obstruction (pickwickian syndrome).**

   2. **Abnormal ventilation during sleep** is manifested by apnea or hypopnea.

  B. Clinical features

   1. Patients complain of **daytime sleepiness, loud snoring,** or **cardiovascular effects of their nocturnal hypoxemia** (arrhythmias, pulmonary hypertension, and cor pulmonale).

   2. On physical examination, **obesity, narrowing of the airways due to tonsillar hypertrophy,** or other mechanical **conditions** can be found.

C. Laboratory findings

 1. A **polysomnographic study** with arterial oxygen saturation monitoring may show a positive result for apnea.

 2. On **hematologic evaluation**, erythrocytosis is common.

D. Treatment

 1. Treatment consists of a **weight reduction program, nighttime nasal administration of continuous positive airway pressure (CPAP)** and strict **avoidance of both alcohol** and **hypnotic medications.**

 2. **Surgical approaches** are worth consideration if symptoms are severe.

3

Cardiology

Stan Willenbring
Rebecca Lovell Scott

I. MAJOR PRINCIPLES OF CARDIAC CARE

A. Three factors are needed to **maintain adequate pressure** in the cardiovascular system.

  1. A functioning pump

  2. Sufficient fluid volume

  3. Resistance

B. All cardiac pathologies result from **abnormalities of electrical or contractile functions of heart muscle, fluid load, or vascular resistance.**

II. SHOCK

A. General characteristics

  1. Shock is **severe cardiovascular failure** caused by **poor blood flow** or **inadequate distribution of flow.**

  2. **Inadequate oxygen delivery to body tissues** results in shock, which, if inadequately treated, leads rapidly to **organ failure** and **death.**

  3. Shock may result from **multiple causes.**

   a. **Hypovolemic shock** is due to **hemorrhage, plasma loss,** or **loss of fluid** and **electrolytes.**

   b. **Cardiogenic shock** may arise from **myocardial infarction, arrhythmias, heart failure, defects in the valves or septum, hypertension, myocarditis,** or **myocardiopathies.**

   c. Causes of **obstructive shock** include **tension pneumothorax, pericardial tamponade, obstructive valvular disease,** and **pulmonary problems.**

   d. Shock due to **poorly regulated distribution of blood volume** includes **septic shock** (see Chapter 4), **anaphylaxis,** and **neurogenic shock.**

B. Clinical features

  1. Signs and symptoms of shock include **low blood pressure, tachycardia, peripheral hypoperfusion, altered mental status, oliguria** or **anuria,** and **metabolic acidosis.**

  2. Patients with cardiogenic shock present with **distended neck veins** and an **abnormal electrocardiogram (ECG).**

C. Laboratory studies

  1. All patients require a **complete blood cell count (CBC), blood type,** and **crossmatch.**

  2. Electrolytes, glucose, urinalysis, and **serum creatinine** may aid in the diagnosis of the cause of shock.

  3. Pulse oximetry or **serial arterial blood gases** should be obtained.

D. Treatment

    1. Specific treatments **depend on the cause** of shock.

    2. The **Trendelenburg** or **supine position with legs elevated** maximizes blood flow to the brain.

    3. **Oxygen and intravenous fluids** are essential.

    4. **Urine flow** should be monitored via indwelling catheter and sustained at **0.5 ml/kg/h** or more.

    5. Patients should have **continuous cardiac monitoring.**

III. HYPERTENSION

  A. General characteristics

    1. **Primary, or essential, hypertension** is the most common form (95% of cases) of high arterial blood pressure and has no identifiable cause.

    2. **Secondary causes** of hypertension include estrogen use, pheochromocytoma, coarctation of the aorta, pseudotumor cerebri, renal disease, renal artery stenosis, and primary hyperaldosteronism.

    3. Essential hypertension is **exacerbated** in **males, blacks, sedentary individuals,** and **smokers.**

    4. Hypertension plays a major role in the genesis and exacerbation of other forms of cardiovascular disease and causes numerous secondary disorders.

  B. Clinical features (Table 3-1)

    1. The essential diagnostic criterion is a **systolic pressure of greater than 140 mm Hg** or a **diastolic pressure greater than 90 mm Hg on 3 occasions.**

    2. Most patients with mild to moderate hypertension are **asymptomatic.**

    3. End-organ damage in severe hypertension includes **heart failure, renal failure,** and **retinal hemorrhage.**

  C. Laboratory studies

    1. ECG may reveal **left ventricular hypertrophy** or **heart failure** (Figure 3-1).

    2. Chest radiograph or ECG may show **ventricular hypertrophy** (Figure 3-2).

    3. **Decreased hemoglobin** or **hematocrit** or **elevations in blood urea nitrogen (BUN), creatinine, glucose (serum** or **urine)** may indicate related renal disease or diabetes.

    4. A **lipid profile** is important for ascertaining associated atherosclerosis.

  D. Treatment

    1. Nonpharmacologic therapies include **weight loss, exercise, cessation of smoking, limiting of alcohol and sodium,** and **improved stress reduction.**

Table 3-1.
Classification of Blood Pressure for Adults Age 18 Years and Older

Category	Systolic	Diastolic
Normal	<130	<85
High normal	130–139	85–89
Hypertension*		
Stage 1 (mild)	140–159	90–99
Stage 2 (moderate)	160–179	100–109
Stage 3 (severe)	180–209	110–119
Stage 4 (very severe)	>210	>120

From Joint National Committee. The fifth report of the Joint National Committee on Detection, Evaluation, and Treatment of High Blood Pressure (JNC V). *Arch Intern Med* 1993;153:154–183.
* Based on the average of two or more readings taken at each of two or more visits after an initial screening.

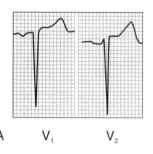

A   V₁   V₂

B   V₅   V₆

Figure 3-1. Electrocardiogram (ECG) findings in left ventricular hypertrophy: (A) Deep S waves in V_1 and V_2; (B) Tall R waves in V_5 and V_6. (From Stein E: *Rapid analysis of electrocardiograms: A self-study program*, 2nd edition. Baltimore, Williams & Wilkins, 1992.)

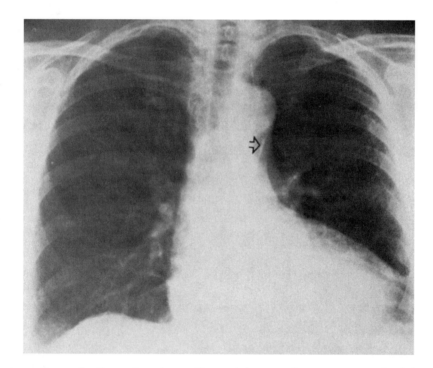

Figure 3-2. Hypertensive cardiovascular disease, frontal view. There is left ventricular prominence and a slight increase in the tortuosity of the aorta at its arch. There is calcification in the descending aorta (*arrow*). (From Daffner RH: *Clinical radiology: The essentials*. Baltimore, Williams & Wilkins, 1993.)

2. **Diuretics** (e.g., furosemide, spironolactone, thiazides) may be used to reduce circulatory volume. **Potassium supplements** may be needed for some patients.

3. **Other drug therapy** includes:

    a. **Central sympatholytic agents** (e.g., clonidine)

    b. **β-Adrenergic antagonists** (e.g., propranolol, atenolol)

    c. **Calcium channel blockers** (e.g., diltiazem, verapamil, nifedipine)

   d. α-Adrenergic antagonists (e.g., prazosin)

   e. Other agents (e.g., hydralazine, minoxidil)

IV. CONGESTIVE HEART FAILURE (CHF)

A. General characteristics

   1. CHF is a **clinical syndrome characterized by dyspnea and abnormal water and sodium retention.**

   2. CHF has **multiple causes,** including myocardial and pericardial disorders, and valvular and congenital abnormalities.

   3. CHF adversely affects **left atrial pressure** and **cardiac output.**

B. Clinical features

   1. Distended neck or **leg veins** reflect venous congestion.

   2. Peripheral edema is common.

   3. Pulmonary edema causes **dyspnea, cough,** and **basilar rales.**

   4. A hallmark of CHF is **paroxysmal nocturnal dyspnea.**

   5. Patients experience **fatigue** and **decreased exercise tolerance.**

   6. Sympathetic activity produces **pallor** and **clammy skin.**

   7. Abdominal tenderness and **hepatomegaly** may result from engorgement of organs.

   8. Nocturia is a common symptom.

C. Laboratory studies

   1. Patients may have **hyponatremia** and **elevated liver enzymes**; those on diuretics may develop **hypokalemia.**

   2. Chest radiograph may show **cardiomegaly** and bilateral or right-sided **pulmonary effusions** (Figure 3-3).

   3. ECG may show **nonspecific changes** (e.g., low voltage).

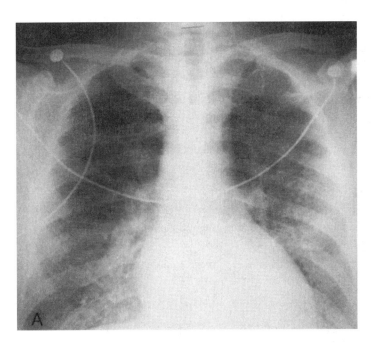

Figure 3-3. Congestive heart failure. Frontal view shows mild pulmonary edema and pulmonary venous engorgement. (From Daffner RH: *Clinical radiology: The essentials.* Baltimore, Williams & Wilkins, 1993.)

D. Treatment

   1. **Preventive nonpharmacologic measures** include **exercise, low sodium diet,** and **stress reduction.**

   2. **Diuretic therapy** reduces fluid volume.

   3. Other drug therapies include **direct inotropic agents** (digitalis), **arterial vasodilators, venous vasodilators,** and **angiotensin-converting enzyme (ACE) inhibitors.**

V. ATHEROSCLEROSIS

A. General characteristics

   1. Atherosclerosis is characterized by **lipid deposition, fibrosis, calcification,** and **plaque formation in the intima of large- and medium-sized vessels.**

   2. Atherosclerosis is associated with **premature coronary** and **peripheral vascular morbidity** and **mortality.**

      a. Atherosclerotic heart disease is the **most common cause of cardiac-related death** and **disability.**

      b. **Men** are affected **4 times as often as women**; however, by the age of 70 years, the ratio is 1:1.

   3. Etiology is closely related to **smoking** and **elevated (more than 200 mg/dl) cholesterol levels.**

   4. **Lipid abnormalities** associated with atherosclerosis may be due to **lifestyle features** or **familial dyslipidemias.**

B. **Clinical features** depend on the location of the vessels involved (e.g., cerebral occlusions lead to cognitive disorders, renal artery blockage leads to kidney failure).

C. Laboratory studies (see Chapter 10)

D. Treatment

   1. **Smoking cessation** is essential.

   2. For **dietary modifications** and other **treatment of dyslipidemias,** see Chapter 10.

VI. ISCHEMIC HEART DISEASE

A. General characteristics

   1. Ischemic heart disease is a syndrome characterized by **insufficient oxygen supply to cardiac muscle** caused by atherosclerotic narrowing or constriction of coronary arteries.

   2. Risk factors include **male sex, increased age, low estrogen state, cigarette smoking, family history of heart disease, hypertension, diabetes, inactivity,** and **abnormal lipids.**

B. Clinical features

   1. Ischemia causes **angina pectoris.** Angina is characterized by **paroxysmal chest pain** often accompanied by a **sensation of smothering** and a **fear of impending death.**

      a. **Stable angina** is exacerbated by physical activity and relieved by rest.

      b. **Prinzmetal's,** or **variant, angina** is caused by vasospasm at rest with preservation of exercise capacity.

   2. **Levine's sign,** a clenched fist over the sternum and **clenched teeth when describing chest pain,** may be seen in patients with ischemia.

   3. Angina pectoris is usually **midsternal**; the pain can **radiate** to the jaw, shoulder(s), arm(s), wrist(s), and the back of the neck, or a combination of these.

C. Laboratory studies

   1. A **stress test with ECG** may reveal angina on exertion.

   2. **Horizontal** or **down-sloping ST-segment depression** in the ECG is among the most sensitive clinical signs.

   3. **Angiography** is the most definitive method of identifying specific occluded coronary vessels.

D. Treatment

1. Preventive treatment includes **exercise, weight reduction,** a **diet low in fat and cholesterol, smoking cessation,** and **careful control of diabetes** and **hypertension**.

2. **Sublingual nitroglycerin** is the primary pharmacotherapy for acute anginal attacks.

3. **Anticoagulants** (e.g., aspirin, dipyridamole) reduce the possibility of infarction due to emboli.

4. **β-Adrenergic antagonists** and **calcium channel blockers** decrease cardiac muscle oxygen demand.

5. **Angioplasty** or **coronary artery bypass surgery** provides long-term relief of ischemia in suitable patients.

VII. MYOCARDIAL INFARCTION (MI)

A. General characteristics

1. MI is a result of **prolonged myocardial ischemia,** usually as a result of **thrombus formation** on a preexisting atherosclerotic plaque or an **embolic crisis**.

2. Signs and symptoms, prognosis, and complications depend on the size and location of the infarct.

3. One fifth of patients will die before reaching a hospital, usually of **ventricular fibrillation**.

B. Clinical features

1. The patient usually develops **prolonged (more than 30 minutes) severe anterior chest pain,** which can lead to arrhythmias, hypotension, shock, and heart failure.

2. **Diaphoresis, weakness, anxiety, restlessness, syncope, dyspnea, nausea,** and **vomiting** are often present.

3. Patients may be **brady- or tachycardic,** or **hypo- or hypertensive**.

4. **Low-grade fever** may develop.

5. Lung fields may be **clear** or show **rales and wheezing**.

6. **Jugular venous distention, soft heart sounds,** and an S_4 gallop may be present.

7. **Pericardial friction rubs** may appear after 24 hours.

8. **Dressler's syndrome** (postmyocardial infarction syndrome) includes **pericarditis, fever, leukocytosis,** and **pericardial** or **pleural effusion**.

C. Laboratory studies

1. **Peaked T waves, ST-segment elevations (or depressions), Q waves, and T-wave inversions** classically occur over hours to days, but are not present in all cases (Figure 3-4).

2. The location of cardiac damage may be determined by examination of changes on the ECG (Table 3-2).

3. Serial **cardiac enzymes** [isoenzyme of creatine kinase containing M and B subunits (CK-MB), troponin T, troponin I] demonstrate characteristic elevations (Table 3-3).

4. **Echocardiography** may show abnormalities of cardiac wall motion; Doppler studies may show postinfarction ventricular septal defect or mitral regurgitation.

D. Treatment

1. **Thrombolytic therapy** [with tissue plasminogen activator (TPA), streptokinase, or urokinase] is of greatest benefit within 1–3 hours, but may be initiated up to 12 hours after symptoms begin.

2. **Acute percutaneous transluminal coronary angioplasty (PTCA)** or **coronary artery bypass grafting (CABG)** may be performed at specialized centers.

3. General measures include administration of **aspirin,** admission to a **coronary care unit, bed rest, low-flow oxygen therapy, sublingual nitroglycerin,** and **analgesia** with **morphine** or **meperidine**.

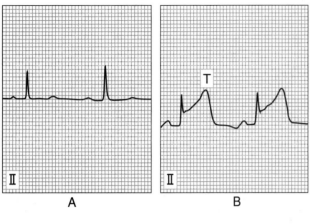

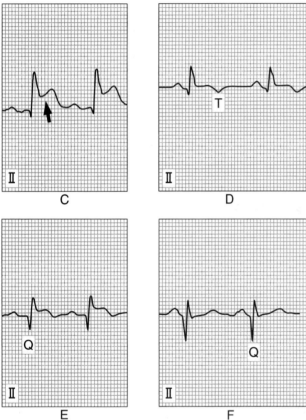

Figure 3-4. Evolutionary changes of a Q wave infarction as seen from lead II. Note: examples not necessarily from the same patient. (A) Normal. (B) T wave becomes tall, then (D) inverts symmetrically; (C) ST segment elevates (arrow); (E) Significant Q waves develop; (F) Healed infarction. Q waves persist while ST segment and T wave return to normal. (From Mulholland GC, Brewer BB: *Improving your skills in 12-lead ECG interpretation.* Baltimore, Williams & Wilkins, 1990.)

Table 3-2.
ECG Localization of AMI

Location	Found in ECG Leads
Inferior	II, III, aVF
Posterior	V_1, V_2
Anteroseptal	V_1, V_2
Anterior	V_1, V_2, V_3
Anterolateral	V4, V5, V6

AMI = acute myocardial infarction; ECG = electrocardiogram.

Table 3-3.
Cardiac Markers in Acute Myocardial Infarction (AMI)

Marker	Timing of Initial Elevation;	Peak Elevation; and	Return to Normal Level	Sampling Schedule
Myoglobin	1–4 hours;	6–7 hours;	24 hours	Often, beginning 1–2 hours after onset of chest pain
Cardiac troponin I	3–12 hours;	24 hours;	5–10 days	12 hours after onset of chest pain
Cardiac troponin T	3–12 hours;	12–48 hours;	5–14 days	12 hours after onset of chest pain
Total CK	3–5 hours;	24 hours;	28–72 hours	May not be drawn due to many false positives; CK-MB more sensitive
CK-MB	3–12 hours;	24 hours;	48–72 hours	Three times, each 12 hours apart
LDH	10 hours;	24–48 hours;	10–14 days	Once, at least 24 hours after onset of chest pain

CK = Creatine kinase; *CK-MB* = isoenzyme of creatine kinase containing M and B subunits; *LDH* = lactate dehydrogenase.

VIII. CONGENITAL HEART ANOMALIES

A. **General characteristics**

    1. Congenital heart anomalies are classified as either **cyanotic** or **noncyanotic.**

        a. **Cyanotic types** all involve **right-to-left shunts.**

            (1) **Tetralogy of Fallot** consists of a subaortic septal defect, right ventricular outflow obstruction, overriding aorta, and right ventricular hypertrophy.

            (2) **Pulmonary atresia** occurs most often with an intact ventricular septum; the pulmonary valve is closed; an atrial septal opening and patent ductus arteriosus are present.

            (3) **Hypoplastic left heart syndrome** is actually a group of defects with a small left ventricle and normally placed great vessels.

            (4) **Transposition of the great vessels** is most commonly complete transposition of the aorta and pulmonary artery.

        b. **Noncyanotic types** include **atrial septal defect, ventricular septal defects, patent ductus arteriosus, coarctation of the aorta,** and others.

            (1) **Atrial septal defect ostium secundum** type is the most common of four types and involves an opening between the right and left atria.

            (2) **Ventricular septal defects** may be muscular, perimembranous, or outlet openings between the ventricles.

            (3) **Patent (persistent) ductus arteriosus** is a failure to close or delay in closing of the channel bypassing the lungs and allowing placental gas exchange during the fetal state.

            (4) **Coarctation of the aorta** involves narrowing in the proximal thoracic aorta.

    2. Congenital heart anomalies are the **most common congenital structural malformations.**

B. **Clinical features** (Table 3-4)

C. **Laboratory studies.** Evaluation of most cardiac anomalies involves **chest radiograph, ECG, echocardiography, cardiac catheterization,** and **angiography.**

D. **Treatment** of most congenital heart anomalies is **surgical.**

Table 3-4.
Comparison of Findings in Various Congenital Defects

Anomaly	Murmur	Other Physical Findings	Important Clinical Information
		CYANOTIC DEFECTS	
Tetralogy of Fallot (6%–10% of significant congenital heart defects)	Crescendo/decrescendo holosystolic at LSB, radiating to the back	Cyanosis, clubbing, increased right ventricular impulse at LLSB, loud S_s	Polycythemia usually present; Tet spells (hypercyanotic spells) include extreme cyanosis, hyperpnea, and agitation and are a medical emergency
Pulmonary atresia (1%–3% of congenital heart disease)	Depends on presence or absence of tricuspid regurgitation	Cyanosis with tachypnea at birth; tachypnea without dyspnea; hyperdynamic apical impulse; single S_1 and S_s	Sudden onset of severe cyanosis and acidosis requires emergency treatment
Hypoplastic left heart syndrome (7%–9% of significant congenital heart defects)	Variable, not diagnostic	Shock, early heart failure, respiratory distress, single S_s; presentation varies with specific syndrome	Occurs more often in males; accounts for 25% of cardiac deaths before age 7 days
Transposition of the great vessels (2nd most common congenital cardiac defect in neonates; 5%–7% of all congenital heart defects)	Systolic murmur if associated VSD; systolic ejection murmur if pulmonary stenosis	Cyanosis in newborn is most common sign; tachypnea without respiratory distress; if large VSD, symptoms of congestive failure & poor feeding; single loud S_s; absent LE pulses if aortic arch obstruction	
		NONCYANOTIC DEFECTS	
Atrial septal defect (about 7% of congenital heart disease; secundum most common type)	Systolic ejection murmur 2nd LICS; early to mid-systolic rumble	Failure to thrive, fatigability, RV heave, wide fixed split S_s	
Ventricular septal defect (most common of all congenital heart defects)	Systolic murmur at LLSB; others depending on severity of defect	Depends on size of defect from asymptomatic to signs of congestive failure	Outlet VSDs more common in Japanese and Chinese
Patent ductus arteriosus (12%–15% of significant congenital heart disease; higher in premature infants)	Continuous ("machinery") murmur in patients with isolated PDA	Wide pulse pressure, hyperdynamic apical pulse	
Coarctation of the aorta	Systolic, LUSB and left interscapular area; continuous murmur may be present	Infants may present with CHF; older children may have systolic hypertension or murmur	Differences between arterial pulses and blood pressure in upper and lower extremities pathognomonic

CHF = congestive heart failure; *LE* = lower extremity; *LICS* = left intercostal space; *LLSB* = left lower sternal border; *LSB* = left sternal border; *LUSB* = left upper sternal border; *PDA* = patent ductus arteriosus; *RV* = right ventricle; *VSD* = ventricular septal defect.

IX. VALVE DISORDERS

A. Aortic and mitral valve disorders

1. General characteristics

   a. **Aortic stenosis** narrows the valve opening, impeding the ejection function of the left side of the heart.

   b. **Aortic regurgitation** results in volume overloading of the left ventricle.

   c. **Mitral stenosis** impedes blood flow between the left atrium and ventricle.

   d. **Mitral regurgitation** causes backflow and volume overload of the left atrium.

   e. **Progressive heart failure** leads to **pulmonary hypertension** and **congestion**.

   f. The most frequent etiologies of both mitral and atrial valve disorders are **congenital defects** or **rheumatic heart disease**; others include **connective tissue disorders, infection,** or **senile degeneration**.

   g. Most patients present as **adults after extended periods of asymptomatic conditions**.

2. Clinical features (Table 3-5)

   a. The most common presenting symptoms include **dyspnea, fatigue,** and **decreased exercise tolerance**.

   b. Patients may also have **cough, rales, paroxysmal nocturnal dyspnea** or **hemoptysis,** and **hoarseness**.

   c. Carotid pulses are typically thready in aortic stenosis; **aortic regurgitation** produces **widened pulse pressures**.

3. Laboratory studies

   a. ECG is **not definitive** in establishing the diagnosis.

   b. Chest radiograph

      (1) With **aortic valve disorders**, chest radiograph may show **left-sided atrial enlargement** and **ventricular hypertrophy**.

      (2) With **mitral disorders,** chest radiograph may show **atrial enlargement alone**.

   c. **Echocardiogram** or **cardiac catheterization** is the only definitive method of identifying structural or functional abnormalities.

4. Treatment

   a. The only effective long-term treatments are **surgical repair** or **replacement of the defective valve** or **balloon valvuloplasty**.

   b. Patients with good exercise tolerance may be managed medically with **diuretics** and **vasodilators** to treat pulmonary congestion and **digoxin** or β-**blockers** to treat dysrhythmias.

   c. **Anticoagulant therapy** is recommended for the prevention of thromboemboli.

   d. **Antibiotics** may be indicated for prevention of endocarditis and recurrent rheumatic fever.

Table 3-5.
Comparison of Findings in Aortic and Mitral Valve Disorders

Valve Disorder	Murmur (location, radiation, intensity, pitch, quality)	Aids to Hearing Murmur	Associated Findings
Aortic stenosis	Located at 2nd RICS, radiates to the neck and LSB, medium pitch, harsh, often loud with a thrill	Patient sitting and leaning forward	
Aortic regurgitation	Located at 2nd–4th LICS, radiates to apex and RSB, grade 1–3 intensity, high-pitched and blowing	Patient sitting and leaning forward; full exhalation	Midsystolic or Austin Flint murmur suggests large flow; arterial pulses large and bounding
Mitral stenosis	Located at apex, little or no radiation; grade 1–4 intensity, low-pitched	Patient in left lateral position; full exhalation	S_1 accentuated; opening snap follows S_2
Mitral regurgitation	Located at apex, radiates to left axilla; soft to loud intensity, medium-to high-pitched, blowing		S_2 often decreased; apical impulse prolonged

LICS = left intercostal space; *LSB* = left sternal border; *RICS* = right intercostal space; *RSB* = right sternal border.

Table 3-6.
Comparison of Findings in Tricuspid Regurgitation and Pulmonic Stenosis

Valve Disorder	Murmur (location, radiation, intensity, pitch, quality)	Aids to Hearing Murmur	Associated Findings
Tricuspid regurgitation	Holosystolic murmur; located at LLSB, radiates to right sternum and xyphoid area; variable intensity, medium-pitch, blowing	Increases slightly with inspiration	JVP often elevated
Pulmonic stenosis	Midsystolic crescendo–decrescendo; located at 2nd and 3rd LICS, radiates to left shoulder and neck; soft to loud intensity, possibly associated with thrill; medium-pitched, harsh quality		Early pulmonic ejection sound is common

JVP = jugular venous pressure; LICS = left intercostal space; LLSB = left lower sternal border.

B. Tricuspid and pulmonic valve disorders

   1. General characteristics

   a. Patients with **congenital anomalies** of the tricuspid and pulmonic valves usually present in **infancy or childhood**; adults may present with **tricuspid** or **pulmonic stenosis** resulting from **rheumatic scarring** or connective tissue disease.

   b. **Tricuspid regurgitation** (TR) may be intrinsic or functional.

   c. In all cases, right-sided pressure overload leads to **right-sided cardiomegaly, systemic venous congestion,** and **right-sided heart failure.**

   2. Clinical features (Table 3-6)

   a. Patients usually present with **exercise intolerance.**

   b. Systemic venous congestion is reflected in **jugular venous distention, peripheral edema,** and **hepatomegaly.**

   3. Laboratory studies

   a. Chest radiograph may show a **prominent right heart border** with **dilation of the superior vena cava.**

   b. **ECG findings** may show **right axis deviation, P-wave abnormalities** associated with right atrial enlargement or the **prominent R** and **deep S waves** of right ventricular hypertrophy.

   c. **Echocardiogram** or **cardiac catheterization** is the only definitive method of identifying structural or functional abnormalities.

   4. Treatment

   a. **Sodium restriction** and **diuretic therapy** decrease fluid volume and right atrial filling pressure.

   b. Underlying conditions causing pulmonary hypertension are treated with **arterial vasodilators** or **positive inotropic agents.**

   c. Definitive treatment includes **surgical repair, valvuloplasty,** or **replacement with porcine** or **synthetic prostheses.**

X. ARRHYTHMIAS

A. Supraventricular arrhythmias

   1. General characteristics

   a. Arrhythmias may be triggered by **abnormal automaticity (impulse formation), abnormal impulse conduction, reentry phenomena,** or **abnormal triggers.**

   b. Sinus bradycardia [heart rate slower than 50 beats per minute (BPM)] may be normal in athletes; in others, it **represents sinus node pathology with increased risk for ectopic rhythms.**

    c. **Paroxysmal supraventricular tachycardia (PSVT)** is the most common paroxysmal tachycardia.

    d. **Atrial fibrillation** is the most common **chronic arrhythmia**; it is called **"holiday heart"** when precipitated by excessive alcohol use and withdrawal.

    e. **Atrial flutter** usually occurs in patients with chronic obstructive pulmonary disease, CHF, atrial septal defect, and coronary artery disease.

    f. **Junctional rhythms** occur in patients with myocarditis, coronary artery disease, and digitalis toxicity.

2. Clinical features

    a. Patients may present with **palpitations, angina, fatigue,** and **other symptoms of heart failure.**

    b. Patients may also be completely **asymptomatic.**

3. Laboratory studies. Characteristic ECG findings assist in the diagnosis of supraventricular arrhythmias (Figure 3-5).

4. Treatment

    a. Nonpharmacologic treatments may include **surgical** or **radio frequency ablation of the abnormal site, cardioversion,** and **electrical pacing.**

    b. **Antiarrhythmic drugs** are divided into **5 classes.**

        (1) **Class I** drugs are the **sodium channel blockers** (e.g., lidocaine, procainamide, mexiletine).

        (2) **Class II** drugs are the **β-blockers.**

        (3) **Class III** drugs are the **slow potassium channel blockers** (e.g., bretylium).

        (4) **Class IV** drugs are the **calcium channel blockers.**

        (5) **Class V** drugs are the **direct inotropic agents.**

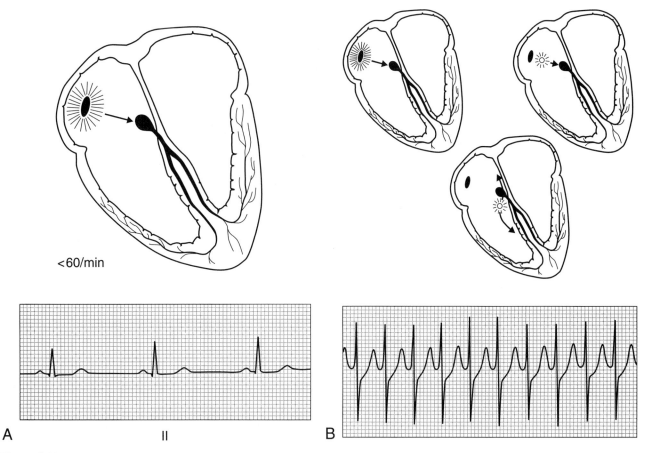

Figure 3-5. Electrocardiogram (ECG) findings in supraventricular arrhythmias. (A) Sinus bradycardia. (B) Supraventricular tachycardia. (C) Atrial fibrillation. (D) Atrial flutter. (E) Junctional rhythm, P waves. (Adapted from Stein E: *Rapid analysis of electrocardiograms: A self-study program,* 2nd edition. Baltimore, Williams & Wilkins, 1992.)

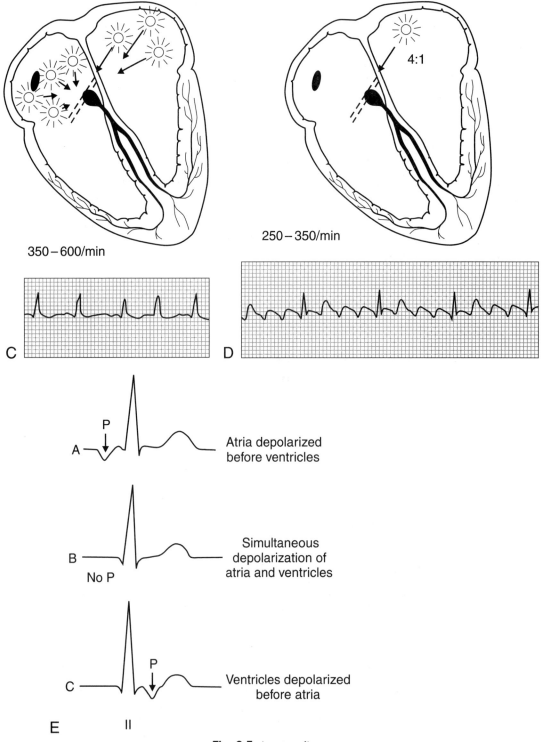

350 – 600/min

250 – 350/min

C

D

A — Atria depolarized before ventricles

B — Simultaneous depolarization of atria and ventricles (No P)

C — Ventricles depolarized before atria

E

II

Fig. 3.5. *(continued)*

B. Ventricular arrhythmias

1. General characteristics

a. Premature ventricular contractions (PVCs) may lead to sudden death in persons with underlying heart disease.

b. Ventricular tachycardia (V tach) is defined as **3 or more consecutive PVCs.** It may be **sustained** or **nonsustained.**

c. In **ventricular fibrillation,** no effective pumping action exists; without intervention death ensues.

Table 3-7.
Antiarrhythmic Drugs

Class	Action	Indications	Examples
Ia	Sodium channel blockers; depress phase 0 depolarization; slow conduction; prolong repolarization	Supraventricular tachyardia; ventricular tachycardia; prevention of ventricular fibrillation; symptomatic ventricular premature beats	Guanidine; procainamide; disopyramide; moricizine
Ib	Shorten repolarization	Ventricular tachycardia; prevention of ventricular fibrillation; symptomatic ventricular premature beats	Lidocaine; mexiletine; phenytoin
Ic	Depress phase 0 repolarization; slow conduction	Life-threatening ventricular tachycardia; refractory supraventricular tachycardia	Flecainide; propafenone
II	β-blocker; slows AV conduction	Supraventricular tachycardia	Esmolol; propranolol; acebutolol
III	Prolongs action potential	Refractory ventricular tachycardia; supraventricular tachycardia; prevention of ventricular tachycardia; ventricular fibrillation	Amiodarone; bretylium (indicated for V-fib and V-tach only)
IV	Slow calcium channel blockers	Supraventricular tachycardia	Verapamil; diltiazem
V	Adenosine: slow conduction time through AV node, interrupt reentry pathways; digoxin: direct action on cardiac muscle and indirect action on cardiovascular system via autonomic nervous system	Supraventricular tachycardia	Adenosine; digoxin

AV = atrioventricular.

2. Clinical features

    a. Patients with **PVCs** may be asymptomatic or may be aware of **skipped beats or palpitations.**

    b. Patients with **V tach** may be asymptomatic or experience **syncope.**

    c. **Ventricular fibrillation** is a common complication of myocardial infarction.

3. **Laboratory studies.** Characteristic ECG findings assist in the diagnosis of ventricular arrhythmias (Figure 3-6).

4. Treatment

    a. PVCs may be treated with β-**blockers** if symptomatic.

    b. In V tach with severe hypotension or loss of consciousness, **cardioversion** may be necessary.

    c. The preferred pharmacologic interventions are **class I** or **class III drugs,** although class II drugs appear to work well with exercise-induced V tach (Table 3-7)**.**

    d. In many types of ventricular arrhythmias, patients with an identifiable site of arrhythmic origin may be treated with surgical or radio frequency ablation.

    e. Some patients may be appropriate for implantable cardioverter-defibrillators.

XI. CONDUCTION DISTURBANCES

A. General characteristics

    1. **Sick sinus syndrome** is found most often in the elderly but may occur even in infancy. It may result from underlying cardiac disease, collagen or metastatic disease, or surgical injury. It may be reversible when caused by digitalis, quinidine, β-blockers, or aerosol propellants.

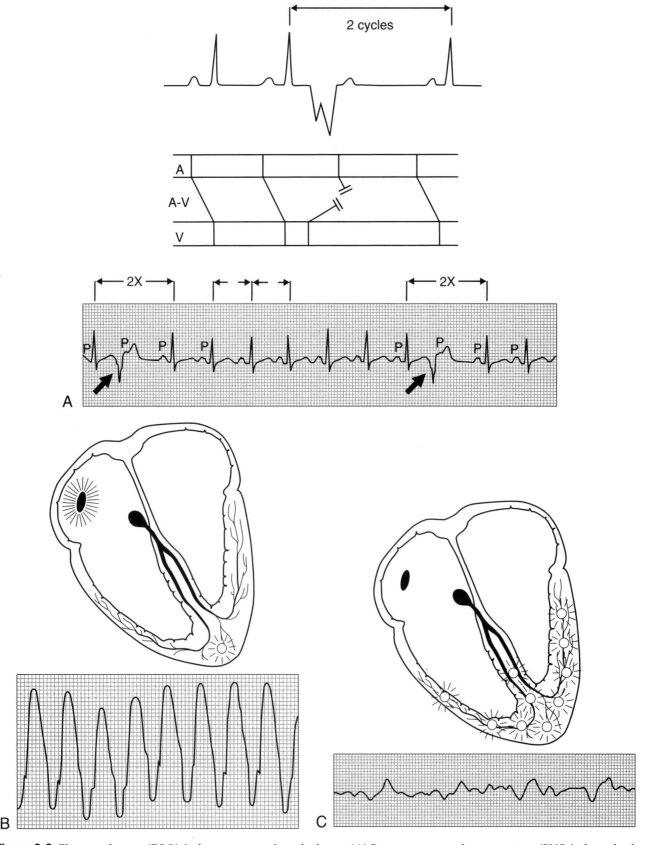

Figure 3-6. Electrocardiogram (ECG) findings in ventricular arrhythmias. (A) Premature ventricular contractions (PVCs), shown by the arrows, are frequently identified by the accompanying compensatory pause. (B) Ventricular tachycardia. The illustration shows sustained tachycardia; it can also be intermittent. (C) Ventricular fibrillation. (Adapted from Stein E: *Rapid analysis of electrocardiograms: A self-study program*, 2nd edition. Baltimore, Williams & Wilkins, 1992.)

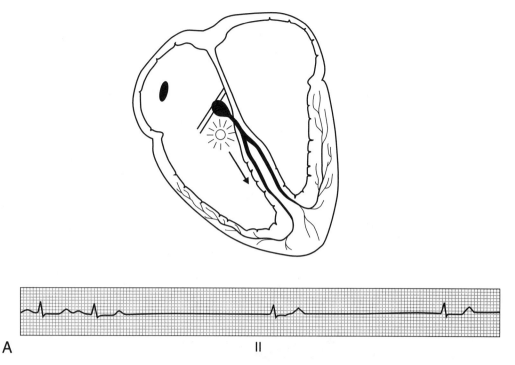

Figure 3-7. Electrocardiogram (ECG) findings in conduction disturbances. (A) Sinus arrest. (B) First degree AV block. (C) Second degree AV block. (D) Second degree AV block (Mobitz I block). (E) Second degree AV block. (F) Third degree (complete) AV block. (Adapted from Stein E: *Rapid analysis of electrocardiograms: A self-study program*, 2nd edition. Baltimore, Williams & Wilkins, 1992.)

   2. Atrioventricular (AV) block is characterized by refractory conduction of impulses from the atria to the ventricles through the AV node, the bundle of His, or both.

B. Clinical features

   1. Most patients with **sick sinus syndrome** are **asymptomatic**, but may have **syncope, dizziness, confusion, heart failure, palpitations,** or **angina.**

   2. AV conduction block produces **weakness, fatigue, light-headedness,** and **syncope.**

C. Laboratory studies. ECG changes associated with conduction disturbances are found in Figure 3-7.

D. Treatment

   1. Most symptomatic patients with sick sinus syndrome require **permanent pacing.**

   2. The only effective long-term treatment for AV conduction disorders is **cardiac pacing.**

XII. CARDIOMYOPATHIES

A. General characteristics. Cardiomyopathies are categorized by their effects on the left ventricular wall thickness, chamber size, and function.

   1. Dilated cardiomyopathies are most common (95%) and are associated with reduced strength of ventricular contraction resulting in dilation of the left ventricle. The myocardium is thinner than normal. **Hypertension** and **excessive alcohol consumption** are the most common predisposing factors; infection, age, or chemotherapy toxicity may also play a role.

   2. Hypertrophic obstructive cardiomyopathy (HCM; 4%) is characterized by massive hypertrophy, particularly of the septum. HCM is almost exclusively a **genetically transmitted disorder.** Sudden cardiac death occurs in HCM patients under 30 years of age at a rate of 2%–3% annually.

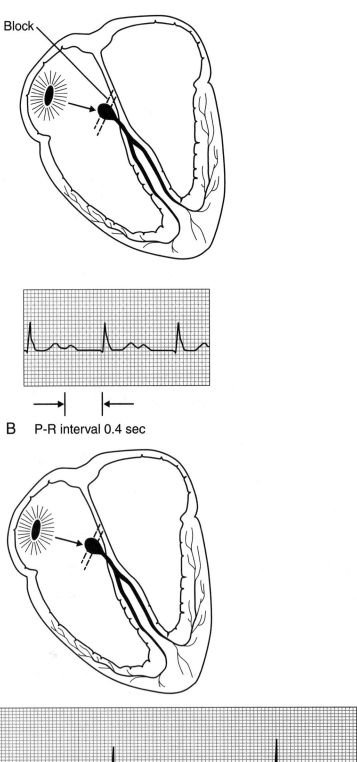

B   P-R interval 0.4 sec

C   2:1 AV block

Fig 3.7. (continued)

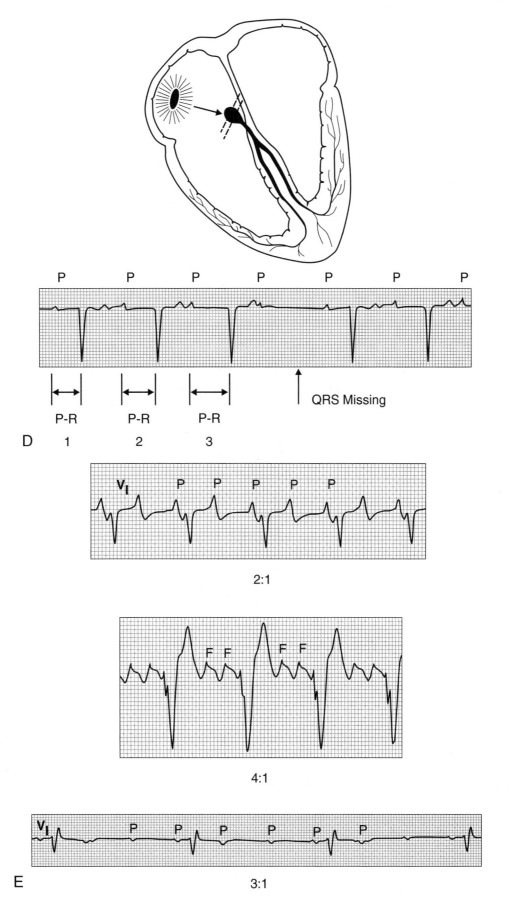

Fig 3.7. (*continued*)

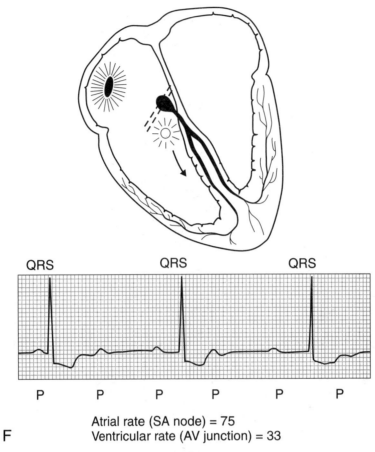

QRS   QRS   QRS

P   P   P   P   P   P

Atrial rate (SA node) = 75
Ventricular rate (AV junction) = 33

F

Fig 3.7. (*continued*)

3. **Restrictive cardiomyopathy** (1%) occurs as the result of **fibrosis or infiltration of the ventricular wall** due to collagen-defect diseases or idiopathic causes. The left ventricular walls are thickened but the cavity is not dilated.

B. Clinical features

1. Patients with **dilated cardiomyopathies** have **fatigue, dyspnea, chest pain, weight gain, venous** and **hepatic congestion,** and **narrowed pulse pressure.**

2. **HCM** patients may present with **dyspnea, angina, fatigue,** or **syncope, or may be asymptomatic.** A harsh **crescendo–decrescendo systolic murmur** is accentuated by the Valsalva maneuver or abrupt standing and diminished by isometric handgrip or in the squatting position.

3. **Restrictive cardiomyopathy** patients present with **decreased exercise tolerance;** in advanced disease, heart failure and pulmonary congestion may produce dyspnea, elevated jugular venous pressure, and prominent third and fourth heart sounds.

C. Laboratory studies

1. Dilated cardiomyopathies

   a. ECG may show **sinus tachycardia** and **nonspecific ST- and T-wave changes.**

   b. Chest radiograph in long-standing disease shows **cardiomegaly.**

   c. Echocardiography or **cardiac catheterization** may be required to rule out valvular disorders.

2. HCM

    a. **Chest radiograph** often reveals a normal cardiac silhouette with a prominent left ventricle.

    b. ECG abnormalities include **nonspecific ST- and T-wave changes** and **abnormal Q waves**.

    c. **Cardiac catheterization** may be necessary to rule out valvular disease or in the anticipation of surgical intervention.

3. Restrictive cardiomyopathy

    a. **Chest radiograph** may show enlarged cardiac silhouette.

    b. **Echocardiography** or **cardiac catheterization** may demonstrate rapid diastolic inflow with early cessation of diastolic filling.

    c. **Endomyocardial biopsy** may be necessary to differentiate restrictive disease from other forms of cardiomyopathy or pericarditis.

D. Treatment

  1. **Dilated cardiomyopathies** are treated with **positive inotropic drugs, arterial vasodilators, diuretics, venous vasodilators,** and **ACE inhibitors. Anticoagulant therapy** is needed to prevent systemic emboli, which are found in 30% of patients.

  2. In **HCM,** β-blockers and **calcium channel blockers** alleviate angina but do not decrease the incidence of sudden death. Patients may require **surgical reduction** of the ventricular wall.

  3. **Restrictive cardiomyopathy** requires **combined diuretic therapy** and **ACE inhibitors. Corticosteroid therapy** may arrest underlying disorders.

XIII. PERICARDIAL DISORDERS

A. General characteristics

  1. **Pericarditis** most often occurs as the result of **infection (viral or bacterial), autoimmune disease, radiation therapy,** or **chemotherapy toxicity.**

  2. **Pericardial effusion** (secondary to pericarditis, uremia, or cardiac trauma) produces restrictive pressure on the heart.

  3. **Cardiac tamponade** occurs when fluid **compromises cardiac filling** and **impairs cardiac output.**

B. Clinical features

  1. The **primary presenting symptom** of pericarditis is **pleuritic chest pain relieved by sitting upright** and **leaning forward;** a **friction rub** is characteristic.

  2. **Pericardial effusions** may be **painful or painless,** often accompanied by **cough** and **dyspnea.**

  3. In infectious conditions, patients may be **febrile.**

C. Laboratory studies

  1. Elevated white blood cell profiles indicate infection, necessitating **blood** and **pericardial fluid cultures.**

  2. **Chest radiograph** or **echocardiogram** is useful to determine the extent of **cardiac effusion** (Figure 3-8)**.**

D. Treatment

  1. In the presence of hemodynamic compromise, **pericardiocentesis** is necessary to relieve fluid accumulation.

  2. Strictly inflammatory conditions may be treated with **steroidal** or **nonsteroidal anti-inflammatory drugs** (NSAIDs); infectious conditions require **antibiotic therapy.**

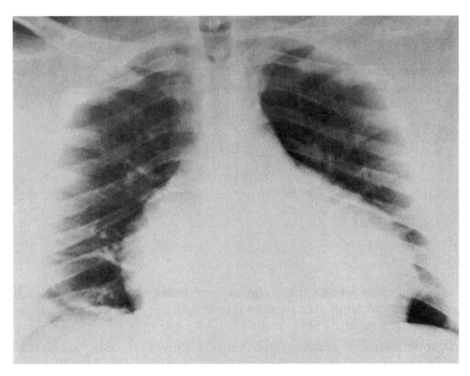

Figure 3-8. Chest radiograph, frontal view, showing pericardial effusion. There is massive enlargement of the patient's cardiac silhouette ("water bottle heart"). (From Daffner RH: *Clinical radiology: The essentials.* Baltimore, Williams & Wilkins, 1993.)

XIV. INFECTIVE ENDOCARDITIS

A. General characteristics

   1. Most infective endocarditis is due to *Streptococcus viridans, Staphylococcus aureus,* and **enterococci.**

   2. In intravenous drug users, *S. aureus* is the most common cause, and the **tricuspid valve** is involved most often.

   3. Prosthetic valve endocarditis is most often caused by *S. aureus*, gram-negative organisms, and fungi in the first 2 months after implantation.

   4. Most patients with endocarditis have an **underlying cardiac defect** that provides a nidus for disease.

   5. Infection may result from **direct intravascular contamination** or from **bacteremia.**

B. Clinical features

   1. Most patients present with **fever and nonspecific symptoms** (e.g., cough, dyspnea, arthralgias, and gastrointestinal complaints).

   2. Approximately 90% of patients will have a **murmur,** although this may be absent in right-sided infections.

   3. **Classic features** include **palatal, conjunctival,** or **subungual petechiae; splinter hemorrhages; Osler nodes; Janeway lesions;** and **Roth spots.**

C. Laboratory studies

   1. Three sets of **blood cultures** over 24 hours should be obtained prior to starting antibiotics.

   2. **Chest radiograph** may demonstrate any associated cardiac abnormality.

   3. The ECG has no specific diagnostic features.

   4. **Echocardiography** may identify the specific valve(s) involved; **transesophageal echo** is particularly useful.

   5. The **criteria** shown in Table 3-8 are used for diagnosis of infective endocarditis.

Table 3-8.
Clinical Criteria for Infective Endocarditis

Patient must have two major or one major and three minor or five minor criteria for the diagnosis to be made on clinical grounds.

Major Criteria
Positive blood culture
Evidence of endocardial involvement

Minor Criteria
Predisposition
Fever > 38°C
Vascular phenomena
Immunologic phenomena
Microbiological evidence
Echocardiogram

For details, see Durack DT, Lukes AS, Bright DK. New criteria for diagnosis of infective endocarditis. Am J. Med. 96:200, 1994.

D. Treatment

1. Antibiotic prophylaxis prior to dental work or surgical procedures should be used in patients with predisposing cardiac abnormalities.

2. Antibiotic treatment should include coverage of staphylococci, streptococci, and enterococci, pending blood culture results.

3. Valve replacement, especially of the aortic valve, may be necessary.

XV. PERIPHERAL VASCULAR DISORDERS

A. Peripheral arterial disease

1. General characteristics

a. Peripheral arterial disease is usually due to **atherosclerosis.**

b. It results in lower extremity **ischemia and pain,** causing significant limitation of activity.

2. Clinical features

a. Lower leg pain with exercise, relieved by rest, is usually the first symptom.

b. Severe disease results in **numbness, tingling,** and **ischemic ulcerations.**

3. Laboratory studies

a. Doppler flow studies are used to determine systolic pressures in the posterior tibial and dorsalis pedis arteries.

b. An **ankle-to-brachial index** less than 0.8 indicates significant disease.

c. Angiography is used to locate stenotic sites.

4. Treatment

a. Cigarette smoking is contraindicated.

b. Lower extremity revascularization must be preceded by a thorough cardiac evaluation.

c. Pentoxifylline may improve exercise tolerance.

B. Varicose veins

1. General characteristics

a. Fifteen percent of adults develop varicosities, **particularly women who have been pregnant.**

b. Inherited defects play a major role.

2. Clinical features

    a. Dilated, tortuous veins develop superficially in the lower extremities, particularly in the distribution of the **long, saphenous vein.**

    b. Varicosities may be asymptomatic or associated with **aching** and **fatigue.**

    c. **Distal edema, abnormal pigmentation,** and **skin ulceration** may develop.

3. **Laboratory studies** are not usually necessary; however, **Doppler sonography** may be used to locate incompetent valves prior to surgery.

4. Treatment

    a. **Elastic stockings** give external support to veins.

    b. **Surgical stripping** should be limited to varicosities and incompetent valves only.

    c. **Sclerotherapy** is appropriate for small veins.

C. Thrombophlebitis and deep venous thrombosis (DVT)

    1. General characteristics

        a. Thrombophlebitis involves **partial or complete occlusion of a vein** and **inflammatory changes.**

        b. Superficial thrombophlebitis may occur spontaneously or following trauma.

        c. DVT occurs most often in the **lower extremities** and **pelvis.**

        d. DVT is associated with **major surgical procedures (especially total hip replacement), prolonged bed rest, use of oral contraceptives,** and **cancer-associated hypercoagulable states.**

    2. Clinical features

        a. Superficial thrombophlebitis presents with **erythema, tenderness,** and **induration of the involved vein;** it is most common in the long saphenous vein.

        b. Half of DVT patients have no early signs or symptoms; **classic findings of DVT** include **swelling** of the involved calf, **heat** and **redness** over the site, and a **positive Homan's sign (calf pain on dorsiflexion of the foot).**

    3. Laboratory studies

        a. **Duplex ultrasonography** is the study of choice for DVT.

        b. **Venography** is the **most accurate** method of DVT diagnosis, but is **associated with increased risk.**

    4. Treatment

        a. Superficial disease is treated with **bed rest, heat, elevation of the extremity,** and **NSAIDs.**

        b. **Prevention of DVT in bedridden patients** is accomplished by elevation of the foot of the bed, leg exercises, and compression hose; in high-risk patients, anticoagulation may be appropriate.

        c. Preferred treatment of DVT is **anticoagulation with heparin for 7–10 days and oral anticoagulants for a total of 3 months.**

D. Chronic venous insufficiency (CVI)

    1. General characteristics

        a. CVI is characterized by **loss of wall tension in veins** resulting in **stasis of venous blood** often associated **with thrombophlebitis.**

        b. In most cases, chronic venous insufficiency is associated with **history of deep thrombophlebitis, leg injury,** or **varicose veins.**

        c. Prevention is accomplished by **early aggressive treatment** of acute thrombophlebitis.

    2. Clinical features

        a. **Progressive edema** is followed by **skin** and **subcutaneous changes.**

        b. **Itching, dull pain with standing,** and pain with **ulceration** is common.

        c. Skin is **shiny, thin,** and **atrophic,** with **dark pigmentary changes.**

        d. Medial or anterior **ulcers occur just above the ankle.**

3. Laboratory studies. See XV D 1 a for laboratory studies for the common causes of insufficiency.

4. Treatment

    a. General therapeutic measures include **elevation of the legs, avoidance of extended sitting or standing**, and **support hose.**

    b. Stasis dermatitis should be treated with wet compresses and hydrocortisone cream.

    c. Ulcerations may be treated with wet compresses, compression boots, elastic stockings, and, occasionally, skin grafting.

XVI. PULMONARY EMBOLUS (PE)

A. General characteristics

    1. Thromboemboli from the peripheral vasculature or the heart **lodge in pulmonary arteries, occluding blood flow to the lung.**

    2. Occlusion produces a **ventilation–perfusion mismatch** and causes **right-sided heart failure.**

    3. The most prominent risk factors include **immobilization, lower limb** or **abdominal trauma (including surgery), heart failure, sedentary lifestyle,** and **certain malignancies.**

B. Clinical features

    1. PE is characterized by sudden onset of **dyspnea, accompanied by chest pain, tachypnea,** and **tachycardia.**

    2. Patients may also have **cough, hemoptysis, palpitations,** and **wheezing.**

C. Laboratory studies

    1. Chest radiograph and **ECG findings** are usually normal unless the underlying cause is preexisting cardiac disease.

    2. Ventilation–perfusion lung scan or **pulmonary angiography** is the most reliable method for diagnosis.

    3. Most patients with acute PE have a **respiratory alkalosis.**

D. Treatment

    1. Prevention includes identifying patients at risk and treating them **prophylactically with pressure stockings** and **anticoagulants.**

    2. Supplemental oxygen aids in normalizing arterial saturation, decreasing tachypnea, and making the patient more comfortable.

    3. Anticoagulation therapy (heparin, warfarin) is the primary treatment for PE, with frequent monitoring of bleeding or coagulation times.

    4. Thrombolytic therapy may be indicated in severe PE.

    5. Some patients may benefit from a **vena cava filter.**

XVII. AORTIC ANEURYSMS

A. General characteristics

    1. An aortic aneurysm is a **weakness and subsequent dilation of the vessel wall usually due to genetic defect or atherosclerotic damage of the intima.**

    2. Atherosclerosis is the **most common cause** of aortic aneurysms, although some exist as congenital defects or as a result of syphilis.

    3. Aneurysms may occur in the **abdominal (90%)** or **thoracic (10%) aorta.**

B. Clinical features

    1. Abdominal aortic aneurysm may be **asymptomatic** and present as a **pulsating abdominal mass,** sometimes accompanied by abdominal or back pain.

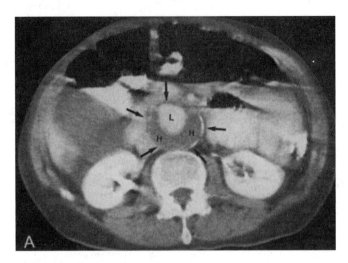

Figure 3-9. Abdominal aortic aneurysm. A computed tomography (CT) scan through the abdomen shows a large abdominal aortic aneurysm (*arrows*). Note the central enlarged lumen (*L*) and the more peripheral hematoma (*H*) and the calcification of the wall on the left side. (From Daffner RH: *Clinical radiology: The essentials.* Baltimore, Williams & Wilkins, 1993.

    2. Thoracic aortic aneurysms may be **asymptomatic** or cause **substernal, back,** or **neck pain; dyspnea, stridor, and cough; dysphagia; hoarseness;** or **symptoms of superior vena caval syndrome.**

C. Laboratory studies

    1. **Abdominal ultrasound** is the study of choice for abdominal aneurysms; this may be followed by **computed tomography (CT) scanning, aortography,** or **magnetic resonance imaging (MRI)** (Figure 3-9).

    2. **Thoracic aneurysms** may require **aortography** for diagnosis; **CT and MRI** are preferred to ultrasound.

D. **Treatment.** The only effective treatment is surgical repair.

4

Hematology

Rebecca Lovell Scott

I. ANEMIAS

A. General characteristics

1. **Anemias** are conditions involving **hemoglobin concentrations** or **packed red blood cell concentrations** at levels **below normal** (Table 4-1).

2. Anemias may be caused by **increased red cell destruction, decreased red cell production, bleeding,** or may be **secondary to a systemic disease.**

3. Anemias present in many forms, including **hypochromic-microcytic anemias** (iron deficiency anemia, thalassemia, and sickle cell anemia), **normochromic-normocytic anemias,** and **macrocytic anemias** (Figure 4-1).

B. Clinical features

1. Many patients have **few signs** or **symptoms.** The most common are **fatigue, headache,** and **exertional dyspnea.**

2. **Acute anemia of rapid onset** may cause **tachycardia, orthostatic hypotension, faintness,** and **pale, cold extremities.**

3. **Chronic anemia** may cause findings **associated with hyperkinetic circulation** (e.g., large pulse volume, tachycardia).

4. **Pronounced anemia** may cause **pallor, cheilosis, jaundice, beefy red tongue,** and **koilonychia.**

C. Laboratory studies (Table 4-2)

1. Hemoglobin (Hgb)

2. Hematocrit (Hct)

3. Red cell indices

4. Red cell distribution width (RDW)

5. Peripheral smear

6. Corrected reticulocyte count

D. Hypochromic-microcytic anemias [mean corpuscular volume (MCV) less than 80]

1. Iron deficiency anemias

a. General characteristics

(1) Iron deficiency anemias **result from an inadequate supply of iron for synthesis of hemoglobin. Iron deficiency** is the **most common cause of hypochromic-microcytic anemias.**

(2) In an adult, **blood loss,** particularly from the **gastrointestinal tract,** is usually the cause of the iron deficiency.

(3) **Low dietary intake** of iron may occur in children and pregnant women.

(4) Menstruation should not automatically be assumed to cause a woman's iron deficiency.

Table 4-1.
Values for Normal Adult Blood

Parameter	Male	Female
Hemoglobin	13.6–17.5 g/dl	12.0–15.5 g/dl
Hematocrit	39%–49%	35%–45%
Red blood cells	4.6–6.3 million/mm^3	4.2–5.4 million/mm^3

dl = deciliter.

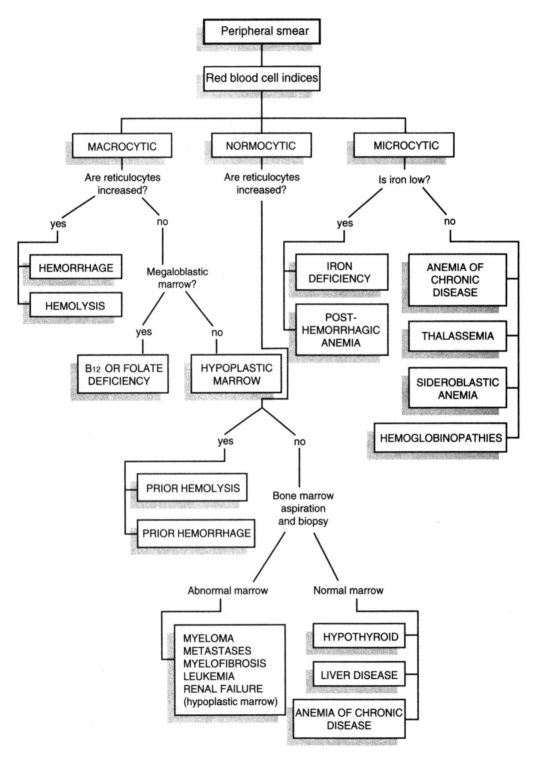

Figure 4-1. Diagnostic approach to anemias. (From Nirula R: *High-Yield Internal Medicine*. Baltimore, Williams & Wilkins, 1997, p 166.)

Table 4-2.
Red Blood Cell Studies

Parameter Value	Normal
MCH	26–34 pg
MCV	80–100 fl
MCHC	31–36 g/dl
RDW	11.5%–14.5%
Corrected reticulocyte count	0.5%–2.5%

dl = deciliter; *fl* = femtoliter; *MCH* = mean corpuscular hemoglobin; *MCV* = mean corpuscular volume; *MCHC* = mean corpuscular hemoglobin concentration; *pg* = picogram; *RDW* = red cell distribution width.

   b. Clinical features

      (1) Lack of iron causes **few specific complaints. General complaints** in severe iron deficiency (hematocrit less than 25%) include **pallor, lethargy, irritability, anorexia, and poor weight gain in infants.**

      (2) **Pica** is a hallmark of iron deficiency.

   c. Laboratory findings

      (1) **Hgb and Hct** are decreased. The **peripheral smear** shows **hypochromic, microcytic red cells.**

      (2) **A plasma ferritin level less than 10 ng/ml in women** and **30 ng/ml in men** is diagnostic.

      (3) **Serum iron** is decreased; **total iron binding capacity** (TIBC) is elevated.

   d. Treatment

      (1) **Ferrous sulfate,** 325 mg twice a day, should be given with meals but not simultaneously with milk.

      (2) **Therapy should be continued** up to 6 months or more to replenish tissue stores.

2. Thalassemia syndromes

   a. General characteristics

      (1) Thalassemia syndromes are **hereditary anemias** caused by **genetically transmitted abnormalities.**

      (2) They may be caused by **congenitally decreased or absent synthesis of the α or β globin chains.**

   b. Clinical features

      (1) Deficits range from **silent carrier status to profound anemia.**

      (2) *α*-Thalassemia may have mild symptoms, or none. It exists in 2 forms: **Hgb H disease** and **Bart's Hgb,** which leads to hydrops fetalis.

      (3) Problems of *β*-thalassemia begin at **4–6 months** when the switch from fetal to adult Hgb occurs and include **severe anemia, growth retardation, fractures, splenomegaly, and jaundice. Most patients with** *β*-thalassemia die before reaching the age of 30 years.

   c. Laboratory findings reveal **persistence of Hgb F.**

      (1) Peripheral smear shows **target cells; small, pale red blood cells (RBCs); and nucleated erythroblasts.**

      (2) **Serum iron** and ferritin levels are well above normal.

      (3) **Hgb level** is usually **between 3–6 g/dl** in the untreated state.

   d. **Treatment** consists of **transfusions to keep hemoglobin concentrations at least 12 g/dl.**

3. Sickle cell anemia (SS disease)

   a. General characteristics

      (1) **Sickle cell anemia** is a **hereditary** form of anemia in which **abnormal crescent-shaped erythrocytes** are present.

        (2) RBCs containing primarily **Hgb S** sickle under deoxygenated conditions.

        (3) In the United States this disease is most often seen in blacks.

    b. Clinical features

        (1) Problems begin in **infancy** when **Hgb F levels fall.**

        (2) By childhood or adolescence, vascular occlusions produce **painful crises, organ swelling and dysfunction,** and **infarction.**

        (3) Patients with SS disease are at increased risk for **cholelithiasis** and infection with **encapsulated organisms (i.e.,** *Streptococcus pneumoniae***).**

        (4) Avascular necrosis of the femoral head is common.

    c. Laboratory findings

        (1) Electrophoresis demonstrates **Hgb S in red cells.**

        (2) Peripheral smear shows **sickled cells, nucleated RBCs,** and an **elevated reticulocyte count.**

    d. Treatment

        (1) Symptomatic treatment includes administration of **analgesics, fluid,** and **oxygen.**

        (2) Patients should receive **pneumococcal vaccine.**

  4. Other hypochromic-microcytic anemias

    a. Sideroblastic anemias are a group of disorders in which hemoglobin synthesis is reduced.

    b. Some anemias associated with systemic or chronic disease

    c. Some anemias associated with copper deficiency

E. Normochromic-normocytic anemias (MCV 80–100)

  1. General characteristics

    a. These anemias are **caused by organ failure** or **impaired marrow function due to systemic disease.**

        (1) The organ failure causing these anemias may be associated with **kidney, endocrine, thyroid,** or **liver disease.**

        (2) The impaired marrow function causing these anemias may be associated with **infection, aplastic anemia, infiltrative marrow disease (myelophthisic syndromes),** and **pure red cell aplasia.**

  2. Clinical features

    a. Anemia associated with chronic disease is **usually mild** and **remits with treatment of the disease.**

    b. Clinical features are **consistent with the underlying disease.**

  3. Laboratory studies are ordered according to the underlying disease.

  4. Treatment

    a. The underlying disease must be treated.

    b. Additional treatment includes **administration of corticosteroids.**

    c. Refractory anemias require **immunosuppressive therapy** or **plasmapheresis.**

F. Macrocytic anemias (MCV more than 100)

  1. General characteristics

    a. This group includes anemias caused by **acute hemorrhage** and **hemolysis.**

    b. Macrocytic anemias also include **deficiencies leading to megaloblastic states (e.g., deficiency of folic acid or vitamin B_{12}).**

2. Folic acid deficiency anemia

  a. General characteristics

   (1) Folic acid deficiency is caused by **poor intake, defective absorption, pregnancy, hemolytic anemias, alcohol abuse,** and **consumption of folic acid antagonists.**

   (2) The daily requirement of folic acid is 50–100 g.

  b. Clinical features

   (1) **Sore tongue (glossitis)**

   (2) **Gastrointestinal problems** (e.g., poorly localized pain, intermittent constipation and diarrhea)

  c. Laboratory findings

   (1) **Hypersegmented polymorphonuclear cells** are pathognomonic for megaloblastic maturation.

   (2) **Howell-Jolly bodies** are typical.

   (3) **Red blood cell folate levels** are **decreased.**

  d. Treatment

   (1) **Dietary** or **oral replacement** with folic acid is the first line of treatment.

   (2) **Alcohol** and **folic acid metabolism antagonists** should be **avoided.**

   (3) **Malabsorption** must be **reversed.**

3. Vitamin B_{12} deficiency

  a. General characteristics

   (1) **Pernicious anemia** is the most common cause.

   (2) **Irreversible neurologic damage** can be caused by uncorrected deficiency. **Folate administration can mask the deficiency but does not correct it.**

  b. Clinical features

   (1) The physical examination will be unremarkable in most patients; **sore tongue (glossitis)** may be present.

   (2) Neurologic findings include **stocking-glove paresthesias, loss of fine touch and vibratory sensation, clumsiness,** and **ataxia.**

  c. Laboratory studies should include a **Schilling test** for pernicious anemia.

  d. Treatment

   (1) Supplemental vitamin B_{12} should be administered **intramuscularly** for **pernicious anemia.**

   (2) **Reversible causes** of **malabsorption** should be treated.

4. Hemolytic anemias

  a. General characteristics

   (1) Hemolytic anemias are those **characterized by accelerated red blood cell destruction.**

   (2) **Genetic disorders** are the cause of some hemolytic anemias.

   (3) Types

    (a) **Extravascular** hemolytic disorders include **hereditary spherocytosis, warm immune hemolytic anemia, cold agglutinin disease,** and **hemolysis caused by liver disease.**

    (b) **Intravascular** hemolytic disorders include **fragmentation syndromes, red cell enzyme defects such as glucose-6-phosphate dehydrogenase (G6PD) deficiency,** and **paroxysmal nocturnal hemoglobinuria.**

  b. Clinical features

   (1) **Both extravascular and intravascular disorders** present with **jaundice, gallstones, pallor,** and **symptoms related to decreased oxygen delivery to the tissues.**

   (2) Infection with **parvovirus B19** can lead to a **transient aplastic crisis.** Patients are at risk for infection with **salmonella** and **pneumococcus.**

   c. Laboratory findings

      (1) An **elevated reticulocyte count** is the hallmark of hemolytic anemia.

      (2) **Peripheral smear** may reveal **immature red cells, nucleated red cells,** or **morphologic changes.**

      (3) **Plasma hemoglobin** may be **increased,** often accompanied by **hemoglobinuria.**

      (4) **Unconjugated (indirect) bilirubin** is elevated.

   d. **Treatment** depends on the underlying disorder.

II. POLYCYTHEMIA VERA

A. General characteristics

   1. Polycythemia vera is a **slowly progressive disease** characterized by **increased numbers of red blood cells** and **increased total blood volume.**

   2. Unregulated expansion of red cell mass causes **hyperviscosity,** which leads to **decreased cerebral blood flow.**

   3. **Secondary causes** of erythrocytosis include **chronic hypoxia** and **renal tumors.**

B. Clinical features

   1. Diagnostic criteria are **splenomegaly, normal arterial oxygen saturation,** and an **elevated red cell mass.**

   2. Patients may present with **symptoms of increased blood viscosity (i.e., headache, dizziness, fullness in the head and face, weakness, fatigue); burning, pain,** and **redness of the extremities**; and, rarely, stroke.

   3. **Pruritus after bathing** is characteristic.

   4. **Plethora, systolic hypertension,** and **splenomegaly** may be found on physical examination.

C. Laboratory findings

   1. Patients **without splenomegaly** must have 2 of the following to establish the diagnosis: **thrombocytosis, leukocytosis, elevated leukocyte alkaline phosphatase, elevated serum B_{12}** or **B_{12}** binding capacity.

   2. **Peripheral smear** shows **neutrophilic leukocytosis, increased basophils,** and **large, bizarre platelets.**

   3. Red cell morphology is usually normal; **erythropoietin levels** are generally **low.**

D. **Treatment** is generally **phlebotomy** or **hydroxyurea.**

III. MALIGNANCIES

A. Leukemias

   1. General characteristics

      a. Leukemias are diseases characterized by **unrestrained growth of leukocytes and leukocyte precursors** in the tissues.

      b. Leukemias are classified **according to cell type** and may be **myeloid** or **lymphoid.**

      c. They may also be classified as either **acute** or **chronic.**

      d. **Risk factors** include a **positive family history, exposures to ionizing radiation, benzene,** and certain **alkylating agents.**

   2. Acute leukemias

      a. General characteristics

         (1) There are **two types** of acute leukemias: **acute lymphocytic leukemia (ALL)** or **acute myelogenous leukemia (AML).**

         (2) The incidence **increases with age.** In children, ALL is more common than AML.

(3) Fifty percent of children with ALL are cured with chemotherapy.

(4) Only 10%–30% of patients with AML survive for more than 5 years disease-free, despite chemotherapy.

b. Clinical features

(1) **Children** and **young adults** present with **fatigue, abrupt onset of fever, lethargy, headache,** and **bone pain.**

(2) **Older adults** have a **slow progressive onset** with **lethargy, anorexia,** and **dyspnea.**

(3) Symptoms of **anemia, thrombocytopenia, gingival hyperplasia, rashes,** or **cranial nerve palsies** occur in most patients.

(4) **Lymphadenopathy** and **splenomegaly** are more common with ALL than AML.

c. Laboratory findings

(1) **Blasts** comprise **30% of nucleated cells** in the bone marrow.

(2) **Auer rods (rod-shaped structures in cell cytoplasm)** signify **myeloid** leukemia.

(3) **White blood cell counts** are **usually,** but not always, **high.**

(4) **Bone marrow biopsy confirms** the diagnosis.

d. Treatment

(1) **Induction (remission-inducing) chemotherapy** is targeted toward eradication of most of the leukemic cells.

(2) **Consolidation therapy** destroys the remainder.

(3) **Increased serum urate levels** may be caused by the treatment. **Allopurinol** and **diuretics** may be needed to prevent uric acid stones.

3. Chronic leukemias

a. General characteristics

(1) The **cause of chronic lymphocytic leukemia (CLL) is unknown** but some cases are familial.

(2) CLL is the **most prevalent** of all leukemias. It is **twice as common in men** as in women. Incidence **increases with advancing age.**

(3) The **B-cell form** accounts for 95% of CLL.

b. Clinical features

(1) **Chronic myelogenous leukemia (CML)**

(a) CML presents in **young to middle-aged adults.** CML occurs in **3 phases: chronic, accelerated,** and **acute (blast crisis).** CML **inevitably transforms into acute disease.**

(b) Symptoms include **fatigue, anorexia, weight loss,** and **excessive sweating.** Most patients also have **splenomegaly.**

(c) The symptoms of CML develop gradually. It generally runs a mild course until the blast crisis phase.

(2) **CLL**

(a) CLL has an **indolent course. It is often harmless,** but is resistant to cure.

(b) Clinical manifestations of CLL include **peripheral lymphocytosis** and **lymphocytic invasion of bone marrow, liver, spleen,** and **lymph nodes.**

(c) Patients may have **recurrent infections, splenomegaly,** and **lymphadenopathy.**

c. Laboratory findings

(1) The **Southern blot test** is used to detect the **Philadelphia chromosome,** which is pathognomonic for CML. This chromosome is present in **95% of patients.**

(2) **Peripheral smear**

(a) In **CML,** this smear reveals **anemia, thrombocytosis,** and **leukocytosis.**

(b) In **CLL,** this smear reveals large numbers of **mature small lymphocytes;** smudge cells are **pathognomonic.**

    d. Treatment

        (1) CML: The **standard therapy for the acute phase** has been hydroxyurea. **Recombinant alpha interferon** has largely replaced it as initial treatment of choice.

        (2) CLL: Treatment of **CLL** is usually **palliative.**

B. Hodgkin's disease

  1. General characteristics

    a. **Hodgkin's disease** refers to a **group of cancers** characterized by **enlargement of lymphoid tissue, spleen, and liver,** and the presence of **Reed-Sternberg cells.**

    b. Hodgkin's is most common **between the ages of 15–45 years and after age 60.**

    c. Among adults 15–45 years of age, it is **more common in men.**

  2. Clinical features

    a. Patients usually present with **cervical, supraclavicular, and mediastinal lymphadenopathy.**

    b. **Nodular sclerosis** is commonly seen in **young women.**

    c. **Stage A** designation indicates a **lack of constitutional symptoms. One third** of patients present with **constitutional ("B") symptoms,** associated with poorer prognosis.

  3. Laboratory studies

    a. The **Ann Arbor staging system** is used to stage Hodgkin's and non-Hodgkin's lymphoma (Table 4-3).

    b. **Basic staging** includes **computed tomography (CT) scans of neck, chest, abdomen, and pelvis** and **biopsy of the bone marrow.**

    c. **Reed-Sternberg cells** confirm the diagnosis.

  4. Treatment

    a. **Chemotherapy cures** more than **50% of patients even with advanced stage disease.**

    b. **Radiation therapy** cures **90% of stage I disease.**

    c. **Adriamycin, bleomycin, vinblastine, and dacarbazine (ABVD)** have fewer side effects than **nitrogen mustard, vincristine, procarbazine, and prednisone (MOPP).**

C. Non-Hodgkin's lymphoma

  1. General characteristics

    a. Lymphomas are a group of **malignancies** that arise from **cells residing in lymphoid tissue.**

    b. About **90% of cases are derived from B lymphocytes.**

    c. The incidence of B-cell lymphomas is higher in patients with **HIV and other immunodeficiencies.**

Table 4-3.
Staging for Hodgkin's Disease—The Ann Arbor Criteria

Stage	Criterion
I	Single LNR (I) or a single ELS (I_E)
II	Two or more LNRs on the same side of the diaphragm (II) or a solitary ELS and one or more LNRs on the same side of the diaphragm (II_E)
III	LNR on both sides of the diaphragm (III); with spleen involvement (III_S) or solitary involvement of an ELS (III_E) or both (III_{ES}); III_1 = upper abdomen; III_2 = lower abdomen
IV	Diffuse involvement of ELSs with or without node involvement
	Presence of constitutional symptoms (fever, night sweats, loss of 10% of body weight) = B; absence = A

ELS = extralymphatic site; *LNR* = lymph node region.

     d. The incidence of lymphoma has been **rising about 1%–2% per year since the 1950s.**

     e. Peak incidence occurs between the ages of **20 and 40 years.**

     f. These lymphomas are divided into **clinically indolent** or **aggressive groups:**

        (1) **Indolent lymphomas** tend to **convert to aggressive disease.**

        (2) One third of **aggressive lymphomas** are **curable with chemotherapy.**

  2. Clinical features

     a. **Diffuse, painless, persistent lymphadenopathy is** the **most common presentation.**

     b. Common **extralymphatic sites** are the gastrointestinal tract, skin, bone, and bone marrow.

     c. Fever, night sweats, weight loss, pruritus, and fatigue are **less likely** than with Hodgkin's.

  3. **Laboratory studies.** Persistent, unexplained enlarged nodes should be biopsied.

  4. Treatment

     a. **Radiation therapy** may cure indolent lymphomas but it usually plays a limited role.

     b. **Aggressive lymphomas** require aggressive **combination chemotherapy.** Relapses may be cured with bone marrow or peripheral stem cell transplantation.

IV. HUMAN IMMUNODEFICIENCY VIRUS (HIV) INFECTION AND ACQUIRED IMMUNODEFICIENCY SYNDROME (AIDS)

  A. General characteristics

    1. HIV is a **retrovirus** that **infects and later destroys CD4+** (T helper lymphocytes).

    2. The definition of a case of **AIDS is a specific opportunistic infection** or a **CD4+ count of less than 200/L** (or CD4+ cells less than 14% of lymphocytes) **in an HIV-infected person** (Table 4-4).

    3. HIV has **3 main routes of transmission.**

      a. **Sexual intercourse**

      b. **Exposure to blood or other infected body fluids**

      c. **Mother-to-child exposure in utero, during childbirth,** or **through infected breast milk**

    4. The mean time period from HIV exposure to development of a case of AIDS is **11 years.**

  B. Clinical findings

    1. Acute HIV infection

      a. Newly infected patients may have no clinical signs; more than half develop **an acute retroviral syndrome** (a febrile flu-like illness) **2–4 weeks postexposure.**

      b. A **symmetric, erythematous, maculopapular rash** is seen in 70% of patients with the retroviral syndrome.

      c. **Neurologic involvement** is common.

    2. Asymptomatic infection

      a. Most infected people remain **asymptomatic for several years;** some develop **persistent generalized lymphadenopathy.**

      b. **CD4+ count is 500/L or higher.**

      c. **Immune system deterioration** continues.

      d. After 5–8 years, an **accelerated decline of CD4+ lymphocytes** and **increased viral load** predict development of AIDS within 2 years.

    3. Symptomatic infection

      a. An **increasing range of infections** occur; patients may also develop an increasing number of symptoms related to various autoimmune conditions, but these are **not life-threatening.**

Table 4-4.
CDC AIDS Case Definition for Surveillance of Adults and Adolescents

Definitive AIDS diagnoses (with or without laboratory evidence of HIV infection)
1. Candidiasis of the esophagus, trachea, bronchi, or lungs
2. Cryptococcosis, extrapulmonary
3. Cryptosporidiosis with diarrhea persisting > 1 month
4. Cytomegalovirus disease of an organ other than liver, spleen, or lymph nodes
5. Herpes simplex virus infection causing a mucocutaneous ulcer that persists longer than 1 month, or bronchitis, pneumonitis, or esophagitis of any duration
6. Kaposi's sarcoma in a patient < 60 years of age
7. Lymphoma of the brain (primary) in a patient < 60 years of age
8. *Mycobacterium avium* complex or *Mycobacterium kansasii* disease, disseminated (at a site other than or in addition to lungs, skin, or cervical or hilar lymph nodes)
9. *Pneumocystis carinii* pneumonia
10. Progressive multifocal leukoencephalopathy
11. Toxoplasmosis of the brain

Definitive AIDS diagnoses (with laboratory evidence of HIV infection)
1. Coccidioidomycosis, disseminated (at a site other than or in addition to lungs or cervical or hilar lymph nodes)
2. HIV encephalopathy
3. Histoplasmosis, disseminated (at a site other than or in addition to lungs or cervical or hilar lymph nodes)
4. Isosporiasis with diarrhea persisting > 1 month
5. Kaposi's sarcoma at any age
6. Lymphoma of the brain (primary) at any age
7. Other non-Hodgkin's lymphoma of B cell or unknown immunologic phenotype
8. Any mycobacterial disease caused by mycobacteria other than *Mycobacterium tuberculosis,* disseminated (at a site other than or in addition to lungs, skin, or cervical or hilar lymph nodes)
9. Disease caused by extrapulmonary *M. tuberculosis*
10. *Salmonella* (nontyphoid) septicemia, recurrent
11. HIV wasting syndrome
12. CD4 lymphocyte count below 200 cells/μL or a CD4 lymphocyte percentage below 14%
13. Pulmonary tuberculosis
14. Recurrent pneumonia
15. Invasive cervical cancer

Presumptive AIDS diagnoses (with laboratory evidence of HIV infection)
1. Candidiasis of esophagus: (a) recent onset of retrosternal pain on swallowing and (b) oral candidiasis
2. Cytomegalovirus retinitis: a characteristic appearance on serial ophthalmoscopic examinations
3. Mycobacteriosis: specimen from stool or normally sterile body fluids or tissue from a site other than lungs, skin, or cervical or hila- lymph nodes, showing acid-fast bacilli of a species not identified by culture
4. Kaposi's sarcoma: erythematous or violaceous plaque-like lesion on skin or mucous membrane
5. *Pneumocystis carinii* pneumonia: (a) a history of dyspnea on exertion or nonproductive cough of recent onset (within the past 3 months); (b) chest x-ray evidence of diffuse bilateral interstitial infiltrates or gallium scan evidence of diffuse bilateral pulmonary disease; (c) arterial blood gas analysis showing an arterial oxygen partial pressure of < 70 mm Hg or a low respiratory diffusing capacity of < 80% of predicted values or an increase in the alveolar-arterial oxygen tension gradient; and (d) no evidence of a bacterial pneumonia
6. Toxoplasmosis of the brain: (a) recent onset of a focal neurologic abnormality consistent with intracranial disease or a reduced level of consciousness; (b) brain imaging evidence of a lesion having a mass effect or the radiographic appearance of which is en- hanced by injection of contrast medium; and (c) serum antibody to toxoplasmosis or successful response to therapy for toxo- plasmosis
7. Recurrent pneumonia: (a) more than one episode in a 1-year period and (b) acute pneumonia (new symptoms, signs, or radiologic evidence not present earlier) diagnosed on clinical or radiologic grounds by the patient's physician
8. Pulmonary tuberculosis: (a) apical or miliary infiltrates and (b) radiographic and clinical response to antituberculosis therapy

CDC = Centers for Disease Control.

      b. CD4 + count is 200–499/L.

      c. Pulmonary infection may develop and present as increasing cough and shortness of breath.

      d. Weight loss, fever, and night sweats are common.

   4. Active AIDS

      a. AIDS-associated malignancies and opportunistic infections occur.

      b. CD4 + counts fall below 200/L.

c. Patients with CD4+ counts **under 50/L** may develop disseminated infections and severe wasting syndromes, peripheral neuropathies, and dementia.

d. **Median survival is 12–18 months.**

C. Laboratory studies

   1. **Enzyme-linked immunosorbent assay (ELISA)** test is used for **screening 6–12 weeks postinfection** and is highly sensitive.

   2. The **Western blot test** is the **confirmatory test.**

   3. **CD4 lymphocyte counts fall** as the disease progresses.

D. Treatment

   1. Management is based on **clinical features** and **serial CD4+ counts.**

   2. Prophylaxis

      a. **Pneumococcal vaccine** should be given every 6 years. At-risk patients require prophylaxis for **tuberculosis, hepatitis B, chickenpox,** and **measles.**

      b. **Trimethoprim-sulfamethoxazole, aerosolized pentamidine,** and **oral dapsone** are used to prevent *Pneumocystis carinii* infection.

      c. **Rifabutin, clarithromycin,** or **azithromycin** is given to prevent *Mycobacterium avium* complex infection, and **ganciclovir** is given to patients with very low CD4+ counts **after cytomegalovirus (CMV) exposure.**

      d. **Zidovudine** [formerly azidothymidine (AZT)] is used to reduce **mother-to-infant transmission.**

   3. **Antiretroviral therapy** should be started when the CD4+ count is less than 500/L.

      a. **Combination therapy** is considered most effective. Available agents include **reverse transcriptase inhibitors** and **HIV protease inhibitors.**

         (1) **Reverse transcriptase inhibitors** include zidovudine, didanosine (ddI), zalcitabine [dideoxycytidine (ddC)], lamivudine (3TC), and stavudine (d4T).

         (2) **Protease inhibitors (e.g., saquinavir, ritonavir, and indinavir)** must be given in combination with other agents to prevent resistance.

      b. **Other treatment** is geared toward the specific autoimmune problem, infection, or malignancy.

V. BLEEDING DISORDERS

A. General characteristics

   1. Bleeding disorders involve **excessive or repetitive bleeding** or **bleeding at unusual sites.**

   2. Bleeding disorders may be classified as either **congenital** or **acquired.**

   3. **Common inherited coagulation deficiency states** include **hemophilia A** and **von Willebrand's disease.** (see V G)

B. **Clinical features** will vary somewhat with the cause of the bleeding.

   1. **Congenital** disorders usually involve **single defects** related to **vascular integrity, platelet function, coagulation,** or **fibrinolytic systems.**

   2. **Acquired** disorders more commonly involve **more than one system,** usually **the liver, kidneys, collagen vascular system,** or **immune system.**

      a. **Abnormal bleeding** is seen with **neoplasia, infection, malabsorption, shock,** and **obstetrical complications.**

      b. **Drugs** associated with bleeding include **nonsteroidal anti-inflammatory drugs (NSAIDs), aspirin,** certain **antibiotics,** and **anticoagulants.**

C. Laboratory studies

    1. Initial assessment includes:

        a. Platelet count

        b. Peripheral smear

        c. Bleeding time

        d. Prothrombin time (PT), partial thromboplastin time (PTT), or activated partial thromboplastin time (APTT)

        e. Thrombin clotting time (TT)

    2. Special studies should be done as indicated.

D. Thrombocytopenia

    1. General characteristics

        a. Thrombocytopenia is an **abnormal decrease in the number of platelets in the blood.**

        b. It may be caused by **impaired production, increased destruction, sequestration, or dilution.**

            (1) **Acute idiopathic thrombocytopenic purpura (ITP)** is found most commonly in **children of both sexes** and is associated with a preceding viral upper respiratory infection.

            (2) **Chronic ITP** may occur at any age and is 10–50 times **more common in women**; it often coexists with other **autoimmune diseases.**

        c. It is the **most common cause of abnormal bleeding.**

    2. Clinical features

        a. Acute ITP is characterized by **the abrupt appearance of petechiae and purpura on the skin and mucous membrane.**

        b. Chronic ITP patients are **asymptomatic, but have petechiae on the skin and mucous membranes.**

    3. Laboratory findings

        a. Acute ITP shows **decreased platelets (10,000–20,000/L), eosinophilia,** and **mild lymphocytosis.**

        b. In chronic ITP, **platelet** count is 25,000–75,000/L.

    4. Treatment

        a. Acute ITP usually **resolves spontaneously;** some patients require **corticosteroids** or **splenectomy.**

        b. Chronic ITP may be treated with **corticosteroids, intravenous gamma globulin, immunosuppressive agents,** and splenectomy (occasionally); **danazol** for older women.

        c. Platelet antagonists (i.e., aspirin) should be **avoided.**

E. Platelet consumption syndromes

    1. General characteristics. There are **3 major types** of platelet consumption syndromes.

        a. Thrombotic thrombocytopenic purpura (TTP), **rare but often fatal,** is found in previously healthy people, **more commonly young women.**

        b. Hemolytic-uremic syndrome (HUS) is identical to TTP, but is found in **children rather than adults.**

        c. Disseminated intravascular coagulation (DIC) causes generalized hemorrhage in patients with **severe underlying systemic illness.**

    2. Clinical features

        a. TTP is characterized by **severe thrombocytopenia with purpura, microangiopathic hemolytic anemia, fever, abnormal neurologic signs,** and **renal dysfunction.**

        b. HUS is identical to TTP but **limited to the kidney.**

        c. In DIC, **skin and mucous membrane bleeding and shock** are more common, and **thrombosis** less often predominates.

3. Laboratory findings

    a. TTP and HUS: red cell fragmentation, normal leukocytes, polychromatophilia, and **reduced platelets;** the **Coombs' test** is negative (hemolysis is not immune related).

    b. DIC: **thrombocytopenia, schistocytes, and fragmented red cells;** PT, APTT, PTT, and **bleeding times** are prolonged; **excessive fibrinogen-fibrin degradation products** are found in serum.

4. Treatment

    a. TTP and HUS: Combined **treatment** with **corticosteroids, plasmapheresis** and **fresh frozen plasma** has improved prognosis.

    b. DIC: The treatment is **prompt and aggressive treatment of the underlying cause.**

F. Disorders of platelet dysfunction

    1. General characteristics

        a. **Congenital** or **acquired** abnormalities may cause these disorders.

        b. Acquired platelet dysfunction

            (1) The **most common causes** of acquired platelet dysfunction are **aspirin** and other **NSAIDs.**

            (2) It is also seen with use of certain **drugs, uremia, alcoholism, myeloproliferative diseases,** various **vitamin deficiencies,** and other conditions.

    2. **Clinical features** are **prolonged bleeding time** and **hemorrhage.**

    3. **Laboratory findings** indicate that there is a **normal number of platelets** but **platelet function study results are abnormal.**

    4. Treatment

        a. In **drug-related** cases, the drug should be discontinued.

        b. **Dialysis** may help patients with uremia.

        c. **Transfusion with platelets** is necessary for serious bleeding.

G. Disorders associated with coagulation protein defects

    1. Hemophilia A (factor VIII deficiency or classic hemophilia)

        a. General characteristics

            (1) Hemophilia A is a **hereditary** disease characterized by **excessively prolonged coagulation time.**

            (2) It is the **most common severe congenital coagulopathy,** after von Willebrand's disease (see V G 2).

            (3) It is X-linked recessive and occurs in about 20/100,000 **male births.**

            (4) **Recent genetic mutation** causes one third of all cases of hemophilia A.

        b. Clinical features

            (1) **Severely affected patients** have repeated, spontaneous, hemorrhagic episodes with **hemarthroses, epistaxis, intracranial bleeding, hematemesis, melena, microscopic hematuria,** and **bleeding into the soft tissue and gingiva.**

            (2) **Less severely affected patients** may experience excessive bleeding following trauma or surgery.

        c. Laboratory findings

            (1) APPT or PTT is prolonged; PT, bleeding time, and **platelet count are normal.**

            (2) **Factor VIII activity** and **factor VIIIc** are **reduced,** but **factor VIII antigen** is **normal.**

        d. Treatment

            (1) **Fresh frozen plasma** or **cryoprecipitates** treat bleeding and should be given prior to surgery or dental procedures.

            (2) **Desmopressin** may elevate factor VIII levels in patients with mild to moderate disease.

2. von Willebrand's disease

   a. General characteristics

      (1) von Willebrand's disease is a **congenital bleeding disorder.** It is **the most common severe congenital coagulopathy.**

      (2) This disease involves **factor VIII deficiency** and it is usually inherited in an **autosomal dominant pattern.**

      (3) Both **men and women** may be affected.

      (4) It occurs in **6 major types.**

   b. Clinical features

      (1) **Bleeding** occurs in **nasal, sinus, vaginal,** and **gastrointestinal mucous membranes.**

      (2) **Spontaneous hemarthrosis** and **soft tissue bleeds** are less common.

   c. Laboratory findings indicate that **bleeding time** is **prolonged** and **factor VIII levels** are **decreased.**

   d. Treatment includes **fresh frozen plasma, cryoprecipitate,** or **desmopressin.**

3. **Hemophilia B,** also known as **factor IX deficiency** or **Christmas disease,** is a heterogeneous group of disorders similar to hemophilia A, but occurring less frequently.

4. Vitamin K-dependent factor deficiencies

   a. General characteristics

      (1) These are the **most common acquired coagulopathies.**

      (2) Deficiencies may be secondary to **liver failure, malabsorption, malnutrition,** and **use of some drugs.**

   b. Clinical features

      (1) **Features of the primary disorder** are evident.

      (2) **Soft tissue bleeding** may occur.

   c. Laboratory findings

      (1) PT/PTT are **prolonged; bleeding time** is **normal.**

      (2) **Liver enzymes** may be **elevated.**

      (3) Levels of **vitamin K** and **factors II, VII, IX,** and **X** are **decreased.**

   d. Treatment

      (1) Treatment is directed at the **underlying cause.**

      (2) **Parenteral vitamin K** restores factor production.

      (3) Treat hemorrhage with **fresh frozen plasma.**

VI. THROMBOTIC DISORDERS AND HYPERCOAGULABLE CONDITIONS

A. General characteristics

   1. **Predisposing factors** in patients who present with **thrombus** include:

      a. Age less than 40 years

      b. Venous thrombosis in the neck, arms, abdomen, or central nervous system

      c. Recurrent thrombosis

      d. Family history of thrombosis

      e. Repeated thrombosis despite adequate anticoagulation (which suggests a neoplasm)

   2. The common congenital defects are **autosomal-dominant** (except cystathionine-synthase deficiency).

   3. Acquired hypercoagulable states are associated with **malignancy** (Trousseau's syndrome), **pregnancy, nephrotic syndrome, ingestion of certain medications** (especially oral contraceptive agents and pure estrogen compounds), **immobilization**, **myeloproliferative disease**, **ulcerative colitis** and **Crohn's disease**, **Behcet's syndrome**, **intravascular devices**, **DIC**, **hyperlipidemia** (particularly familial type II hyperbetalipoproteinemia), **paroxysmal nocturnal hemoglobinuria**, **TTP-HUS**, **hyperviscosity syndrome**, and **antiphospholipid syndrome**.

B. **Clinical features** include typical signs and symptoms of **arterial** or **venous thrombus formation**.

C. **Laboratory testing** for a hypercoagulable state should be conducted by a hematologist.

D. Treatment

    1. Treatment is **heparin** or **thrombolytic therapy** followed by **oral anticoagulation** for prolonged periods.

    2. **No prophylaxis is indicated** in an at-risk person who has **not** had a prior thrombotic event.

    3. At-risk persons **with prior thrombotic events** should be **anticoagulated** for prolonged periods.

VII. ILL-DEFINED PRESENTATIONS

A. Septic shock

    1. General characteristics

        a. **Severe infections**, mostly caused by **gram-negative bacteria**, may cause septic shock.

        b. **Immunodeficient persons** are at **increased risk**.

        c. The **in-hospital mortality rate** is about **50%**.

    2. Clinical features

        a. Patients first develop **hypotension, tachycardia, tachypnea, and hyper- or hypothermia**. They may also be **oliguric, delirious,** or **obtunded**.

        b. Later, **cardiac output decreases, cardiac function is depressed, and vasorelaxation and increased vascular permeability lead to low systemic pressure**.

        c. **Anuria, cholestasis, reduced synthesis of albumin and clotting factors,** and **adult respiratory distress syndrome (ARDS)** may occur.

    3. **Laboratory tests** should be done to identify the **source of infection** based on the presenting symptoms.

    4. Treatment

        a. Treatment is **infusion of isotonic fluids, transfusion with packed red cells for anemia, and administration of a vasopressor agent to maintain systolic arterial pressure above 90 mm Hg**.

        b. **Identification of the source of infection** and **aggressive antibiotic treatment** are imperative.

B. Fever of unknown origin (FUO)

    1. General characteristics

        a. FUO is a fever that has persisted for **at least 3 weeks**, has reached at least **38.3°C (101°F)** on at least two occasions, and whose **cause is not apparent** after routine history and physical examination.

        b. Approximately 85% of FUOs are caused by **infection (40%), tumors (30%),** and **rheumatic diseases (15%)**.

            (1) **Infectious causes** may be **localized** or **generalized**.

            (2) **Tumors** such as adenocarcinomas usually cause fever due to a related infection; other malignancies, including **lymphoma and leukemia**, may present with fever.

            (3) The **chief rheumatic diseases** causing FUO are **giant cell arteritis, Still's disease, periarteritis nodosa, Wegener's granulomatosis, lymphomatoid granulomatosis,** and **Takayasu's disease**.

            (4) **Miscellaneous causes** of FUO include **Crohn's disease, allergic reactions to drugs, allergic reactions to inhaled substances,** and **granulomatous diseases with or without small vessel vasculitis**.

            (5) **Factitious fever** and other psychiatric conditions account for **5% or more** of patients with FUO.

2. **Clinical features** are dependent on the cause of FUO.

3. **Laboratory findings**

   a. **Urinalysis, complete blood count, erythrocyte sedimentation rate, blood chemistry panels,** and a **chest radiograph** should be done routinely on every FUO patient.

   b. **CT scan of the chest and abdomen** and repeated **blood cultures** should also be given to every patient.

4. Treatment

   a. A patient who is febrile, anemic, and has lost significant amounts of weight should be started on a powerful **NSAID.**

   b. If the patient does not improve within 2 weeks of treatment with an NSAID, consider **corticosteroids** or **antituberculous therapy.**

   c. In most cases where a diagnosis is not found, the fever eventually **subsides spontaneously.**

5

Gastroenterology

Susan LaLecheur

I. DISEASES OF THE ESOPHAGUS

A. Reflux esophagitis

1. General characteristics

a. **Reflux esophagitis** is the **recurrent reflux of gastric contents into the distal esophagus.**

b. Commonly called **"heartburn,"** reflux esophagitis is experienced by **10% of the normal population** at least once per week.

c. In a minority of patients, reflux causes **erosion** of the esophagus that leads to **Barrett's esophagitis** (replacement of normal squamous epithelium with metaplastic columnar epithelium), which can predispose to malignancy.

d. **Factors that protect the esophagus** include gravity, lower esophageal sphincter tone, esophageal motility, salivary flow, gastric emptying, and tissue resistance.

2. Clinical features

a. **Heartburn** is the most common presenting feature.

b. **Hoarseness, cough, hiccuping,** and **atypical chest pain** are atypical reflux symptoms.

3. Laboratory studies

a. **Barium swallow** may identify a **large hiatal hernia** (small hernias generally do not contribute to the disease).

b. **Endoscopy** is indicated when symptoms are severe or do not respond to medical therapy.

c. **Endoscopy with biopsy** describes the presence and extent of mucosal damage.

d. **pH monitoring** (to monitor reflux) can be done with an intraesophageal electrode.

4. Treatment

a. **Lifestyle modifications** should be implemented on presumptive diagnosis, with further work-up if symptoms persist. Appropriate lifestyle modifications include **cessation of smoking, avoidance of eating at bedtime, avoidance of large meals,** and **avoidance of foods that cause irritation.**

b. Pharmacotherapy

(1) **Antacids or alginic acid** (Gaviscon) may be used for mild symptoms.

(2) **Histamine (H_2) blockers** may be used, but usually in larger doses than would be used for peptic ulcer disease (see II C 5 b).

(3) **Prokinetic drugs** (e.g., **bethanechol, metoclopramide, cisapride**) increase gastric emptying, and can be combined with H_2 **blockers.**

(4) An **acid-suppressant proton pump inhibitor** (e.g., **omeprazole, lansoprazole**) may be tried as a last resort.

(5) **Anticholinergic, β-adrenergic,** and **calcium channel-blocking agents** decrease lower esophageal sphincter pressure and therefore **should be avoided.**

B. Infectious esophagitis

1. General characteristics

a. Infectious esophagitis is **rare, except in immunocompromised persons.**

b. Causes

(1) Fungal. *Candida* should be considered, especially if oral thrush is present [see Chapter 12 II C 1 a (1)].

(2) Viral. Cytomegalovirus (CMV) and **herpes simplex virus** are also common causes.

(3) Human immunodeficiency virus (HIV), *Mycobacterium tuberculosis*, Epstein-Barr virus, and *Mycobacterium avium intracellulare* (MAI) are additional, though uncommon, causes of infectious esophagitis.

2. Clinical features. The main clinical feature is **odynophagia** (painful swallowing) or **dysphagia** (difficult swallowing) in an immunocompromised patient.

3. Laboratory findings

a. Endoscopy in patients with CMV or HIV reveals large, deep ulcers. Herpes simplex virus infection is characterized by multiple shallow ulcers. *Candida* infection shows white plaques.

b. Cytology or **culture from endoscopic brushings** is needed for definitive diagnosis.

4. Treatment is specific to the type of infection: fluconazole or **ketoconazole** for *Candida*, **acyclovir** for herpes simplex virus, and **ganciclovir** for CMV.

C. Esophageal dysmotility

1. General characteristics

a. The esophageal motility disorders include **neurogenic dysphagia, Zenker's diverticulum, esophageal stenosis, achalasia, diffuse esophageal spasm,** and **scleroderma.**

b. Dysmotility can be caused by **neurologic factors, intrinsic or external blockage,** or **malfunction of esophageal peristalsis.**

2. Clinical features. Dysphagia is the most common presenting symptom for all motility disorders. Its presentation can help determine the underlying cause.

a. Neurogenic dysphagia causes difficulty with both liquids and solids, and is caused by injury or disease of the brain stem or the cranial nerves involved in swallowing.

b. Zenker's diverticulum is an outpouching of the posterior hypopharynx that can cause regurgitation of undigested food and liquid into the pharynx several hours after eating.

c. Esophageal stenosis causes dysphagia for solid foods. Slow progression of solid food dysphagia indicates a more benign process (e.g., webs or rings), and rapid progression indicates malignancy.

d. Achalasia is a global esophageal motor disorder in which peristalsis is decreased and lower esophageal sphincter tone is increased, causing slowly progressive dysphagia with episodic regurgitation and chest pain.

e. Diffuse esophageal spasm is characterized by dysphagia or intermittent chest pain that may or may not be associated with eating.

f. Scleroderma eventually progresses to involve the esophagus in most patients with the disease, causing decreased esophageal sphincter tone and peristalsis, predisposing the patient to the symptoms and complications of reflux esophagitis.

3. Laboratory findings

a. Barium swallow can reveal both structural and motor abnormalities of the esophagus that may cause dysphagia. Achalasia typically has a "parrot-beaked" appearance on barium swallow—a dilated esophagus tapering to the distal obstruction.

b. Pharyngoscopy or **esophagoscopy** must be done (generally by an otolaryngologist) to clarify the nature of a structural lesion.

c. Esophageal manometry can be used to assess the strength and coordination of peristalsis.

4. Treatment

a. Neurogenic dysphagia must be managed by **treating the underlying disease.**

b. Strictures. Most **benign** strictures can be managed by **dilation,** whereas **malignant strictures** must be resected (see I D 4).

D. Esophageal neoplasms

   1. General characteristics

      a. **Ninety-five percent are squamous cell carcinomas.**

      b. **Local spread to the mediastinum** is common because the esophagus has no serosa.

      c. **Cigarette smoking, alcohol,** and **exposure to other caustic agents** (e.g., nitrosamines, fungal toxins, other carcinogens) are **predisposing factors.**

   2. **Clinical features.** The main clinical feature of esophageal cancer is **progressive dysphagia for solid food** associated with **marked weight loss.**

   3. Laboratory findings

      a. **Endoscopy with brushings** is used for diagnosis.

      b. **Endoscopic sonography** and **computed tomography (CT)** may be used for staging.

   4. **Treatment** of esophageal cancer is **surgical.** Because the disease is often advanced on discovery, it is associated with a low (5%–10%) five-year survival rate.

II. DISEASES OF THE STOMACH

A. Gastritis and duodenitis

   1. General characteristics

      a. Gastritis and duodenitis can be defined as **inflammation of the stomach or duodenum.**

      b. Causes

         (1) **Autoimmune disorders** (e.g., pernicious anemia) and other noninfectious factors cause **type A gastritis, which involves the body of the stomach.**

         (2) *Helicobacter pylori* **(HP) causes type B gastritis, which involves the antrum and body of the stomach.** HP tolerates well the acidity of a normal stomach, and is also associated with peptic ulcer, gastric adenocarcinoma, and gastric lymphoma.

         (3) **Nonsteroidal anti-inflammatory drugs (NSAIDs)** can cause gastric injury by diminishing local prostaglandin production in the stomach or duodenum.

         (4) **Stress** from central nervous system (CNS) injury, burns, sepsis, or surgery can lead to erosion of the stomach or duodenum.

         (5) **Alcohol use** is another leading cause of gastritis.

   2. Clinical features

      a. The clinical features of gastritis generally **reflect the underlying syndrome,** rather than the gastric injury itself.

      b. **Dyspepsia** and **abdominal pain** are common indicators of gastritis.

   3. Laboratory studies

      a. **Endoscopy with biopsy** reveals the location and extent of gastritis, as well as the presence of HP.

      b. **A urea breath test** can be used to detect HP because urea is a product of the bacterial metabolism.

      c. **Specific tests** for underlying conditions [e.g., vitamin B_{12} level, complete blood cell count (CBC) for pernicious anemia] should be used as indicated by history.

   4. **Treatment** of gastritis involves **removing the causative factor** (e.g., NSAID, alcohol) or **treating the underlying cause.**

B. Delayed gastric emptying

   1. General characteristics

      a. Delayed gastric emptying can be defined as **an alteration in gastric motility.**

      b. **Causes** include **myopathic diseases** of the smooth muscles or **neurologic dysfunction.**

2. Clinical features include **nausea** and a **feeling of excessive fullness** after meals.

3. Treatment. **Prokinetic medications** (e.g., cisapride, metoclopramide) can sometimes help speed the movement of food through the stomach.

C. Peptic ulcer disease (PUD)

1. General characteristics

a. PUD describes any **ulcer of the digestive system (e.g., gastric ulcer, duodenal ulcer).**

b. Causes. **HP is a common cause** of PUD. When HP is the cause, the ulcer disease can be eradicated with treatment.

c. Lifetime risk of ulcer disease is **5%–10%**, and men and women are equally affected.

d. Gastric ulcers and HP are both **highly associated with gastric malignancy**. While most patients with HP or a gastric ulcer will not get gastric cancer, almost all patients with cancer have had HP or a gastric ulcer.

2. Differential diagnosis. Dyspepsia, abdominal pain, discomfort, or nausea is often associated with gastric or duodenal ulcers, but can also occur in a variety of other conditions, including **gastritis, malignancy,** and **ischemic heart disease.**

3. Clinical features

a. Abdominal pain or discomfort is the primary clinical feature. The pain may be described as burning or gnawing. The pain of a **duodenal ulcer improves with food,** whereas the pain of a **gastric ulcer worsens,** causing associated weight loss.

b. Bleeding can occur, manifesting as melena.

c. Dyspepsia or nausea may also be reported.

4. Laboratory studies

a. Endoscopy is best for detecting small or healing ulcers, and allows for immediate **biopsy** of gastric ulcers in order to rule out malignancy.

b. Barium radiography is widely used and cheaper, but is less sensitive, with a 30% false-negative rate.

5. Treatment

a. Irritating factors (e.g., smoking, alcohol) **should be avoided.**

b. Antacids, H_2 blockers, or sucralfate generally heal duodenal ulcers within 4–6 weeks, and gastric ulcers within 8 weeks.

c. Combination antibiotic therapy for HP accelerates healing and prevents recurrence. Regimens include **bismuth with metronidazole and tetracycline or amoxicillin, or omeprazole with either clarithromycin or amoxicillin.**

D. Gastric neoplasm

1. Zollinger-Ellison syndrome (ZES)

a. General characteristics

(1) In ZES, a **gastrin-secreting tumor (gastrinoma)** causes **hypergastrinemia,** which results in **refractory PUD.**

(2) Only **1% of cases of PUD are caused by ZES.**

(3) Most gastrinomas are found in the **pancreas** or **duodenum,** but they may be found anywhere or may metastasize.

(4) **About 20%** of gastrinomas are **part of a syndrome known as multiple endocrine neoplasia, type I (MEN-I).**

b. Clinical features

(1) Most commonly, the clinical presentation is **indistinguishable from that of PUD** (see II C 3), although ZES is usually more advanced or refractory to treatment.

(2) **Abdominal pain** may be accompanied by a **secretory diarrhea** that improves with H_2 blockers (e.g., ranitidine, cimetidine) or proton pump inhibitors (e.g., omeprazole, lansoprazole).

(3) **Occult** or **frank bleeding** causing **anemia** may be present.

c. Laboratory findings

(1) **A fasting gastrin level of greater than 150 pg/ml** indicates hypergastrinemia.

(2) A **secretin test** is needed to confirm ZES. Patients are given 2 units/kg secretin intravenously. In most patients with ZES, the gastrin levels will increase by more than 200 pg/ml.

(3) **Endoscopy, CT,** or **magnetic resonance imaging (MRI)** may help in localizing the tumor.

d. Treatment

(1) **Omeprazole** controls gastrin secretion.

(2) **Surgical resection** of the gastrinoma **should be attempted** when possible.

2. Gastric adenocarcinoma

a. General characteristics

(1) This is **among the most common types of cancer worldwide,** but is less common in the United States.

(2) Gastric adenocarcinoma is **twice as common in men** as in women.

(3) It **almost never occurs** in a patient **younger than 40 years of age.**

(4) With **early diagnosis,** an **80% cure rate** can be accomplished; if the muscularis propria is involved, the cure rate is 50%; if there is lymphatic spread, the cure rate is 10%.

b. Clinical features

(1) **Dyspepsia** and **weight loss** associated with anemia and occult gastrointestinal (GI) bleeding in a patient older than 40 years of age are common presenting complaints.

(2) **Progressive dysphagia** may be caused by a neoplasm impinging on the esophagus.

(3) **Postprandial vomiting** may be caused by a neoplasm near the pylorus.

(4) **Signs of metastatic spread include left supraclavicular lymphadenopathy** (Virchow's node) or **an umbilical nodule** (Sister Mary Joseph's nodule).

c. Laboratory studies

(1) **Iron deficiency anemia** is the most common finding.

(2) **Liver enzymes** may be elevated with hepatic metastases.

(3) **Endoscopy with cytology** should be done on any patient older than 40 years of age with dyspepsia that is unresponsive to therapy.

(4) **Abdominal CT** is used after the diagnosis has been made, to determine the extent of disease.

d. Treatment is curative or palliative **resection of the tumor,** though chemotherapy or radiation may provide some palliative benefit.

3. **Carcinoid tumors of the stomach** rarely occur in response to hypergastrinemia, and are generally benign and self-limited.

4. Gastric lymphoma

a. General characteristics

(1) Gastric lymphomas account for fewer than 2% of gastric malignancies but the stomach is **the most common extranodal site for non-Hodgkin's lymphoma.**

(2) **The risk** of gastric lymphoma is **6 times greater if HP infection is present.**

b. Clinical features are the same as for gastric adenocarcinoma.

c. Laboratory findings differ from those of gastric adenocarcinoma only in pathology of the lesion.

d. Treatment is resection with or without radiation or chemotherapy.

III. DISEASES OF THE SMALL INTESTINE

A. Diarrhea

1. Diarrhea is **increased frequency or volume of stool** (i.e., 3 or more liquid or semisolid stools daily for at least 2–3 consecutive days).

2. **Causes** of diarrhea may be **infectious** (Table 5-1), **toxic**, or **dietary** (e.g., laxative use) or other **GI disease.**

3. **Patient history.** The history should include all **current medications** as well as **illness among others who have shared meals** with the patient.

4. **Clinical features**

   a. Secretory diarrhea (large volume without inflammation) indicates pancreatic insufficiency, ingestion of preformed bacterial toxins, or laxative use.

   b. Inflammatory diarrhea indicates invasive organisms or inflammatory bowel disease.

   c. Antibiotic-associated diarrhea is almost always caused by *Clostridium difficile* colitis, which in the most severe cases causes the classic pseudomembranous colitis.

5. **Laboratory findings**

   a. White blood cells in stool denote an inflammatory process.

   b. Cultures for bacterial agents, microscopy for parasites, or **toxin identification** (if enterotoxic *Escherichia coli* or *C. difficile* is suspected) can identify infectious agents in stool.

6. **Treatment**

   a. Supportive therapy is sufficient for most patients with viral or bacterial diarrhea.

   b. Antibiotics may be indicated for patients with severe diarrhea and systemic symptoms (e.g., *Shigella, Campylobacter,* severe cases of *C. difficile*).

   c. Treatment of the underlying cause is required for noninfectious diarrhea.

B. Small bowel obstruction

1. **Clinical features**

   a. Obstruction presents with **abdominal pain, distention, vomiting of partially digested food,** and **obstipation.**

   b. Bowel sounds are **high-pitched** and **come in rushes.**

2. **Treatment is surgical,** with large bowel obstruction more urgent than small bowel obstruction.

C. Malabsorption

1. **General characteristics**

   a. Malabsorption **may involve a single nutrient,** as with pernicious anemia (vitamin B_{12}) or lactase deficiency (lactose), or **may be global,** as with celiac disease or AIDS.

   b. Malabsorption **may be caused by problems in digestion, absorption,** or **impaired blood** and **lymph flow.**

2. **Clinical features**

   a. Diarrhea is usually the primary complaint, and may be accompanied by **bloating and abdominal discomfort. Weight loss** and **edema** may also be present.

   b. Steatorrhea may occur.

   c. Specific deficiencies may cause **bone demineralization, tetany, bleeding,** or **anemia.**

3. **Laboratory findings**

   a. If a **72-hour fecal fat test** is normal, specific defects such as pancreatic insufficiency or abnormal bile salt metabolism should be considered.

   b. A D-xylose test will distinguish maldigestion (e.g., pancreatic insufficiency, bile salt deficiency) from malabsorption.

   c. Specific tests may be used to detect **vitamin B_{12}, calcium,** or **albumin** deficiencies.

Table 5-1.
Foodborne and Waterborne Causes of Diarrhea

Agent	Source	Onset	Nausea and Vomiting	Diarrhea	Fever	Duration	Therapy
Norwalk virus	Food, water	1–3 days	Yes	Watery	Low-grade	1–2 days	Hydration
Rotavirus	Person-to-person	1–3 days	Yes	Watery	Low-grade	5–8 days	Hydration
Staphylococcus aureus (Toxin)	Food, after cooking	1–7 hours	Yes, rapid onset	Cramping, some diarrhea	Uncommon	Acute (4–6 hours), total (1–2 days)	Supportive
Clostridium perfringens (Toxin)	Food, before cooking	8–14 hours	Uncommon	Cramping, watery	Rare	<24 hours	Supportive
Vibrio species (Cholera)	Water	2–3 days	Some	Profuse, watery	Rare	days	Hydration
Enterotoxic *Escherichia coli*	Food	5–15 days	Some	Cramping, watery	Low-grade	1–5 days	Hydration, Bismuth/ASA loperamide
Giardia lamblia	Water, person-to-person	5–25 days	Nausea	+/– diarrhea, bloating	None	Until treated	Metronidazole 250mg twice a day for 10 days
Cryptosporidia	Water, outbreaks	2–10 days	Yes	Watery	Possible	30 days (unless HIV)	Supportive, HIV treatment
Cyclospora	Imported, uncooked foods	1 week	Nausea, anorexia	Watery	Low-grade	Weeks	Trimethoprim soulfamethazole with Bactrim twice a day for 7 days
Salmonella (Invasive)	poultry	6–72 hours	Nausea, some vomiting	Purulent	Yes, septicemia common	4–7 days	Hydration
Enterohemorrhagic *E. coli* (Invasive)	Undercooked ground beef	12–60 hours	No	Purulent, bloody, cramping	Yes	5–10 days	Supportive unless severe
Shigella (Invasive)	Fecal–oral	1–6 days	No	Purulent, bloody, cramping	Yes	1–7 days	Supportive
Campylobacter (Invasive)	Undercooked poultry	2–5 days	Some	Purulent, bloody, cramping	Yes	2–5 days	Supportive

ASA = acetylsalicylic acid.

  4. **Therapeutic trials** of the following can help in both diagnosis and treatment:

   a. **A lactose-free diet** for lactase deficiency

   b. **A gluten-free diet** for celiac disease

   c. **Pancreatic enzyme replacement** for pancreatic insufficiency

   d. **Tetracycline** for bacterial overgrowth

D. Crohn's disease (regional enteritis)

  1. General characteristics

   a. Crohn's disease is an **inflammatory bowel disease** for which there is **some genetic predisposition** although the **cause is unknown.**

   b. Crohn's **may involve both the small and large bowel.** Most commonly, the terminal ileum and right colon are involved.

   c. **Complications** include **fistulas, abscesses,** and **predisposition to colonic cancer.**

   d. The success or failure of treatment is variable. The disease usually waxes and wanes throughout life.

  2. Clinical features

   a. **Abdominal cramps** and **diarrhea** in a **patient younger than 40 years** are the most common complaints.

   b. **Low-grade fever, polyarthralgia,** and **anemia** are frequently encountered.

   c. **Blood may be present in stool.**

  3. Laboratory findings

   a. A **double-contrast barium enema** or **CT scan** will show cobblestone filling defects with segmental areas of involvement.

   b. **Contrast studies** and **sigmoidoscopy should be avoided** in patients with fulminant disease because of the possibility of inducing toxic megacolon.

  4. Treatment

   a. **Oral corticosteroids** may be used in combination with **aminosalicylate anti-inflammatory agents** such as 5-aminosalicylic acid (mesalamine)**.**

   b. **Metronidazole** or **tetracycline** may be added if deep fissure or fistula is present.

E. Irritable bowel syndrome (IBS)

  1. General characteristics

   a. IBS can be defined as **hypersensitivity to intestinal distention.**

   b. IBS is **the most common cause of chronic** or **recurrent abdominal pain** in the United States.

   c. IBS generally remains an **intermittent, lifelong problem.**

   d. IBS is **more common in women** than men.

   e. **The differential diagnosis** includes lactose intolerance, cholecystitis, chronic pancreatitis, intestinal obstruction, chronic peritonitis, and carcinoma of the pancreas or stomach.

  2. Clinical features

   a. **Physical examination is generally normal,** but may include, on occasion, a tender, palpable sigmoid colon, and hyperresonance on percussion over the abdomen.

   b. **Abdominal pain** may occur anywhere, or may be localized to the **hypogastrium** or **left lower quadrant,** and may be **worsened by food intake.** Pain is associated with **bowel distention** from accumulation of gas, and associated spasm of the smooth muscle.

   c. **Constipation, diarrhea,** or **alternating constipation and diarrhea may occur.**

   d. **Dyspepsia** is common.

   e. **Onset of symptoms is often insidious, generally appearing in early adulthood.**

3. Laboratory findings are generally normal. Stool should be tested for blood, bacteria, parasites, and lactose tolerance (or milk restriction) and a barium enema should be performed.

4. Treatment involves a **high fiber diet** and **bulking agents** such as psyllium hydrophilic mucilloid.

IV. DISEASES OF THE COLON, RECTUM, AND ANUS

A. Constipation

1. General characteristics

  a. Constipation is **a decrease in stool volume and increase in stool firmness accompanied by straining. Normal bowel function** ranges from 3 stools per day to 3 stools per week.

  b. Patients **more than 50 years of age** with new-onset constipation **should be evaluated for colon cancer.**

2. Treatment

  a. In most cases an **increase in fiber** (to 10–20 grams daily) and **fluid intake** (up to 1.5–2 liters), and **increased exercise** will resolve the problem.

  b. A patient with constipation lasting more than 2 weeks or refractory to modifications in diet, exercise, and fluid intake should have a work-up to detect the underlying cause. If a **treatable underlying cause** is found, constipation will resolve with treatment of the disease process.

B. Diverticular disease

1. General characteristics

  a. Diverticulosis can be described as **large outpouchings of the diverticula** in the colon. **Diverticulitis** is defined as **inflammation of the diverticula.**

  b. Sixty percent of people older than 60 years have **diverticula,** or **outpouchings from the colon,** of whom 20% become symptomatic.

  c. Twenty percent of patients with acute diverticulitis are younger than 40 years.

  d. In patients with diverticulosis, diverticulitis and its complications **can be prevented** with a **high-fiber diet.**

2. Clinical features

  a. Diverticulitis **generally presents with sudden-onset abdominal pain, usually in the left lower quadrant or suprapubic region,** with or without fever. **Symptoms may range from mild disease to severe infection with peritonitis.**

  b. Diverticular bleeding generally presents as sudden-onset, large-volume hematochezia. It resolves spontaneously, although continuous or recurrent bleeding are indications for surgery.

  c. Nausea and **vomiting** are common.

3. Laboratory findings

  a. Occult blood in the stool and **mild to moderate leukocytosis** may occur with diverticulitis.

  b. Barium enema should be avoided during an acute episode, as it may lead to perforation and peritonitis.

4. Treatment

  a. Low-residue diet and **broad-spectrum antibiotics** plus **metronidazole** (500 mg 3–4 times daily) are appropriate for patients with mild diverticulitis.

  b. Hospitalization for intravenous administration of antibiotics, bowel rest, and analgesics **is often required.**

  c. Surgical management may be necessary in severe cases.

C. Ulcerative colitis

1. General characteristics

  a. Ulcerative colitis must be **differentiated from inflammatory infectious conditions** (see Table 5-1) **and from Crohn's disease** (Table 5-2).

Table 5-2.

Differentiation of Crohn's Disease and Ulcerative Colitis

	Crohn's Disease	**Ulcerative Colitis**
Onset	Gradual	Sudden or gradual
Distribution of disease	Right-sided, skips areas	Distal to proximal, continuous
Symptoms	Diarrhea and pain	Bloody, pus-filled diarrhea, tenesmus
Complications	Fistulas (common), toxic megacolon, colon cancer	Toxic megacolon, colon cancer

  b. The disease generally **starts distally, at the rectum,** and **progresses proximally.**

  c. Onset is **generally gradual,** but may be abrupt.

 2. Clinical features

  a. Tenesmus and **bloody, pus-filled diarrhea** are common presenting symptoms.

  b. **Lower left quadrant pain** may be present.

  c. **Weight loss, malaise,** and **fever** may occur in more severe disease.

 3. Laboratory findings

  a. **Anemia, increased sedimentation rate,** and **decreased serum albumin** are common.

  b. **Sigmoidoscopy** is the best method of diagnosis, although an **abdominal plain film** might show colonic dilatation.

  c. **Colonoscopy** and **barium enema should be avoided** because of the risks of perforation and toxic megacolon, respectively.

 4. **Topical** or **oral aminosalicylates** and **corticosteroids** are the mainstays of treatment.

D. Anal fissure

 1. Anal fissures are **linear lesions in the rectal wall,** leading to **severe pain on defecation** often accompanied by **bright red blood per rectum.**

 2. **Treatment includes bulking agents** and **topical styptic** such as silver nitrate (1%–2%) or gentian violet solution (1%).

E. Hemorrhoids

 1. **General characteristics.** Hemorrhoids are **varices of the hemorrhoidal plexus.**

 2. **Clinical features** include **rectal discomfort, pruritus, rectal bleeding,** or **mucoid discharge.**

 3. **Treatments** range from **dietary changes** and **stool softeners** to **surgical repair,** depending on severity.

F. Colorectal cancer

 1. General characteristics

  a. Colorectal cancer is the **second leading cause of cancer death** in the United States after lung cancer.

  b. Ninety percent of cases occur in persons older than 50 years.

  c. **The prognosis is good in early disease.** There is a 75%–100% 5-year survival rate when the cancer does not penetrate the colon and there is no lymphatic spread. However, the 5-year survival rate drops to 5% when there are distant metastases.

 2. Clinical features

  a. Colorectal cancer is **slow growing** and **symptoms often appear late in the disease.**

  b. **Fatigue** and **weakness** may occur if chronic blood loss has led to anemia.

  c. **Changes in stool size** and shape may be noted, as may **frank blood in the stool.**

3. Laboratory findings

  a. Occult blood in the stool is the best early marker and is used for screening adults over 40 years of age. **Flexible sigmoidoscopy** is also used in those over 40 or 50 years of age.

  b. Carcinoembryonic antigen (CEA) may be used to monitor, although not to detect, colorectal cancer.

  c. Sigmoidoscopy, colonoscopy, and **barium enema** may all be used to visualize colonic masses, while a **chest radiograph** and **CT scan** can be used to detect metastases.

4. Treatment is by **surgical resection, accompanied by chemotherapy** in those with any extension through the serosa or with lymphatic spread.

V. DISEASES OF THE APPENDIX AND PANCREAS

A. Appendicitis

  1. General characteristics

  a. Appendicitis occurs when **obstruction of the appendix, by fecalith or other cause, leads to inflammation and infection.**

  b. Patients are usually **between 10 and 30 years of age.**

  c. Appendicitis affects 10% of the population of the United States, making it **the most common abdominal surgical emergency.**

  d. Perforation and peritonitis (see VIII A) occur in about **20% of patients** with appendicitis, causing high fever, generalized abdominal pain, and increased leukocytosis.

  2. Clinical features

  a. The **initial symptom is intermittent periumbilical** or **epigastric pain.**

  b. In about 12 hours, **pain localizes to the right lower quadrant (McBurney's point),** becomes constant, and is worsened by movement, leading to rebound tenderness on examination.

  c. Nausea and anorexia are common. Vomiting may occur but is generally isolated and begins subsequent to the onset of pain. Diarrhea may occur but is not common.

  d. A **low-grade fever is common,** although a high fever is unlikely.

  e. Obturator sign (i.e., patient is supine and attempts to raise leg against resistance) **and psoas sign** (i.e., patient is supine and attempts to flex and internally rotate the right hip with the knee bent) **are generally positive,** indicating inflammation adjacent to those muscles.

  f. Variability in anatomy can cause unusual presentations of appendicitis, with symptoms reflecting the location of the appendix.

  3. Laboratory findings

  a. Leukocytosis (usually 10,000–20,000 cells/μL) is characteristic. Higher levels suggest perforation and peritonitis.

  b. Some **microscopic hematuria** and **pyuria** may be seen.

  c. Abdominal CT may be used in some cases to confirm the diagnosis and to locate an abnormally placed appendix.

  4. Treatment consists of **appendectomy,** with **broad-spectrum antibiotics administered prior to surgery** if there is any reason to suspect perforation.

B. Acute pancreatitis

  1. General characteristics

  a. The **most common cause is alcohol abuse,** but **cholelithiasis, hyperlipidemia, trauma, drugs, hypercalcemia,** and **penetrating PUD** may also cause pancreatitis.

  b. The **range of presentation is wide,** from mild episodes of deep epigastric pain with nausea and vomiting, to the sudden onset of severe pain, with shock.

    c. The **differential diagnosis** for acute pancreatitis **includes other processes that cause abdominal pain** (e.g., gastritis, PUD, cholecystitis).

2. Clinical features

    a. The **classic presentation is epigastric pain radiating to the back.**

    b. **Nausea and vomiting are common.**

    c. **Fever, leukocytosis,** and **sterile peritonitis** may occur.

    d. **Severe hypovolemia, adult respiratory distress syndrome,** and **tachycardia greater than 130 beats per minute indicate a grave prognosis.**

3. Laboratory studies

    a. **Serum amylase.** Elevation in amylase occurs, but may be transient and can return to normal after 48–72 hours.

    b. **Serum lipase** is more sensitive and specific than amylase for acute pancreatitis, but only with elevations of threefold or greater.

    c. The **white blood cell count** is generally elevated, and hemoconcentration may occur with third spacing of fluid.

    d. **Liver enzymes may increase** as a result of biliary obstruction.

    e. **Mild hyperbilirubinemia** and **bilirubinuria, hyperglycemia,** and **hypocalcemia** may occur.

    f. **Poor prognosis** is indicated by a **leukocyte count greater than 16,000 cells/ml,** a **blood glucose level greater than 200 mg/dl,** a **lactate dehydrogenase (LDH) level greater than 350 IU/dl** (normal level is 20–50 IU/dl), **aspartate aminotransferase (AST) greater than 250 IU/dl** (normal level is less than or equal to 120 IU/dl), a **falling hematocrit,** and a **falling calcium level.**

4. Treatment

    a. **Oral intake must be stopped** to prevent continued secretion of pancreatic juices.

    b. **Fluid volume must be restored** and maintained.

    c. **Parenteral hyperalimentation should be started early** to prevent nutritional depletion.

    d. **The patient must be closely monitored for complications** including pancreatic pseudocyst, renal failure, pleural effusion, hypocalcemia, and pancreatic abscess.

C. Chronic pancreatitis

1. General characteristics

    a. **Ninety percent of cases of chronic pancreatitis** in the United States are **caused by alcohol abuse,** with some cases caused by cholelithiasis, PUD, hyperparathyroidism, and hyperlipidemia.

    b. Some chronic cases can resolve **if alcohol consumption is decreased.**

    c. The **classic triad of pancreatic calcification, steatorrhea,** and **diabetes mellitus occurs in only 20% of patients.**

2. **Clinical features** are **the same as those of acute pancreatitis,** with the addition of **fat malabsorption** and **steatorrhea** late in the disease. Fecal fat will be elevated if malabsorption is present.

3. Laboratory studies

    a. The **amylase level** may be elevated early, but will decrease with each episode of pancreatitis, and ceases to be a useful marker.

    b. An **abdominal plain film** reveals calcification in 20% of patients.

4. **Treatment** is as for acute pancreatitis. **Surgical removal of part of the pancreas** can **control pain.** The **only definitive treatment** for chronic pancreatitis is to **address the underlying cause,** which is **most commonly alcohol.**

D. Pancreatic neoplasm

    1. General characteristics

        a. Pancreatic cancer is the **fifth leading cause of cancer death** in the United States.

        b. Only about 10% of those with pancreatic cancer can be cured surgically.

        c. **Chronic pancreatitis** increases the risk 10- to 15-fold, and **smoking** increases the risk slightly.

    2. Clinical presentation

        a. **Abdominal pain** occurs in most patients. The pain can **radiate** depending on the location of the tumor.

        b. **Jaundice** may be seen in patients with cancer of the pancreatic head.

    3. **Diagnostic studies** include **CT** (to search for metastases) and **angiography** (to look for vascular invasion).

    4. **Treatment** is **surgical resection** (modified Whipple procedure) in those without metastases. Subsequent radiation and chemotherapy are controversial.

VI. DISEASES OF THE BILIARY TRACT

A. Acute cholecystitis

    1. Acute cholecystitis is **caused by obstruction of the bile duct, generally by a stone, leading to chronic inflammation.**

    2. Clinical presentation

        a. Colicky epigastric or **right upper quadrant pain** becomes steady and **increases** in intensity.

        b. **Right shoulder** or **subscapular pain** may occur.

        c. Nausea, vomiting, and **low-grade fever** are common.

        d. **Constipation** and **mild paralytic ileus** may occur.

    3. Laboratory findings

        a. After 24 hours, bilirubin levels increase in **blood** and **urine.**

        b. **Leukocytosis** is common.

        c. Gallstones are found in **95% of patients** with cholecystitis; although only 20% are radioopaque, the remainder are generally **visible by sonography.**

        d. **Hepatobiliary imaging [hepato-iminodiacetic acid (HIDA) scan]** can be used for confirmation of the diagnosis.

B. Choledocholithiasis

    1. **General characteristics.** By age 75, 35% of women and 20% of men have gallstones. **Only 30% of people with gallstones develop symptomatic disease.**

    2. **Treatment.** Generally, **only the complications of choledocholithiasis should be treated,** as most people with gallstones will never develop disease. Complications include **cholecystitis, pancreatitis,** and **acute cholangitis.**

VII. DISEASES OF THE LIVER

A. Hepatitis

    1. General characteristics

        a. Hepatitis can describe **acute** or **chronic hepatocellular damage.**

        b. The **most common cause of acute hepatitis is viral,** with toxins (e.g., alcohol) as the second most common cause.

    c. **Chronic hepatitis** most often **results from viral infection (hepatitis B, D)** but is often caused by **inherited disorders** (e.g., Wilson's disease, alpha-antitrypsin deficiency), **autoimmune disease of the liver,** or **hepatic effects of systemic disease.**

2. Viral hepatitis

    a. General characteristics

        (1) The **severity of the disease is highly variable,** ranging from asymptomatic to fulminant, generally fatal infection.

        (2) **Hepatitis A and E are transmitted by fecal-oral contamination** and can be prevented by maintaining a sanitary water supply and hand washing.

        (3) **Hepatitis B, C, and D are transmitted parenterally** or by mucous membrane contact.

    b. Clinical features

        (1) **Fatigue, malaise, anorexia, nausea, tea-colored urine,** and **vague abdominal discomfort** are common presenting complaints.

        (2) **Hepatitis A and E are self-limited** and **mild,** without long-term sequelae.

        (3) **Hepatitis B and C can have a highly variable presentation,** ranging from asymptomatic to fulminant.

        (4) **Hepatitis D** is only seen **in conjunction with B** and is associated with **a more severe course.**

    c. Laboratory findings

        (1) **Aminotransferase elevations** are seen in all types of acute hepatitis indicating hepatocellular damage.

        (2) **Bilirubin greater than 3.0 mg/dl** will be associated with scleral icterus, if not frank jaundice.

        (3) **Immunoglobulin M (IgM) antibody to hepatitis A virus (anti-HAV) can be detected** with the onset of clinical disease (after a 15–40 day incubation period), but then it disappears after several months. HAV IgG indicates resolved hepatitis A.

        (4) **Hepatitis B serum antigen (HBsAg) indicates ongoing infection** of any duration, while **antigen against hepatitis B serum antigen (anti-HBs) indicates immunity by past infection or vaccination.** (Figure 5-1)

        (5) **Hepatitis B core antibody (anti-HBc) is present between the disappearance of HBsAg** and the **appearance of anti-HBs,** indicating **acute hepatitis.**

        (6) **Hepatitis B envelope antigen (HBeAg) indicates active infection that is highly contagious,** while **anti-Hbe indicates a lower viral titer.**

        (7) **Hepatitis C or D are generally detected by their antibodies,** which for C generally indicates ongoing infection, as it does for D if hepatitis B infection is ongoing.

3. Toxic hepatitis

    a. Toxic hepatitis may be **caused by numerous agents,** including alcohol, acetaminophen, carbon tetrachloride, isoniazid (INH), halothane, phenytoin, and many others.

    b. **Both diagnosis and treatment are accomplished by discontinuing the suspected agent.** Acetylcysteine can be used for acetaminophen toxicity.

    c. **Toxic hepatitis may be reversible,** depending on the amount of the toxin. If the patient survives the acute episode, prognosis is good.

B. Cirrhosis

1. General characteristics

    a. Cirrhosis is **irreversible fibrosis** and **nodular regeneration throughout the liver.**

    b. **Over 45% of cases in the United States are alcohol related,** with the remainder of cases associated with hepatitis B or C, or congenital disorders.

2. Clinical presentation

    a. **Weakness, fatigue,** and **weight loss** are common.

    b. **Nausea, vomiting,** and **anorexia** are usually present.

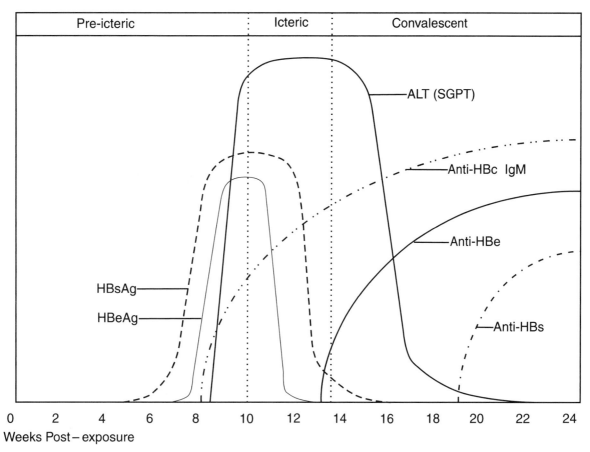

Figure 5-1. Relationship of clinical and laboratory features of hepatitis B. *ALT* = alanine aminotransferase; *anti-HBc* = hepatitis B core antibody; *anti-HBe* = hepatitis B envelope antigen; *anti-HBs* = hepatitis B surface antigen antibody; *HBsAg* = hepatitis B surface antigen; *IgM* = immunoglobulin M; *SGPT* = serum glutamate pyruvate transaminase.

    c. Menstrual changes (generally amenorrhea), **impotence, loss of libido,** and **gynecomastia** occur.

    d. Abdominal pain and **hepatomegaly** are generally present.

    e. Late stage disease includes ascites, pleural effusions, peripheral edema, ecchymoses, esophageal varices, and **signs of hepatic encephalopathy** (e.g., **asterixis, tremor, dysarthria, delirium,** and **eventually, coma**).

  3. Laboratory findings

    a. Laboratory values are often **minimally abnormal until late in the disease.**

    b. Anemia is common, as are **mild aspartate aminotransferase (AST)** and **alkaline phosphatase elevation, increased gamma globulin,** and **decreased albumin.**

  4. Treatment

    a. **Abstinence from alcohol** is the key feature of treatment.

    b. **Salt restriction** and **bed rest** may be sufficient treatment for ascites, although spironolactone 100 mg daily may be added as a diuretic.

    c. **Liver transplant** is indicated in selected patients.

C. **Liver abscess is generally caused by** *Entamoeba histolytica* or by the coliform bacteria. It may occur either **after travel** or **an intra-abdominal infection.** It presents with **fever** and **abdominal pain.**

VIII. OTHER GASTROINTESTINAL DISEASES

  A. **Peritonitis** is a **surgical emergency** presenting with **severe pain, rebound tenderness** and **guarding,** caused by **perforated viscus and inflammation.**

B. **Hernias** of various types can entrap the intestines and cause intestinal blockage. They are treated surgically.

C. **Congenital abnormalities**

   1. **Esophageal atresia** is commonly associated with tracheoesophageal fistula.

   a. Atresia presents **in newborns** as **excessive saliva** and **choking or coughing with attempts to feed.**

   b. **Inability to pass a nasogastric tube** will establish the diagnosis.

   c. **Treatment is surgical,** but pulmonary aspiration should be prevented in the interim by suction and the withholding of feedings.

   2. **Diaphragmatic hernia** causes immediate respiratory distress in the newborn as the affected lung is compressed by pressure of abdominal contents.

   a. **Immediate intubation and ventilation** is required, along with suction of the stomach by nasogastric tube.

   b. **Diagnosis can be made if bowel sounds are heard in the chest.**

   c. Radiography shows **loops of bowel in the involved hemithorax, with displacement of the heart** and mediastinal structures.

   3. **Hypertrophic pyloric stenosis** is caused by hypertrophy of the pyloric muscle and generally develops within the first 4–6 weeks of life.

   a. **Projectile vomiting without bile** is the presenting symptom.

   b. **A movable "olive" mass** may be palpated deep in the epigastrium.

   c. **Barium swallow** will reveal **delayed gastric emptying** and **"string sign"** or the **long narrow pyloric lumen.**

   d. **Treatment is surgical** (pyloromyectomy).

   4. **Bowel atresia** can occur in the ileum (most common), duodenum, jejunum, or colon, and presents with signs of obstruction within the first few days of life.

   5. **Hirschsprung's disease** (congenital megacolon) is caused by congenital absence of Meissner's and Auerbach's autonomic plexuses enervating the bowel wall.

   a. Symptoms may include **constipation** or **obstipation, vomiting,** and **failure to thrive.**

   b. Treatment is **surgical resection** of the affected bowel.

D. **Abdominal aortic aneurysm** is often asymptomatic and is caused by atherosclerosis.

   1. **A pulsatile mass may be felt** on examination.

   2. **A mass larger than 5 cm,** a rapidly expanding mass, or a symptomatic abdominal aortic aneurysm **requires surgical intervention.**

6

Nephrology and Urology

Robert J. McNellis

I. RENAL FAILURE

A. Acute renal failure (ARF)

    1. General characteristics

        a. ARF refers to a syndrome of **rapidly deteriorating kidney function** with the **accumulation of nitrogenous wastes.**

        b. Of the many conditions that can cause ARF, two diseases account for 70%–75% of all cases: **reduced renal perfusion** (prerenal) and **acute tubular necrosis.**

        c. **Causes** of ARF are given in Table 6-1 .

        d. ARF occurs in 5% of hospitalized patients, and in 10%–15% of intensive care unit (ICU) patients. Fifty percent of cases of ARF in hospitals are iatrogenic.

    2. Clinical features

        a. Symptoms include **nausea, vomiting, diarrhea, pruritus, drowsiness, dizziness, hiccups, shortness of breath, anorexia,** and **hematochezia.**

        b. Signs include **change in mental status, edema, weakness, dehydration, rash, jugular venous distention, costovertebral angle tenderness (CVAT), uriniferous odor,** and **ecchymosis.**

    3. Laboratory studies

        a. **Urinalysis** will reveal **proteinuria, hematuria,** and **epithelial cells.**

        b. Urine electrolytes

            (1) **Renal causes:** increased urine sodium (Na), fractional excretion of Na (FE_{Na}) more than 2%, and decreased blood urea nitrogen (BUN) to plasma creatinine (Cr) ratio ($< 15:1$)

            (2) **Prerenal causes:** decreased urine sodium, FE_{Na} less than 1%, and elevated BUN to plasma Cr ratio ($> 20:1$)

        c. **Many other abnormal laboratory findings** are associated with loss of renal function, most importantly **azotemia, decreased creatinine clearance,** and **hyperkalemia.** Other blood chemistries and hematologic tests are abnormal depending on the severity of disease.

    4. Treatment

        a. Treatment involves **correction of underlying hemodynamic abnormalities.**

        b. **Hemodialysis** should be implemented **when glomerular filtration rate (GFR) is 10% of normal** (normal GFR = 125 mm/hr).

        c. **Reversible causes** must be corrected by restoring circulating volume in the hypovolemic patient, improving perfusion in the hypotensive patient, or removing obstructions to renal blood flow or urine flow.

        d. **Medical therapy** may include intravenous saline, mannitol, or furosemide, depending on the cause. Doses should be adjusted for decreased renal function.

Table 6-1.

Causes of Acute Renal Failure

Prerenal causes
  Hypovolemia
  Hypotension
  Ineffective circulating volume (CHF, cirrhosis, nephrotic syndrome, early sepsis)
  Aortic aneurysm
  Renal artery stenosis

Renal causes
  Tubular or interstitial (acute tubular necrosis, nephrotoxins)
  Glomerular (rapidly progressive glomerulonephritis, pregnancy, SLE)

Postrenal causes
  Obstruction (hydronephrosis)

CHF = congestive heart failure; *SLE* = systemic lupus erythematosus.

Table 6-2.

Causes of Chronic Renal Failure

Primary glomerular diseases

Secondary glomerular diseases
  Diabetes mellitus
  Sickle cell anemia

Tubulointerstitial renal diseases
  Chronic pyelonephritis
  Tuberculosis

Hereditary diseases (polycystic kidney disease)

Vascular diseases (renal artery obstruction)

Obstructive nephropathies
  Nephrolithiasis
  Prostate disease

B. Chronic renal failure (CRF) and insufficiency

   1. General characteristics

   a. Definitions

   (1) Chronic renal failure is defined as **slowly progressive and irreversible reduction in GFR.**

   (2) Chronic renal insufficiency describes **mild to moderate decrease in GFR without presence of uremic symptoms.**

   b. Hypertension and diabetes mellitus are the **most common causes** (Table 6-2).

   c. CRF is a serious disease with a mortality rate of 50%, even with careful treatment.

   2. Clinical features

   a. Uremic symptoms are insidious, and include **fatigue, malaise, anorexia, vomiting, metallic taste, dyspnea, orthopnea, impaired mentation, insomnia, irritability, muscle cramps, restless legs, weakness, pruritus, ecchymosis,** and **altered consciousness.**

   b. Signs include **cachexia, weight loss, muscle wasting, pallor, hypertension, sensory deficits, asterixis,** and **Kussmaul's respirations.**

   3. Laboratory findings

   a. BUN and **creatinine** are elevated.

   b. Hemoglobin and hematocrit, serum electrolytes, and urinalysis are abnormal.

4. Treatment

    a. **Medical therapy** requires **careful drug dosing to adjust for decreased renal function, vitamin D supplements**, and medications as needed for **symptomatic problems.**

    b. **Dietary management** includes restriction of **protein intake, adequate caloric intake**, and limitation of **water, sodium,** and **potassium.**

    c. **Hemo-** or **peritoneal dialysis** should be scheduled as needed.

II. GLOMERULONEPHROPATHIES

A. Glomerulonephritis (GN)

    1. General characteristics

        a. GN generally refers to **damage of the renal glomeruli** by deposition of **inflammatory proteins** in the glomerular membranes as the **result of an immunologic response.**

        b. The **major causes of GN** are listed in Table 6-3. Causes are divided into **focal GN,** which is characterized by involvement of less than half of the glomeruli, and **diffuse GN,** which affects most glomeruli.

        c. Sixty percent of cases are in **children from 2–12 years of age. Prognosis is excellent in children** and worse in adults, especially with pre-existing renal disease.

    2. Clinical features

        a. **Hematuria** is present, with urine often tea-colored.

        b. **Oliguria or anuria** is present.

        c. **Edema** of the **face and eyes** occurs in the morning, and edema of the **feet and ankles** occurs in the afternoon and evening.

        d. **Hypertension** is also a common, but not essential, clinical finding.

    3. Laboratory findings

        a. **Antistreptolysin O (ASO) titer** is **increased** in 60%–80% of cases because a common cause of GN is poststreptococcal infection.

        b. **Urinalysis** reveals **red blood cell (RBC) casts, red and white blood cells,** and **proteinuria.**

        c. **Serum complement (C3) levels** are decreased.

        d. **Renal biopsy** may be done to determine exact diagnosis or severity of disease.

Table 6-3.
Causes of Glomerulonephritis (GN)

	Children	**Adults**
Focal	Benign hematuria	IgA nephropathy
GN	IgA nephropathy	Hereditary nephritis
	Henoch-Schönlein purpura	SLE
	Mild postinfectious glomerulonephritis	
	Hereditary nephritis	
Diffuse	Postinfectious glomerulonephritis	SLE
GN	Membranoproliferative glomerulonephritis	Membranoproliferative glomerulonephritis
		Rapidly progressive glomerulonephritis
		Postinfectious glomerulonephritis
		Vasculitis

IgA = immunoglobulin A; SLE = systemic lupus erythematosus.

4. Treatment

   a. Dietary management. Salt and **fluid** intake should be decreased.

   b. Dialysis should be performed if symptomatic azotemia is present.

   c. Medical therapy. Use medications as appropriate for hyperkalemia, pulmonary edema, peripheral edema, acidosis, streptococcal infection, and hypertension.

B. Nephrotic syndrome

   1. General characteristics

      a. Nephrotic syndrome comprises glomerular proteinuria (> 3 gm/day), **hypoalbuminemia, lipiduria, hypercholesterolemia,** and **edema.**

      b. This syndrome **can affect adults or children,** depending on the underlying cause (Table 6-4). It commonly occurs with GN.

      c. Prognosis varies with specific cause. **Complete remission is possible if underlying disease is treatable.**

   2. Clinical features

      a. Symptoms include **abdominal distention, anorexia, puffy eyelids, oliguria, scrotal swelling, shortness of breath,** and **weight gain.**

      b. Signs include **ascites, edema, hypertension, orthostatic hypotension, retinal sheen,** and **skin striae.**

   3. Laboratory findings

      a. Urinalysis shows **proteinuria, lipiduria, glycosuria, hematuria,** and **foamy urine.**

      b. Microscopic examination of the urine shows **RBC casts, granular casts, hyalinuria,** and **fatty casts.**

      c. Blood chemistry shows **hypoalbuminemia** and **azotemia.**

      d. Serum complement (C3) levels are low.

   4. Treatment

      a. Dietary management. Salt and **fluid** intake should be restricted, and **judicious use of diuretics** is recommended.

      b. Infections should be treated aggressively.

      c. Anticoagulants should be used if thromboses are present.

      d. Excessive sunlight should be **avoided,** because skin photosensitivity is common.

      e. Nephrotoxic drugs (e.g., nonsteroidal anti-inflammatories, aminoglycoside antibiotics) should be **avoided.**

Table 6-4.
Causes of Nephrotic Syndrome

Primary Renal Disease	Secondary Renal Diseases
Focal glomerulonephritis	Post-streptococcal glomerulonephritis
Focal glomerulosclerosis	SLE
IgA nephropathy	Malignancy
Membranoproliferative glomerulonephritis	Toxemia of pregnancy
Membranous glomerulopathy	Drugs and nephrotoxins
Mesangial proliferative glomerulonephritis	Lymphomas and leukemias
Minimal change disease	
Rapidly progressive glomerulonephritis	
Congenital nephrotic syndrome	

IgA = immunoglobulin A; SLE = systemic lupus erythematosus.

f. Some patients will respond to **steroid therapy**.

g. Frequent relapsers or steroid nonresponders may try **cyclophosphamide** or **cyclosporine**.

III. NEPHROLITHIASIS

A. General characteristics

1. **Nephrolithiasis (renal calculi)** occur throughout the urinary tract and are common causes of **pain, infection, and obstruction.**

2. The stones are caused by **increased saturation of urine with stone-forming salts.** The stones are typically **formed in the proximal tract** and **pass distally.** They lodge at the ureteropelvic junction, the ureterovesicular junction, or the ureter at the level of the iliac vessels.

3. **Nephrolithiasis commonly occurs in the third decade,** with the typical age range from 30–50 years.

4. **Four major types of stones exist.**

a. **Calcium**—80% of stones are formations of calcium crystals, and these stones are radiopaque. More male patients than female patients have calcium stones.

b. **Uric acid**—5% of stones are formed by precipitation of uric acid, and these stones are radiolucent.

c. **Cystine**—2% of stones are due to an impairment of cystine transport. These stones are radiolucent.

d. **Struvite**—less than 2% of stones are formed by the combination of calcium, ammonium, and magnesium. Formation is increased by urinary tract infections, so this type of stone is more common in female patients than male patients. These stones are radiopaque.

5. Patients usually have complete return to health, but recurrences are common, up to 50% in 5 years.

B. Clinical features

1. Clinical features of nephrolithiasis include **back pain** and **renal colic** that waxes and wanes.

2. The pain can **radiate to the groin, testicles, suprapubic area,** or **labia.**

3. Some cases **may be asymptomatic.**

4. Symptoms include **hematuria, dysuria, urinary frequency, fever, chills, nausea,** and **vomiting.**

5. Signs include **diaphoresis, tachycardia, tachypnea, hypertension due to pain, costovertebral angle tenderness,** and **abdominal distention of ileus.**

C. Laboratory findings

1. **Urinalysis** reveals microscopic or gross **hematuria.**

2. **Urine culture** should be taken to rule out infection.

3. **Plain film of the abdomen** will usually **identify radiopaque stones,** which make up approximately 85% of urinary stones.

4. **Renal ultrasound** can identify stones at the ureterovesical junction.

5. An **intravenous urogram** is indicated if the diagnosis remains uncertain.

D. Treatment

1. **Stones measuring less than 5 mm**

a. These are **likely to pass spontaneously** and, in an otherwise healthy individual, **may be managed on an outpatient basis.**

b. The patient should **drink plenty of fluids.**

     c. Strain urine to catch the stone and save it for analysis.

     d. Use an adequate supply of oral analgesics.

     e. Follow-up weekly or biweekly to monitor progress.

  2. Stones measuring 5–10 mm

     a. These are less likely to pass spontaneously. These should be considered for early elective intervention if no other complicating factors (e.g., infection, high-grade obstruction, solitary kidney) are present.

     b. Treat as above.

     c. Elective lithotripsy or ureteroscopy with stone extraction may be used.

  3. Stones measuring more than 10 mm

     a. These are not likely to pass spontaneously, and these patients are more likely to have complications.

     b. The patient should be treated on an inpatient basis.

     c. Vigorous hydration should be maintained.

     d. Intravenous antibiotics should be administered if signs of infection are present.

     e. Ureteral stent or percutaneous nephrostomy should be used if renal function is jeopardized.

     f. Urgent treatment with extracorporeal shock wave lithotripsy (ESWL) preceded by ureteroscopic fragmentation may also be used.

  4. Medications should be administered, including morphine or meperidine for pain, hydrochlorothiazide to increase urine production, and allopurinol for uric acid stones.

IV. ELECTROLYTE DISORDERS

  A. Hypernatremia

    1. General characteristics

      a. In this condition, water content of body fluid is deficient in relation to sodium content (serum Na > 150 mEq/L).

      b. Causes include sodium excess, water deficit, hypotonic fluid loss, urinary loss, gastrointestinal loss, or insensible loss.

      c. It occurs commonly in the elderly and may occur in infants with diarrhea. It is commonly associated with diabetes insipidus.

    2. Clinical features

      a. Neurologic manifestations include thirst, restlessness, irritability, disorientation, delirium, convulsions, and coma.

      b. Other findings include dry mouth and dry mucous membranes, lack of tears and decreased salivation, flushed skin, fever, oliguria and anuria, hyperventilation, and hyperreflexia.

    3. Laboratory findings

      a. Diabetes insipidus. Low urine sodium and polyuria usually indicate diabetes insipidus. Antidiuretic stimulation will not increase urine osmolality in diabetes insipidus.

      b. Hyperosmolar coma may be indicated by elevated serum glucose, decreased urine output, and increased urine osmolality.

    4. Treatment

      a. Hypernatremia should be treated on an inpatient basis.

      b. The underlying cause must be treated.

      c. Free water may be administered orally, which is the preferred route, or intravenously as a 5% dextrose solution.

d. Hypovolemia should be treated first, then hypernatremia.

e. Dialysis should be implemented if sodium is more than 200 mEq/L.

f. Use caution during treatment because rapid correction of hypernatremia can cause pulmonary edema.

B. Hyponatremia

1. General characteristics

  a. Hyponatremia is defined as **plasma sodium concentration less than 135 mEq/L.**

  b. Hyponatremia is the **most common electrolyte disorder seen** in the general hospital population.

  c. Types and their occurrence

   (1) Hyponatremia with hypervolemia occurs in the setting of congestive heart failure (CHF), nephrotic syndrome, renal failure, and hepatic cirrhosis.

   (2) Hyponatremia with euvolemia occurs with hypothyroidism and syndrome of inappropriate antidiuretic hormone (SIADH) release.

   (3) Hyponatremia with hypovolemia occurs with renal or nonrenal sodium loss.

2. Clinical features

  a. Symptoms include **lethargy, disorientation, muscle cramps, anorexia, hiccups, nausea, vomiting,** and **seizures.**

  b. Signs include **weakness, agitation, hyporeflexia, orthostatic hypotension, Cheyne-Stokes respirations, delirium, coma,** or **stupor.**

3. Laboratory findings

  a. Serum sodium is less than 135 mEq/L.

  b. Plasma osmolality is usually decreased except in cases of fluid redistribution due to hyperglycemia or proteinemia.

  c. Urine sodium will be increased or decreased depending on the cause (Table 6-5).

  d. If SIADH is suspected, a **computed tomography (CT) scan may be done to rule out central nervous system (CNS) disorder** and a **chest radiograph may be done to rule out lung pathology.**

4. Treatment

  a. Treat hypovolemia on an inpatient basis, especially if symptomatic or serum sodium is less than 125 mEq/L.

  b. Treat the **underlying cause.** This usually requires **fluid restriction. Monitor volume status.**

  c. In severe symptomatic hyponatremia with sodium less than 120 mEq/L, hypertonic saline may be used very cautiously. **Overly rapid correction can cause** central pontine myelinolysis resulting in **neurologic damage. Serum sodium levels should be checked hourly and neurologic status closely monitored.**

  d. In chronic hyponatremia unresponsive to fluid restriction, demeclocycline may be used to induce nephrogenic diabetes insipidus.

C. Disorders of potassium

1. Hyperkalemia

  a. General characteristics

   (1) Hyperkalemia refers to an **elevated serum potassium level.**

   (2) It may result from **cellular redistribution from intercellular to extracellular compartment, potassium retention,** or elevations due to **hemolysis** or **thrombocytosis.**

   (3) It is most commonly **associated with renal failure, angiotensin-converting enzyme (ACE) inhibitors, hyporeninemic hypoaldosteronism, cell death,** and **acidosis.**

Table 6-5.
Differential Diagnosis of Causes of Hyponatremia

Disorder	Plasma Osmolality	Urine Osmolality	ECFV	Urine Sodium
Isotonic hyponatremia (e.g., paraproteinemia, hypertriglyceridemia)	280–295			
Hypertonic hyponatremia (e.g., hyperglycemia)	>295			
Hypotonic hyponatremia	<280			
Excessive water intake (e.g., primary polydipsia)	<280	<100		
Impaired renal diluting ability	<280	>100		
Endocrinopathies (e.g., hypothyroidism, glucocorticoid insufficiency)	<280	>100	Normal	
SIADH (e.g., drugs, tumors, CNS disorders, nausea, pain, stress)	<280	>100	Normal	
Reset osmostat	<280	>100	Normal	
Potassium depletion	<280	>100	Normal	
Thiazide diuretics	<280	>100	Normal	
Renal solute loss (e.g., diuretics, osmotic diuresis, Addison's disease)	<280	>100	Decreased	>20
Extrarenal solute loss	<280	>100	Decreased	<10
Renal failure	<280	>100	Increased	>20
Edematous disorders (e.g., CHF, cirrhosis, nephrotic syndrome)	<280	>100	Increased	<10

CHF = congestive heart failure; CNS = central nervous system; ECFV = extracellular fluid volume; SIADH = syndrome of inappropriate antidiuretic hormones.

b. Clinical features

(1) Severe hyperkalemia can result in **arrhythmia** and **cardiac arrest.**

(2) **Neurologic symptoms** include **numbness, tingling, weakness,** and **flaccid paralysis.**

c. Laboratory findings

(1) **Serum potassium level** is greater than 5 mEq/L.

(2) **Electrocardiogram (ECG) changes** evolve as potassium rises above 6 mEq/L.

(a) Early ECG manifestations are **peaking of the T waves.**

(b) **Flattening of the P wave, prolongation of the PR interval,** and **widening of the QRS complex** are seen with more severe hyperkalemia.

(c) A final event is a **sine wave pattern with cardiac arrest.**

d. Treatment

(1) **Potentially life-threatening hyperkalemia** should be treated first, then the underlying cause discovered. Review the clinical situation, determine the acid–base status, and consider drug-induced conditions.

(2) Potassium-sparing drugs or dietary potassium should be **discontinued.**

(3) **Calcium gluconate** should be given to antagonize the effects of hyperkalemia on the heart.

(4) **Sodium bicarbonate, glucose,** and **insulin** may be administered to drive potassium back into the intracellular compartment. The onset of action is rapid but duration is short, so serial potassium levels should be followed until correction is complete.

(5) **Sodium polystyrene sulfonate (Kayexalate), a cation exchange resin,** is used to remove potassium from the body.

2. Hypokalemia

a. General considerations

(1) Hypokalemia is a decreased serum potassium level.

(2) It can result from a **shift of potassium into the intracellular compartment** or **potassium losses of extrarenal or renal origin.**

(3) It occurs most commonly **with use of diuretics, renal tubular acidosis,** or **gastrointestinal losses.**

b. Clinical features

(1) **Cardiovascular manifestations** are the most important, resulting in **ventricular arrhythmias, hypotension,** and **cardiac arrest.**

(2) **Neuromuscular manifestations** also occur, including **malaise, skeletal muscle weakness, cramps,** and **smooth muscle involvement** leading to ileus and constipation.

(3) Other manifestations include **polyuria, nocturia,** and **hyperglycemia.**

c. Laboratory findings

(1) **Serum potassium** is less than 3.5 mEq/L.

(2) **ECG** may reveal **flattened or inverted T waves, increased prominence of U waves, depression of the ST segment,** and **ventricular ectopy.**

(3) The most helpful tests for etiologic work-up include **blood acid–base parameters, urinary potassium,** and **chloride levels.**

d. Treatment

(1) **Hypokalemia is usually not an emergency** unless cardiac manifestations are present. In **non-emergent** conditions **oral potassium therapy** is preferred, usually with **potassium chloride.**

(2) For emergent situations (serum potassium less than 2.5 mEq/L or arrhythmias) **intravenous replacement is indicated.**

(3) **Hypokalemia potentiates the effects of cardiac glycosides** on myocardial conduction and **may lead to digitalis intoxication.** More aggressive potassium replacement may be required in this situation.

D. Disorders of calcium and phosphorus

1. General considerations

a. **Mechanisms for calcium and phosphorus homeostasis are complex** and carefully maintained by several interrelated and interdependent mechanisms. These involve vitamin D, small intestine, renal tubules, parathyroid hormone (PTH), and bone.

b. **Increased PTH levels** result in **increased serum calcium** and **decreased phosphorus.** Conversely, decreased levels of PTH result in decreased serum calcium and increased phosphorus.

c. **Parathyroid disorders, chronic renal failure,** and **malignancy** are the most common causes of disorders of calcium and phosphorus.

2. Hypercalcemia

a. General characteristics

(1) Hypercalcemia is a **significant elevation in serum calcium.** It must be corrected for changes in serum albumin.

(2) **This is one of the most common disorders of calcium and phosphorus seen,** especially in hospitalized patients with malignancy (e.g., lung cancer; squamous carcinoma of the head, neck, esophagus; female genital tract carcinoma; multiple myeloma; lymphoma; renal cell carcinoma).

(3) Other causes include vitamin D intoxication, hyperparathyroidism, and sarcoidosis.

b. Clinical features. Severity of symptoms depends on calcium level, rapidity of onset of hypercalcemia, state of hydration, and the underlying malignancy, if any.

(1) Symptoms include **anorexia, nausea, constipation, polyuria, polydipsia, dehydration,** and **change in level of consciousness (lethargy, stupor,** and **coma).**

(2) Signs of **intravascular volume depletion** (i.e., orthostatic hypotension and tachycardia) are seen.

c. Laboratory studies

(1) Serum calcium and albumin levels. The **true (corrected) calcium level = 0.8 (4.0 – measured albumin) + measured calcium.**

(2) **Serum phosphorus level.** If elevated, it is suggestive of vitamin D intoxication. If decreased, it suggests primary hyperparathyroidism.

       (3) **Chest radiographs** for pulmonary masses

       (4) **Urinalysis** for hematuria, an early sign of renal cell carcinoma

       (5) **Erythrocyte sedimentation rate (ESR)** may be elevated in monoclonal gammopathy. Protein electrophoresis of serum or urine may be needed to confirm the diagnosis.

       (6) **24-Hour urine collection** for calcium determination. An elevated urine calcium suggests malignant neoplastic or paraneoplastic process. A decreased urine calcium suggests primary hyperparathyroidism.

       (7) **Serum vitamin D levels.** Elevations are consistent with vitamin D toxicity.

    d. Treatment

       (1) **Isotonic saline** should be used for **volume repletion.** Loop diuretics should be used if the patient is hypervolemic after volume repletion.

       (2) **Manage** the **underlying cause.**

V. ACID–BASE DISORDERS.

Disturbances in the Acid–Base Equilibrium are common, especially in critically ill patients. They may be **respiratory** or **metabolic** (characterized by alterations in serum bicarbonate levels).

A. Respiratory acidosis

  1. General characteristics

    a. Acidosis is defined by **increased partial pressure of carbon dioxide (P_{CO_2})** in the blood and **decreased blood pH** (acidemia).

    b. It is the result of alveolar hypotension leading to pulmonary carbon dioxide (CO_2) retention.

    c. The causes of respiratory acidosis include **all disorders that reduce pulmonary function and CO_2 clearance,** such as primary pulmonary disease, neuromuscular disease (myasthenia gravis), primary central nervous system dysfunction (severe brain stem injury), and drug-induced hypoventilation.

  2. Clinical features

    a. Metabolic encephalopathy with headache and drowsiness is the most characteristic change.

    b. If not corrected, initial CNS symptoms may **progress to stupor and coma.**

  3. Laboratory findings

    a. Acute CO_2 retention leads to an **increase in blood P_{CO_2}** with **minimal change in plasma bicarbonate content. Serum electrolyte levels are close to normal.**

    b. After 2–5 days, **renal compensation occurs** (i.e., increased hydrogen ion secretion and bicarbonate production in the distal nephron) and **plasma bicarbonate level steadily increases.**

  4. Treatment

    a. The **underlying disorder** must be identified and corrected.

    b. A blood P_{CO_2} of more than 60 mmHg may be an indication for **assisted ventilation** if CNS or pulmonary muscular depression is severe.

B. Respiratory alkalosis

  1. General characteristics

    a. Alkalosis is defined by **decreased blood P_{CO_2} and increased blood pH** (alkalemia)

    b. Respiratory alkalosis is associated with **excessive elimination of CO_2 via the lungs.**

    c. The causes of respiratory alkalosis include **any disorders associated with inappropriately increased ventilatory rate and CO_2 clearance.**

    d. Anxiety (hysterical hyperventilation) is the **most common cause** of respiratory alkalosis. Other causes include salicylate intoxication, hypoxia, intrathoracic disorders, primary CNS dysfunction, gram-negative septicemia, liver insufficiency, and pregnancy.

2. Clinical features

    a. **Obvious hyperventilation** is usually present, particularly when alkalosis is due to cerebral or metabolic disorders.

    b. The **breathing pattern** in the anxiety-induced syndrome **varies from frequent, deep, sighing respirations to sustained and obvious rapid, deep breathing.**

    c. Acute alkalemia may produce a **tetany-like syndrome,** which may be indistinguishable from acute hypocalcemia.

    d. **Circumoral paresthesias, acroparesthesias, giddiness,** or **light-headedness** may occur.

3. Diagnosis

    a. In acute alkalosis, increased respiratory rate leads to a loss of CO_2 via the lungs, which in turn **increases the blood pH.**

    b. Within hours after an acute decrease in arterial P_{CO_2}, hydrogen ion secretion in the distal nephron decreases, leading to a **decrease in plasma bicarbonate. Serum chloride level also is elevated.**

4. Treatment

    a. The primary goal of therapy is to **correct the underlying disorder.**

    b. Use of CO_2-**enriched breathing mixtures** or **controlled ventilation** may be required in cases of severe respiratory alkalosis (pH $>$ 7.6).

C. Metabolic acidosis

  1. General characteristics

    a. **Metabolic acidosis is an elevation in the normal serum concentration of hydrogen ions** that is initiated either by the **loss of bicarbonate** or by the **addition of hydrogen ions to the serum.**

    b. Conditions that may result in increased hydrogen ions in the serum include **lactic acidosis, diabetic ketoacidosis, starvation ketosis,** and **ethylene glycol, methanol,** and **salicylate intoxication.** These conditions result in an increased anion gap. Hydrogen ions may also be **retained in renal tubular acidosis, renal insufficiency,** and **adrenal insufficiency.**

    c. Conditions that may result in the loss of bicarbonate include **diarrhea, pancreatic or biliary drainage, and ureterosigmoidostomy.** These conditions typically have a normal anion gap.

  2. Clinical features

    a. **Hyperventilation** is the earliest and most recognized sign.

    b. **Ventricular arrhythmias** may occur.

    c. **Neurologic symptoms** occur, ranging from lethargy to frank coma.

  3. Laboratory studies

    a. **Arterial blood gas** measurements will reveal a pH less than 7.35, decreased plasma bicarbonate, and decreased P_{CO_2}.

    b. The **anion gap** should be calculated to determine levels of unmeasured anions. **Anion gap = serum Na − (serum bicarbonate + serum chloride).** Normal value is 12 mEq/L.

  4. Treatment

    a. **Identify** and, if possible, **remove the primary cause** of the metabolic acidosis.

    b. **Insulin therapy** and **volume repletion** are the mainstays of diabetic ketoacidosis therapy.

    c. **Bicarbonate therapy** can be considered to raise pH above 7.20. Blood pH should be carefully monitored since ongoing acid production may increase bicarbonate requirements.

D. Metabolic alkalosis

  1. General characteristics

    a. Metabolic alkalosis is defined as an **increase in serum bicarbonate,** with **no change in P_{CO_2},** causing an increase in **extracellular pH greater than 7.45.**

    b. Metabolic alkalosis and increased serum bicarbonate can be **caused by loss of hydrogen, addition of bicarbonate, or disproportionate loss of chloride.** Metabolic alkalosis is maintained due to impaired renal excretion of bicarbonate.

    c. Common causes of metabolic alkalosis include vomiting, nasogastric tube suctioning, villous adenoma, chloride diarrhea, diuretics, hypercalcemia, milk–alkali syndrome, and chloride and potassium depletion due to excessive steroids.

2. Clinical features

    a. **Neurologic abnormalities**, including paresthesias, carpopedal spasm, and light-headedness, may occasionally progress to confusion, stupor, and coma.

    b. **Symptoms arising from volume depletion** are frequently present. Weakness, muscle cramps, and postural dizziness may develop.

    c. **Abnormalities secondary to potassium depletion** may lead to polyuria, polydipsia, and muscle weakness.

3. Laboratory studies

    a. **Arterial blood gas** measurements reveal **pH greater than 7.45, increased serum bicarbonate, and increased** P_{CO_2}.

    b. **Urine chloride concentrations** can **distinguish between hypovolemic hypochloremic patients** with a decreased urine chloride concentration (< 20 mEq/L) and **volume expanded patients** with mineralocorticoid excess who have urine chloride concentrations greater than 30 mEq/L.

4. Treatment

    a. **Maneuvers that increase renal excretion of bicarbonate** are the most effective therapy for metabolic acidosis.

    b. **Chloride-responsive conditions** (e.g., gastric fluid loss and diuretic therapy) are treated with solutions containing sodium chloride (NaCl) to repair the sodium and chloride deficits.

    c. **Chloride-resistant conditions** (e.g., mineralocorticoid excess) can be successfully treated by removing an adrenal adenoma if present or using spironolactone, an aldosterone antagonist.

VI. RENOVASCULAR DISEASE

A. General characteristics

    1. **Disorders that decrease blood flow to the kidneys will result in the release of renin.** Activation of the renin–angiotensin system leads to vasoconstriction and stimulation of aldosterone resulting in hypertension.

    2. **Atherosclerotic disease** and **fibromuscular dysplasia** are the two most common abnormalities that lead to hypertension.

B. Clinical features

    1. In **comparison to patients with essential hypertension,** patients with renovascular hypertension are **more often of ideal body weight,** have **shorter duration of hypertension, more frequent onset of hypertension before age 50,** less family history of hypertension, **more severe retinopathy,** and **more abdominal and flank bruits.**

    2. Renovascular hypertension is **present in 10% of the renal transplant population,** usually occurring approximately **6 months after transplant.**

C. Laboratory studies

    1. **Radionuclide studies** are more useful than intravenous pyelograms. Use of ACE inhibitors prior to scan will increase sensitivity of study.

    2. **Renal angiogram is the diagnostic gold standard** for visualization of the renal artery, but it is an invasive procedure. Complications include injury to cannulated vessels and neighboring organs, reactions to the contrast agent, and bleeding.

    3. **Ultrasonography of the renal arteries** may detect areas of stenosis.

    4. **Magnetic resonance imaging (MRI)** may be helpful to identify proximal renal artery lesions.

D. Treatment

    1. Medical therapy can be attempted for hypertension with mild renal artery stenosis. Avoid diuretics or ACE inhibitors that decrease glomerular filtration rate. Calcium channel blockers, beta blockers, and vasodilators may be more effective.

    2. Angioplasty has a high cure rate with fibromuscular dysplasia, slightly lower for non-occluded arteriosclerotic lesions.

    3. Surgery can be done to repair lesions if angioplasty is contraindicated.

VII. URINARY TRACT INFECTION

A. Cystitis

    1. General characteristics

        a. Cystitis is an **infection of the bladder** most commonly due to coliform bacteria (especially *Escherichia coli*) and occasionally gram-positive bacteria (enterococci).

        b. The route of infection is typically **ascending from the urethra.**

    2. Clinical features

        a. Irritative voiding symptoms (frequency, urgency, dysuria) are common as well as suprapubic discomfort.

        b. Women may demonstrate **gross hematuria.** Symptoms in women may often appear following sexual intercourse.

        c. Physical examination may elicit **suprapubic tenderness,** but examination is often unremarkable.

    3. Laboratory studies

        a. Urinalysis shows pyuria, bacteriuria, and varying degrees of hematuria.

        b. Urine culture is positive for the offending organism.

        c. Imaging is warranted only if pyelonephritis, recurrent infections, or anatomic abnormalities are suspected.

    4. Treatment

        a. Uncomplicated cystitis in women can be treated with **short-term antimicrobial therapy,** which consists of single dose therapy or 1–3 days of therapy. Trimethoprim–sulfamethoxazole or cephalexin are often effective. Uncomplicated cystitis is rare in men.

        b. Hot sitz baths or **urinary analgesics** (phenazopyridine) may provide symptomatic relief.

B. Urethritis

    1. General characteristics

        a. Urethritis is most commonly **caused by *Neisseria gonorrhoeae*,** a gram-negative diplococcus typically found inside polymorphonuclear cells. Gonococcal urethritis is commonly transmitted during sexual activity and has its greatest incidence in 15- to 29-year-olds. The incubation period is usually 2–8 days.

        b. Approximately half of nongonococcal urethritis is caused by *Chlamydia trachomatis*. **Co-infection with gonorrhea and chlamydia is common,** and postgonococcal urethritis may persist after successful treatment of the gonococcal component.

    2. Clinical features

        a. In men, there is initially **burning on urination** and a **serous or milky discharge.** One to three days later, the urethral pain is more pronounced and the discharge becomes yellow, creamy, and profuse, sometimes blood-tinged. Without treatment, the disorder may regress and become chronic or progress to involve the prostate, epididymis, and periurethral glands with acute, painful inflammation. This may progress to chronic infection resulting in prostatitis and urethral strictures.

        b. Women may have **dysuria, urinary frequency, and urgency, with a purulent urethral discharge. Vaginitis** and **cervicitis** with inflammation are common. Infection may be asymptomatic.

        c. Chlamydial infection discharge tends to be less painful, less purulent, and more watery.

3. Laboratory studies

   a. **Gram stain of urethral discharge in men,** especially during the first week after onset, typically shows gram-negative diplococci in polymorphonuclear leukocytes. Smears are less often positive in women.

   b. **Gonococcal cultures** are essential in all cases where gonorrhea is suspected and gonococci cannot be shown in gram-stained smears.

   c. **Absence of gram-negative intracellular diplococci in urethral discharge** from a man is highly suggestive of **chlamydial infection.**

4. Treatment

   a. Due to the **widespread geographic distribution of penicillin-resistant gonorrhea,** it should no longer be considered first-line therapy.

   b. **Ceftriaxone 125 mg intramuscularly (IM)** is the treatment of choice for gonorrhea.

   c. **Concurrent treatment of chlamydia** should be undertaken by **erythromycin** 500 mg 4 times daily orally, or doxycycline 100 mg twice daily orally for 7 days. A single dose of **azithromycin** 1 g orally is also effective when compliance needs to be assured.

   d. **All sexual partners should be treated.**

C. Pyelonephritis

   1. General characteristics

      a. Acute pyelonephritis is an **infectious inflammatory process involving the kidney parenchyma** and **renal pelvis.**

      b. **Gram negative bacteria** are the most common causative agents, including *E. coli, Proteus, Klebsiella, Enterobacter,* and *Pseudomonas.* The infection usually **ascends from the lower urinary tract.**

      c. Chronic pyelonephritis is the result of **progressive inflammation of the renal interstitium** caused by bacterial infection, vesicoureteral reflux, or both.

   2. Clinical features

      a. Symptoms include **fever, flank pain, shaking chills,** and **irritative voiding symptoms.** Nausea, vomiting, and diarrhea are not uncommon.

      b. **Young children** may have fever and abdominal discomfort.

      c. Signs include **fever** and **tachycardia. Costovertebral angle tenderness** is usually pronounced.

   3. Laboratory studies

      a. **Complete blood count (CBC)** shows leukocytosis and left shift.

      b. **Urinalysis** shows pyuria, bacteriuria, and varying degrees of hematuria. White cell casts may be seen.

      c. **Urine culture** demonstrates heavy growth of the offending agent.

      d. In complicated pyelonephritis, **renal ultrasound** may show hydronephrosis from a stone or other source of obstruction.

   4. Treatment

      a. **Hospital admission** is required for patients with severe infections or complicating factors.

      b. **Intravenous ampicillin and an aminoglycoside** are initiated prior to obtaining sensitivity results. Intravenous antibiotics should be continued for 24 hours after defervescence, and oral antibiotics are then given to complete a **3-week course** of therapy.

      c. In the **outpatient setting,** trimethoprim-sulfamethoxazole or quinolones may be initiated and continued for **3 weeks.**

      d. Failure to respond warrants **ultrasound imaging to exclude complicating factors** that may require prompt intervention.

      e. **Follow-up urine cultures** are mandatory following treatment.

D. Prostatitis

1. General characteristics

a. **Acute bacterial prostatitis** is caused by **ascending infection of gram-negative rods** into the prostatic ducts.

b. **Chronic bacterial prostatitis** may or may not be associated with evolution of an acute bacterial infection.

c. **Non-bacterial prostatitis is the most common** of the prostatitis syndromes, and its cause is unknown. It may represent a noninfectious inflammatory disorder, **perhaps with an autoimmune etiology.** It is a **diagnosis of exclusion.**

d. **Prostatic abscess** is an uncommon complication of acute bacterial prostatitis.

2. Clinical features

a. Acute infection is characterized by **sudden onset of high fever, chills,** and **low back** and **perineal pain.** Chronic infection has more variable symptoms ranging from asymptomatic to acute symptomatology.

b. All forms of prostatitis present with **irritative bladder symptoms** of frequency, urgency, dysuria, and some obstruction.

c. The **prostate** will be **swollen** and **tender.**

3. Laboratory studies

a. **Urinalysis** reveals pyuria.

b. **Prostatic fluid culture** is **positive for** *E. coli* in acute infections. Chronic infection is characterized by recurrence of same organism or enterococcus. **In non-bacterial prostatitis, cultures are negative.**

4. Treatment

a. **Antibiotics** are the most effective treatment for bacterial infections: trimethoprim–sulfamethoxazole or ciprofloxacin for 30 days in acute prostatitis and 4–16 weeks in chronic prostatitis. Antibiotics are not effective in non-bacterial prostatitis.

b. Chronic, recurrent, or resistant prostatitis with or without prostatic calculi may need **transurethral resection of the prostate** for ultimate resolution.

E. Orchitis

1. General characteristics

a. **Ascending bacterial infection from the urinary tract** commonly causes this condition.

b. Orchitis **occurs in 25% of postpubertal males who have mumps infection.**

2. Clinical features

a. **Testicular swelling and tenderness** occurs, usually unilateral.

b. **Fever and tachycardia** are common.

3. Laboratory studies

a. **Urinalysis** reveals pyuria and bacteriuria with bacterial infection.

b. **Cultures** are positive for suspected organisms.

c. **Ultrasonography** is useful if abscess is suspected.

4. Treatment

a. If **mumps** is the etiology, **symptomatic relief with ice and analgesia** should be provided.

b. If **bacteria** is the etiology, the orchitis should be **treated like epididymitis** (see VII F).

c. Carefully evaluate any scrotal masses.

F. Epididymitis

1. General characteristics

a. Epididymitis is infection of epididymis **acquired by retrograde spread of organism through the vas deferens.**

b. In men younger than 35 years of age, **chlamydia and gonococcus** are most common organisms; in men older than 35 years of age, *E. coli* is most common organism.

2. Clinical features

    a. Epididymitis presents with **heaviness** and **dull, aching discomfort in the affected hemiscrotum,** which can radiate up the ipsilateral flank.

    b. The epididymis will be **markedly swollen and exquisitely tender** to touch, eventually becoming a **warm, erythematous, enlarged scrotal mass.**

    c. The patient may have **fever and chills.**

    d. **Testicular torsion must be ruled out.** Prehn's sign is a classic sign although it is not very reliable. The scrotum is lifted onto the symphysis pubis, and epididymal pain is relieved while torsion pain is worsened.

3. Laboratory studies

    a. **Urinalysis** reveals pyuria and bacteriuria.

    b. **Cultures** show positive results for suspect organisms.

4. Treatment

    a. **Doxycycline** 100 mg twice per day orally for 21 days may be administered for gonococcus or chlamydia.

    b. Alternatively, **ciprofloxacin** 500 mg twice per day orally for 21 days may be used.

VIII. BENIGN PROSTATIC HYPERPLASIA (BPH)

A. General characteristics

    1. **Proliferation of the fibrostromal tissue** of the prostate can lead to **compression of the prostatic urethra** creating an obstruction of the urinary outlet.

    2. BPH is a **disease of older men.** The mean age of onset is 60–65 years of age.

B. Clinical features

    1. Symptom complex is referred to as "prostatism," which includes **symptoms of obstruction and irritation.**

    2. **Obstructive symptoms** include decreased force of urinary stream, hesitancy and straining, post-void dribbling, and sensation of incomplete emptying.

    3. **Irritative symptoms** include frequency, nocturia, and urgency.

    4. **Recurrent urinary tract infections** and **urinary retention** also occur.

    5. Digital rectal examination typically reveals **enlarged prostate.**

C. Laboratory studies

    1. **Prostate specific antigen (PSA)** will typically be slightly elevated.

    2. **Other tests** are done to evaluate for renal damage, infection, and prostate or bladder cancer, as suspected.

D. Treatment

    1. **Medications** include alpha blockers and 5-alpha-reductase inhibitors.

    2. **Procedures that may be used to relieve obstruction** include use of balloon dilation, microwave irradiation, and stent placements.

    3. Surgical treatment is **transurethral resection of prostate (TURP)** or **transurethral incision** of prostate.

IX. OBSTRUCTIVE UROPATHY

A. General characteristics

    1. Obstructive uropathy is an **increase in the pressure opposing normal urine flow** that **results in structural changes in the lower urinary tract.** Hydronephrosis describes dilation of the calyces and collecting system of the kidney. Obstructive nephropathy refers to renal parenchymal damage.

2. An obstruction of the urinary tract **may occur at any point between the renal tubules and the urethra.** Obstructions may be **acute** or **chronic, unilateral** or **bilateral,** and **partial** or **complete.**

B. Clinical features

1. Features **vary depending on the site of the obstruction** and the **speed with which the obstruction develops.**

2. Urinary symptoms predominate in obstructive disease of the bladder and urethra. Hesitancy, decreased force of urinary stream, urinary frequency, and dribbling are common in the context of obstruction.

3. Progression of obstruction may lead to **flank pain, renal enlargement,** and, ultimately, signs of **renal impairment.**

C. Laboratory findings

1. Urinalysis results vary but may reveal inappropriately dilute urine, hematuria, or bacteriuria.

2. Urine culture is essential because infection often complicates obstruction, causing serious detriment of urinary function.

3. Blood chemistries are not diagnostic but are helpful in assessing the severity of impaired renal function.

4. Intravenous urogram is most useful for identifying obstruction.

D. Treatment

1. Relief of the obstruction is the definitive therapy. It should be appropriate to the structural nature of the lesion. Methods include **surgery, percutaneous nephrostomy, ureteral stent,** and **nephroscopic stone removal.**

2. Medical management following relief of obstruction is aimed at **correcting post-obstructive diuresis.** Management involves adequate fluid replacement and monitoring of intravascular volume, blood, and urine electrolytes.

X. NEOPLASM

A. Prostate cancer

1. General characteristics

a. Prostate cancer is a **generally slow-growing malignant neoplasm of the adenomatous cells of the prostate gland** that can lead to urinary obstruction and metastatic disease.

b. It comprises 21% of all cancers in men. A disease of aging, it is rarely seen in men less than 40 years old.

c. Etiology is unknown. Risk factors may include genetic predisposition, hormonal influences, dietary and environmental factors, and infectious agents.

2. Clinical features

a. Many cases are **not clinically apparent.**

b. Symptoms of urinary obstruction occur.

c. In advanced disease, patients may present with **bone pain from metastases.**

d. Prostate may be enlarged, nodular, and asymmetric.

3. Laboratory studies

a. PSA is usually elevated in prostate cancer.

b. Pathologic examination of tissue removed for treatment of obstructive prostatic hyperplasia reveals that 10% have malignancy.

c. Transrectal ultrasound reveals hypoechoic lesions in prostate.

d. Biopsy confirms diagnosis of adenocarcinoma and allows histologic grading, which can provide prognostic information.

4. Treatment

a. Appropriate treatment is **dependent on the staging.** Staging is done by abdominal and pelvic CT or MRI, pelvic lymphadenectomy, and bone scan.

    b. Stage A and B disease (tumor confined to the prostate) may be treated with **radical retropubic prostatectomy** or **radiation therapy.**

    c. Stage C disease (tumor with local invasion) is treated **similar to stage A and B** with reduced effectiveness.

    d. Stage D disease (distant metastases) is treated with **hormonal manipulation using orchiectomy, antiandrogens, luteinizing hormone–releasing hormone (LH–RH) agonists, or estrogens.** Chemotherapy has limited usefulness. Palliative treatment is given for advanced disease.

B. Bladder cancer

  1. General characteristics

    a. **Etiologic factors** for bladder cancer include exposure to tobacco; occupational carcinogens in the rubber, dye, printing, and chemical industries; schistosomiasis; and chronic infections.

    b. Uroepithelial tumors account for **3% of cancer deaths in the United States.** Bladder carcinoma is **3 times more common in men** than in women and usually occurs in patients who are **40–70 years of age.**

  2. Clinical features

    a. **Hematuria** is the most common presenting symptom.

    b. **Bladder irritability** and **infection** are other presenting symptoms.

  3. Laboratory findings

    a. CBC and **blood chemistry** should be done to evaluate for infection and renal function.

    b. **Cystoscopy,** nearly 100% accurate, is the definitive diagnostic procedure. Biopsy will confirm pathologic diagnosis.

    c. Radiologic procedures include **intravenous urogram, pelvic and abdominal CT scans, chest radiograph, bone scan,** and **retrograde pyelography** for renal pelvic or ureteral tumors and staging.

  4. Treatment

    a. Treatment is **dependent on the stage.**

    b. Superficial lesions (stage 0, A, and sometimes B1) are treated with **endoscopic resection** and **fulguration,** followed by **cystoscopy** every 3 months. Recurrent or multiple lesions can be treated with intravesical instillation of thiotepa, mitomycin, or bacille Calmette-Guérin (BCG).

    c. **Radical cystectomy** is used for recurrent cancer, diffuse transitional cell carcinoma in situ, or stages B and C invasive cancers.

    d. **Combination chemotherapy** has been used in bladder-sparing trials with or without radiation. The results have been mixed.

XI. MALE REPRODUCTIVE DISORDERS

A. Impotence

  1. General characteristics

    a. Impotence is the **consistent inability to maintain an erect penis with sufficient rigidity to allow sexual intercourse.**

    b. **Normal erections require** intact parasympathetic and somatic nerve supply, unobstructed arterial inflow, adequate venous constriction, hormonal stimulation, and psychological desire. **Disorders of any of these systems may result in impotence.**

    c. **Most cases** of male erectile disorders have an **organic rather than psychogenic** cause. **Nearly all cases will have a psychogenic component.**

    d. This condition affects millions of American men, and its **incidence is age-related.**

  2. Clinical features

    a. The **medical history** must be adequately evaluated.

    b. A **sexual history** should be taken, including detailed information on timing and frequency of sexual relations, partners, presence of morning erections, ejaculation, and masturbation.

c. **Past medical history** should document presence of **hypertension, diabetes, endocrine disease, medications, pelvic surgery,** or **trauma.**

d. Physical examination should look for **penile deformities** (e.g., Peyronie's disease), **testicular atrophy, hypertension, peripheral neuropathy,** and other signs of endocrine, vascular, or neurologic abnormalities.

3. Laboratory findings

a. **CBC, urinalyis, lipid profile, thyroid function tests, serum testosterone, glucose, and prolactin screening** should be done depending on suspected cause.

b. **Measurement of follicle-stimulating hormone (FSH) and luteinizing hormone (LH)** may be required for patients with abnormalities of testosterone or prolactin.

c. **Nocturnal penile tumescence testing** can be done to differentiate between organic and psychogenic impotence. Patients with psychogenic impotence will have normal nocturnal erections of adequate frequency and rigidity.

d. **Direct injection of vasoactive substances** into the penis will induce erections in men with intact vascular systems.

e. Patients who do not achieve erections with injections may have studies to evaluate the arterial and venous vasculature. These might include **ultrasonography of the cavernous arteries, pelvic arteriography,** and **cavernosonography.**

4. Treatment

a. True psychogenic causes can be treated with **behaviorally oriented sex therapy.** Patients with organic causes of impotence may also benefit from counseling.

b. **Testosterone injections** can be offered to men with androgen deficiency in whom prostate cancer has been excluded.

c. **Oral medications** (e.g., yohimbine) have been available for many years. These are thought to have only a placebo effect.

d. **Finasteride (Viagra)** has been shown to improve erections in men with vascular disease. There are potential cardiovascular complications with its use.

e. **Vacuum constriction** devices draw the penis into an erect state and block venous outflow to maintain an erection for intercourse.

f. **Injection therapy or urethral suppositories with vasoactive substances** provide safe, acceptable, and effective treatment. Priapism and fibrosis are occasional adverse reactions.

g. Penile prostheses may be implanted directly into corporal bodies. Prostheses may be rigid, malleable, hinged, or inflatable.

h. Patients with disorders of the arterial system are candidates for **arterial reconstruction.** Disorders of venous occlusion may be managed with ligation of deep veins. Experience with vascular reconstructive surgery has been limited and results have been mixed.

B. Scrotal masses

1. **Epididymitis and orchitis** (See VII E, F.)

2. Hydrocele

a. **General characteristics.** A hydrocele is a mass of the fluid-filled congenital remnants of the tunica vaginalis.

b. Clinical features

(1) **Chronic, nontender,** and **transilluminable lesion** is seen.

(2) The mass may **wax and wane in size;** an **indirect hernia** may be concurrently present.

c. Laboratory studies

(1) **Urinalysis** with microscopic analysis will be **negative.**

(2) **Ultrasonography of the testes** will demonstrate a **fluid-filled lesion.**

d. **Treatment.** Elective repair as clinically indicated is the treatment.

C. Inguinal hernia

1. General characteristics

a. A hernia is **any abnormal protrusion through an abnormal anatomic defect**. Inguinal hernias occur as the result of a congenital or acquired defect in the connective tissue supporting the inguinal area.

b. **Types.** Inguinal hernias can be direct or indirect.

(1) An **indirect inguinal hernia** is a **congenital anatomic defect**. The hernia passes through the internal abdominal inguinal ring along the spermatic cord and exits the abdomen through the external inguinal ring. The hernial sac can extend to the scrotum.

(2) A **direct inguinal hernia** is an **acquired anatomic defect**. The hernia passes through the posterior inguinal wall immediately medial to the inferior epigastric vessels.

c. **Risk factors** include trauma, recurrent Valsalva maneuvers, and dysfunctional connective tissue.

2. Clinical features. Inguinal hernias may be reducible, incarcerated, or strangulated.

a. **Reducible hernias** are characterized by a **nontender mass** that occasionally goes away but will return, especially after a Valsalva maneuver. Most hernias of this type are asymptomatic and are found on routine physical examination.

b. **Incarcerated hernias** will not return to normal position spontaneously or with external manipulation. They usually present with a **soft, nontender mass.**

c. A **strangulated hernia** is an incarcerated hernia that has developed edema with resultant ischemia. It is characterized by a tender mass that is non-reducible, fever, diffuse abdominal tenderness, and signs of small or large bowel obstruction.

3. Laboratory studies

a. Preoperative laboratory studies may include **CBC with differential, electrolytes, BUN, creatinine, glucose, prothrombin time (PT), partial thromboplastin time (PTT), platelets, liver function tests,** and **urinalysis,** as indicated.

b. An **abdominal series** can be performed to look for signs of perforation or obstruction if indicated.

4. Treatment. Hernias are definitively treated with **herniorrhaphy.**

D. Testicular torsion

1. General characteristics

a. The **testis is abnormally twisted on its spermatic cord**, thus **compromising arterial supply and venous drainage** of the testis.

b. This condition is **most common in young males,** especially **with a history of cryptorchidism.**

2. Clinical features

a. Pain and **scrotal swelling** are present.

b. An **acute, tender,** and **nontransilluminable lesion** is seen.

3. Laboratory findings

a. **Doppler ultrasonography** will demonstrate decreased blood flow to the affected spermatic cord and testis.

b. **Radioisotope scan** will demonstrate decreased signal in the affected testes.

4. Treatment

a. This is a **surgical emergency. Manual detorsion** may be attempted by experienced clinicians. Whether it is successful or not, surgery will be required.

b. **Emergent surgical intervention** on the affected testis will need to be followed by **elective surgery on the contralateral testis,** which is also at risk of torsion.

E. Varicocele

 1. General characteristics

 a. Varicocele is the **formation of a venous varicosity in the spermatic vein.**

 b. The **left spermatic vein has an increased incidence** of varicosity because it does not drain directly into the inferior vena cava like the right.

 2. Clinical features

 a. A **chronic, nontender, nontransilluminable mass** is seen, usually on the **left side.**

 b. The lesion has the **consistency of a "bag of worms"** and **decreases in size with elevation of the scrotum or supine position.**

 3. Laboratory studies. No laboratory studies are required.

 4. Treatment. **Surgical repair** can be performed if lesion becomes painful or appears to be a cause of infertility.

F. Testicular cancer

 1. General characteristics

 a. This is the **most common malignancy in young men,** with an average age at diagnosis of 32 years.

 b. Risk factors include **history of cryptorchidism** or a **prior history of testicular cancer.**

 2. Clinical features

 a. Over 90% of patients present with a **painless, solid, testicular swelling.** Occasionally, patients with painful testicular masses are erroneously diagnosed as having epididymitis or orchitis.

 b. **Para-aortic lymph node involvement** can **present as ureteral obstruction.**

 c. Patients may also present with **abdominal complaints from an abdominal mass or pulmonary symptoms** from **multiple nodules.**

 3. Laboratory studies

 a. **Scrotal ultrasound** may reveal a suspicious intratesticular echogenic focus.

 b. **Radiologic studies** include chest radiograph; CT scans of chest, abdomen, and pelvis; excretory urography; venacavogram; bipedal lymphangiography; and bone scans.

 c. Tumors are **classified pathologically as seminomatous or nonseminomatous** (subtypes include embryonal carcinoma, teratoma, yolk sac carcinoma, choriocarcinoma).

 d. Elevated blood levels of α-fetoprotein (AFP) or β-human chorionic gonadotropin (β-hCG) are diagnostic for nonseminomatous germ cell tumors; the majority of seminoma patients have normal levels.

 4. Treatment

 a. Treatment is **dependent on pathology and stage. Orchiectomy is always performed** for diagnostic and therapeutic reasons. Seminomatous tumors are radiosensitive; nonseminomatous tumors are radioresistant.

 b. **Nonseminomatous tumors: Stage I disease** limited to testis can be treated with **nerve-sparing retroperitoneal lymph node dissection** or **rigorous surveillance** without surgery or chemotherapy. **Stage II tumors** can be treated with **surgery or chemotherapy. Stage III disease** should be treated with **surgery and chemotherapy.**

 c. **Seminomatous tumors:** The mainstay of **stage I** disease isolated to the testis is **radiation therapy** to the para-aortic and ipsilateral iliac nodal areas. **Therapy for stage IIa and IIb** adds **increased radiation** to the affected nodes. **Stage IIc and III** are treated with **chemotherapy.**

G. Infectious disease

 1. AIDS (See Chapters 4 and 7.)

 2. Syphilis

 a. General characteristics

 (1) Syphilis is an infection **caused by the spirochete *Treponema pallidum*,** which can affect almost any organ or tissue in the body. **Often called the "great imitator" because it can resemble so many different diseases.**

(2) **Transmission occurs most frequently during sexual contact,** usually genital inoculations but can be extragenital.

(3) **Congenital syphilis is transmitted via the placenta** from mother to fetus after the tenth week of pregnancy.

(4) The epidemiology of syphilis is complex, but generally there has been **rising incidence of the disease in urban areas,** particularly in adolescents and young adults who are drug users.

b. Clinical features

(1) The **natural history** of acquired syphilis is generally divided into 2 major clinical stages: **early (infectious)** and **late (tertiary)** syphilis. The 2 stages are **separated by a symptom-free latent phase** during which the infectious stage may recur.

(2) The **primary lesions** of infectious syphilis are the **chancre** (a painless penile lesion) and **regional lymphadenopathy.** The **secondary lesions** may involve **skin, mucous membranes, bone, central nervous system,** or **liver.** There are relapsing lesions during early latency and congenital lesions. The **lesions of late syphilis are gummatous lesions involving skin, bones, and viscera; cardiovascular disease;** and **nervous system** and **ophthalmic lesions.**

(3) Table 6-6 **outlines the stages of syphilis** and the most common clinical manifestations.

c. Laboratory studies

(1) *T. pallidum* cannot be cultured from patients. Diagnosis is reliant on **serologic testing** and **microscopic examination.**

(2) **Serologic testing.** Nontreponemal antigen tests use a component of normal tissue as antigen to measure nonspecific antibodies in patients with syphilis.

(a) **Venereal Disease Research Lab (VDRL) test** has the widest use. It becomes positive 4–6 weeks after infection, is 99% positive during the second stage, and can be negative in late forms of syphilis. False positives can occur with a wide variety of nontreponemal states.

(b) **Rapid plasma reagin (RPR) test** is a reliable substitute for the VDRL.

(c) **Nontreponemal antibody titers** can be used to assess the effectiveness of treatment. It may take 6 months to see a fourfold decrease in titers with primary or secondary syphilis; late syphilis takes even longer.

(d) **Treponemal antibody tests** use live or killed *T. pallidum* as antigen to detect disease antibodies. The **fluorescent treponemal antibody absorption (FTA-ABS)** is the most widely used. The FTA-ABS test is useful principally in determining whether a positive nontreponemal antigen test is a false posi-

Table 6-6.
Stages of Syphilis and Common Clinical Features

Primary syphilis (2–4 weeks after exposure)
  Chancre: Usually a firm, nontender ulcer with well-defined margins and an indurated base
  Regional nontender lymphadenopathy

Secondary syphilis (3–6 weeks after exposure)
  Diffuse maculopapular rash on palms and soles
  Mucous patches: painless, silver ulcerations on mucous membranes
  Generalized lymphadenopathy
  Symptoms of low-grade fever, malaise, anorexia
  Arthralgias and myalgia
  Disorders of nervous system, eyes, kidney, liver, and bones are also possible

Tertiary syphilis
  Gummas: Granulomatous lesions of the skin, mucous membranes, bones, and other organs
  Cardiovascular complications, especially aortic aneurysm or aortic valve incompetence
  Neurologic complications, including seizures, hemiparesis, tabes dorsalis, Argyll Robertson pupil,
    Romberg sign, Charcot joint, and general paresthesias
  Personality changes, slurred speech, decreased memory

tive or true positive. The test is positive in most patients with primary syphilis and in virtually all with secondary syphilis. Lyme disease may cause a false positive FTA-ABS test.

(3) **Microscopic examination**

(a) In infectious syphilis, *T. pallidum* may be seen in **darkfield microscopic examination** of fresh exudate from the lesions. Spirochetes are usually not found in late syphilis.

(b) **Immunofluorescent staining techniques** can also demonstrate *T. pallidum* in dried smears of exudate.

(4) **Lumbar puncture** with examination of spinal fluid for spirochetes should be done if clinical picture suggests possibility of neurosyphilis. Neurosyphilis needs to be recognized and treated as soon as possible to avoid late sequelae.

d. Treatment

(1) **Benzathine penicillin G,** 2.4 million units IM in one dose, is the treatment of choice of **primary, secondary, and early latent syphilis.**

(2) **Late latent** and **tertiary syphilis** requires 3 weekly injections of **benzathine penicillin G,** 2.4 million units IM.

(3) **Neurosyphilis** is treated with **aqueous penicillin G**, 2–4 million units every 4 hours for 10–14 days. Some experts recommend following this with 3 weekly doses of benzathine penicillin G as above.

(4) **All cases of syphilis should be reported** to the appropriate public health agency for contact tracing. All sexual partners who have been exposed to syphilis in the past 3 months should be treated for early syphilis.

(5) **Careful follow-up** is essential to monitor effectiveness of treatment and identify treatment failures. Follow-up should be performed at **3, 6, 12, and 24 months** after therapy.

(6) **HIV testing** and **treatment for concurrent sexually transmitted diseases** should be undertaken upon diagnosis of syphilis.

H. Male infertility

1. General characteristics

a. **Primary infertility** affects 15%–20% of married couples. Approximately one third of cases result from male factors, one third from female factors, and one third from combined factors.

b. Clinical evaluation is warranted following **at least one year** of unprotected intercourse.

2. Clinical features

a. A **thorough history and physical examination** are critical to the evaluation of male infertility.

b. History should include **prior testicular insults, infections, environmental factors, medications,** and **drugs. Sexual habits, frequency, timing, use of lubricants,** and **prior fertility history are important. Loss of libido, headaches, or visual disturbances may indicate a pituitary tumor.** The past history may reveal **thyroid or liver disease, diabetic neuropathy, pelvic surgery,** or **hernia repair.**

c. **Physical examination should look for signs of hypogonadism.** The scrotal contents should be carefully evaluated for testicular size, varicoceles, and intact vas deferens and epididymis.

3. Laboratory findings

a. **Semen analysis** should be performed after 72 hours of abstinence. The specimen should be analyzed within one hour after collection. **Abnormal sperm concentrations are less than 20 million/ml.** Also examine for adequate semen volume, normal sperm motility, and morphology.

b. **Endocrinologic testing** is warranted if sperm counts are low or there is a clinical basis for suspecting an endocrinologic disorder. Testing should include serum FSH, LH, and testosterone.

c. **Scrotal ultrasound** may detect subclinical varicocele.

4. Treatment

a. **Patient education** regarding timing of sexual intercourse with ovulation and avoidance of spermicidal lubricants should be given.

b. **Underlying infections** or **medication related factors** should be remedied.

c. **Testicular failure** may be treated with chorionic gonadotropin once pituitary disease has been excluded.

d. Patients with **retrograde ejaculation** may be treated with **α-adrenergic agonists.** Postmasturbation urine may be collected for intrauterine insemination.

e. **Surgical repairs** of varicoceles may be done.

f. **Obstruction** can be **corrected surgically** as appropriate.

g. **Assisted reproductive techniques** including intrauterine insemination, in vitro fertilization, and gamete intrafallopian transfer are alternatives for patients who have failed other therapies.

7

Gynecology

Rebecca Lovell Scott

I. MENSTRUAL DISORDERS

A. Dysmenorrhea

1. General characteristics

a. **Primary dysmenorrhea** is **painful menstruation,** caused by **excess prostaglandin secretion leading to painful uterine contractions.** It affects more than half of the women of reproductive age at some point during their reproductive years.

b. **Secondary dysmenorrhea** is **painful menstruation caused by an identifiable clinical condition,** usually a disease of the uterus or pelvis (e.g., endometriosis). It usually affects women over 25 years of age.

2. Clinical features

a. Women with **primary dysmenorrhea** have **cramping** in the **central lower abdomen or pelvis, radiating** to the back or thighs, beginning **before or at the onset of menses** and lasting 1–3 days.

b. **Excess prostaglandin** also causes headache, nausea, vomiting, and diarrhea.

c. Symptoms of **secondary dysmenorrhea** are similar to those of primary dysmenorrhea, but also include **bloating, menorrhagia,** and **dyspareunia.**

3. Laboratory studies

a. Primary dysmenorrhea is diagnosed by **history** and **physical examination.**

b. **Tests** for secondary dysmenorrhea target **possible pelvic pathology.**

4. Treatment

a. Primary dysmenorrhea

(1) Start **nonsteroidal anti-inflammatory drugs (NSAIDs)** just before the expected menses and continue for 2–3 days.

(2) **Oral contraceptives and exercise** also reduce pain.

b. Secondary dysmenorrhea

(1) Any **obvious underlying condition** should be treated and intrauterine devices removed.

(2) **Symptomatic treatment** may be sufficient.

(3) **Hysteroscopy, dilation and curettage (D&C),** and **laparoscopy** allow both diagnosis and treatment.

B. Premenstrual syndrome (PMS)

1. General characteristics

a. PMS **lacks** agreed-upon **diagnostic criteria**.

b. Some research indicates that PMS is caused by an **abnormal response to estrogen and progesterone.**

    c. More than **90% of women** have mild to moderate changes that do not interfere with functioning. One third respond to over-the-counter medications.

    d. Fewer than 4% of women meet criteria for **late premenstrual dysphoric disorder.**

2. Clinical features

    a. Symptoms are **associated with the menstrual cycle** and begin 1–2 weeks before menses (i.e., during the luteal phase) and end 1–2 days after the onset of menses.

    b. A monthly **symptom-free period during the follicular phase** (i.e., from day 1 of the menses to ovulation) must exist (Figure 7-1).

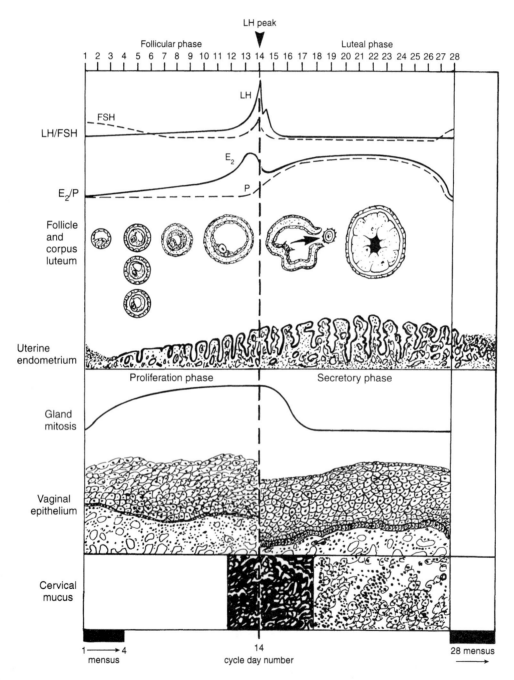

Figure 7-1. Composite changes in tissues and hormones during the reproductive cycle. (From Beckmann CB, Ling FW, Laube, DW, Smith, RP, and Barzansky BM (eds): *Obstetrics and Gynecology, 3rd edition.* Baltimore, Williams & Wilkins, 1998, p 417.)

c. The most common complaints are **mood alteration** and **psychological effects** (e.g., irritability, agitation, anger, insomnia).

d. Symptoms related to **fluid retention** are **edema, weight gain,** and **breast pain.**

e. **Bloating, constipation,** and **backache** may also occur.

3. Tests include **daily charting of symptoms.**

4. Treatment

    a. **Lifestyle modification** includes diet and exercise.

    b. **Drug treatment**

       (1) Some women respond to brief intermittent courses of **anti-anxiety agents;** daily **serotonergic medication;** 25–100 mg **vitamin B_6** daily; **diuretics** and **sodium restriction** for swelling; **bromocriptine** for mastalgia.

       (2) **Oral contraceptives** may improve, worsen, or not change symptomatology.

C. Menopause

  1. General characteristics

    a. By definition, the menopause is the **last menses; perimenopause** is the time surrounding it.

    b. Mean age at natural menopause is **51** years.

    c. The **subjective experience of menopause varies** by individual with cultural expectations and life circumstances.

  2. Clinical features

    a. **Vasomotor symptoms** vary in intensity.

    b. **Urogenital atrophy** may cause poor vaginal lubrication, dysuria, urge incontinence, and other problems.

    c. **Accelerated bone loss** may result in **osteoporosis.**

    d. Estrogen-related cardiovascular protection declines.

  3. Laboratory studies: **Follicle-stimulating hormone (FSH) more than 30 mIU/ml** is diagnostic of menopause.

  4. Treatment

    a. **Hormone replacement therapy (HRT)** appears to prevent or improve **coronary heart disease (CHD), osteoporosis, urogenital atrophy,** and **mortality.**

       (1) **Possible risks** associated with HRT include endometrial and breast cancer, migraine, and gallbladder disease.

       (2) **Contraindications** include undiagnosed vaginal bleeding, acute vascular thrombosis, and a history of estrogen-dependent tumors.

       (3) **Estrogen only, combined estrogen and progestin,** and possibly androgens are available for HRT.

       (4) **Duration of therapy** ranges from 2 years to lifetime.

    b. **Lifestyle modifications** may also ameliorate symptoms.

II. UTERINE DISORDERS

A. Leiomyoma (uterine fibroids)

  1. **General characteristics.** Fibroids are more common in **African-American women** with a positive family history.

  2. Clinical features

    a. Patients have a **firm, enlarged, irregular uterine mass.**

    b. **Menorrhagia or intermenstrual bleeding** is common.

3. **Diagnostic procedures** include **ultrasound, D&C,** and **hysteroscopy.**

4. **Treatment** for symptomatic patients **is myomectomy, hysterectomy,** or **hormone treatment.**

B. Endometrial uterine cancer

   1. General characteristics

      a. **Postmenopausal** women comprise 75% of patients.

      b. These neoplasms are **estrogen-dependent.**

      c. **Prognosis** is influenced by histologic appearance, age (older women have poorer outcomes), and extent of spread.

   2. Clinical features

      a. The cardinal symptom is **inappropriate uterine bleeding.**

      b. A **mucoid** or **watery discharge** may precede bleeding.

   3. The most common **test** is **endometrial sampling.**

   4. Treatment

      a. **Total hysterectomy** combined with bilateral salpingo-oophorectomy is the basis of treatment.

      b. **Radiotherapy** may be indicated.

      c. **Recurrence** is treated with **high-dose progestins.**

III. OVARIAN DISORDERS

A. Ovarian cysts

   1. General characteristics

      a. Cysts are the **most common ovarian growth.**

      b. Most are **functional** cysts (i.e., cysts arising as a result of normal function; not neoplasms).

   2. Clinical features. Cysts may present as **asymptomatic masses** or with **pain** and **menstrual delay.**

   3. Laboratory studies. Cysts are usually **confirmed by ultrasound.**

   4. Treatment

      a. **Follow for 1–2 cycles** in premenopausal women with cysts smaller than 8 cm.

      b. Large or persistent cysts require **laparoscopy.**

      c. Cysts in postmenopausal women are **presumed to be malignant until proved otherwise.**

      d. Oral contraceptives have not been validated in treating functional cysts.

B. Ovarian cancer

   1. General characteristics

      a. High-risk women are **older, nulliparous,** and **white,** and **have a positive family history.**

      b. **Oral contraceptive use** appears to be **protective.**

   2. Clinical features include **ascites, abdominal distention, vague gastrointestinal symptoms,** and a **mass.**

   3. Laboratory studies

      a. **Alpha-fetoprotein (AFP) and carcinoembryonic antigen (CEA)** are elevated.

      b. **CA-125,** a glycoprotein that appears in the blood when natural endometrial protective barriers are destroyed, as with cancer, may be used to follow treatment.

   4. **Treatment** is surgery, plus chemo- and radiotherapy.

IV. CERVICAL DYSPLASIA AND NEOPLASIA

A. General characteristics

1. **Human papillomavirus (HPV) infection** (especially types 16 and 18) is strongly linked to cervical neoplasia.

2. Other risk factors include **early age at first intercourse, multiple sexual partners, low socioeconomic status, African-American race,** and **cigarette smoking.**

B. Clinical features

1. Most women with abnormal Pap smears have **no symptoms.**

2. **Advanced** or **invasive cervical cancer** may cause **abnormal vaginal bleeding** and **tumor** may be seen on clinical examination.

C. Laboratory studies

1. The **Pap smear** is highly effective for screening. Screening should begin **when a woman becomes sexually active** or **reaches 18,** whichever comes first.

2. Abnormal Pap smears (Table 7-1) indicate a need for further diagnostic testing.

a. **Biopsy** is mandatory if a suspicious lesion is seen.

b. **Colposcopy** can determine the location and severity of the lesion.

Table 7-1.
The 1991 Bethesda System for Reporting Cervical and Vaginal Cytologic Diagnoses

Adequacy of the specimen
  Satisfactory for evaluation
  Satisfactory for evaluation but limited by (specify reason)
  Unsatisfactory for evaluation (specify reason)

Descriptive diagnoses
  Benign cellular changes
    Infection
      Trichomonas vaginalis
      Fungal organisms morphologically consistent with *Candida* species
      Predominance of coccobacilli consistent with shift in vaginal flora
      Fungal organisms morphologically consistent with *Actinomyces* species
      Cellular changes associated with herpes simplex virus

Reactive changes
  Reactive cellular changes associated with
    Inflammation (includes typical repair)
    Atrophy with inflammation ("atrophic vaginitis")
    Radiation
    Intrauterine devices
    Other

Epithelial cell abnormalities
  Squamous cells
    Atypical squamous cells of undetermined significance
    Low-grade squamous intraepithelial lesion, encompassing HPV, mild dysplasia, CIN I
    High-grade squamous intraepithelial lesion, encompassing moderate and severe dysplasia, carcinoma in situ/CIN II and CIN III
    Squamous cell carcinoma
  Glandular cells
    Endometrial cells, cytologically benign, in a postmenopausal woman
    Atypical glandular cells of undetermined significance
    Endocervical adenocarcinoma
    Endometrial carcinoma
    Extrauterine adenocarcinoma
    Adenocarcinoma, not otherwise specified

Other malignant neoplasms (specified)

CIN = cervical intraepithelial neoplasia; *HPV* = human papillomavirus.

c. Conization is used when colposcopy results are unsatisfactory or endocervical curettage scrapings indicate severe disease.

D. Treatment

1. Mild lesions may **resolve spontaneously.**
2. **Preinvasive neoplasia** may be treated with electro- or cryocautery, laser therapy, conization, and loop electrosurgical excision procedure (LEEP).
3. **Surgery** is indicated for more severe abnormalities.

V. INFERTILITY

A. General characteristics

1. Infertility is generally defined as a **failure to conceive after 1 year of unprotected intercourse.**
2. Surveys estimate that up to 15% of married couples in the United States are infertile.
3. **Female factors** include older age, ovulatory dysfunction, tubal disease, endometriosis, and cervical abnormalities.
4. **Male factors** include varicocele, obstruction, infection, and hormonal abnormalities (see Chapter 6).

B. Clinical features may be normal.

C. Laboratory studies

1. **Semen analysis** should precede any other testing.
2. **Basal body temperature, ovulation prediction tests,** and **progesterone levels** confirm ovulation.
3. **Luteal phase endometrial biopsy, FSH levels, prolactin,** and **thyroid-stimulating hormone** may be helpful.
4. **Postcoital testing** measures sperm survival.
5. **Hysterosalpingography** determines tubal patency and uterine abnormalities.
6. Other tests that may be useful include **laparoscopy, sperm penetration assay, sperm antibody testing, ultrasonography,** and **hysteroscopy.**

D. Treatment

1. **Clomiphene citrate 50–100 mg for 5 days beginning on day 3, 4, or 5 of the cycle** should be given to anovulatory women.
2. **Artificial insemination** is an alternative for couples with abnormal postcoital tests.
3. Other treatments depend on the cause of the infertility, the couple's resources, and the age of the woman.
4. **Assisted reproductive technologies** include in vitro fertilization, gamete intrafallopian transfer, zygote intrafallopian transfer, and surrogate options.

VI. INFECTIOUS DISEASE

A. Candidiasis

1. **General characteristics.** *Candida albicans* is most often associated with vulvovaginal candidiasis.
2. **Clinical features**

   a. Vulvar candidiasis is characterized by **severe pruritus, erythema of the vulva** and **surrounding skin,** and possibly peripheral pustules.

  b. Patients may experience **dysuria** or **dyspareunia**.

  c. The vagina is **red**, with **curdy, yellow-white discharge**.

 3. Laboratory studies

  a. **Spores and mycelia** on a potassium hydroxide (KOH) preparation are diagnostic.

  b. *Candida* may be cultured in **Sabouraud's medium**.

 4. Treatment

  a. **Topical 1% clotrimazole** or **2% ketoconazole cream** is effective for vulvar candidiasis.

  b. Vaginal **clotrimazole** and **miconazole** are usual treatments, **but econazole, tioconazole,** and **ketoconazole** are all effective.

B. **Vaginitis and vulvovaginitis**

 1. General characteristics

  a. **Vaginitis** may be caused by infection with *Trichomonas vaginalis*, a unicellular flagellated organism, in which case it is called trichomoniasis.

  b. **Bacterial vaginosis** (nonspecific vaginitis) results from infection with *Gardnerella vaginalis* and various anaerobes.

 2. Clinical features

  a. Classic findings of trichomoniasis include a **profuse, frothy, greenish, malodorous discharge with petechial lesions on the cervix** ("strawberry cervix").

  b. Classic findings of bacterial vaginosis include **a gray, homogeneous, foul-smelling discharge**.

 3. Laboratory studies

  a. *T. vaginalis* organisms will be visible on a saline wet mount.

  b. In bacterial vaginosis, the **vaginal pH is above 5**, KOH releases a fishy odor (**positive whiff test**), and wet mount shows **"clue" cells** and absence of lactobacilli.

 4. Treatment

  a. For trichomoniasis, give **single dose metronidazole 2 g orally** to the patient and her partner(s).

  b. For bacterial vaginosis, **metronidazole 500 mg orally twice a day for 7 days, clindamycin 2% cream intravaginally for 7 days,** or **metronidazole gel intravaginally twice a day for 5 days** are 3 effective options.

C. **Gonorrhea and chlamydia** (for a detailed general discussion, see Chapter 6 VII B 1)

 1. General characteristics

  a. Gonorrhea and chlamydia in women are **often asymptomatic**, requiring screening of high-risk women.

  b. **Young age, inconsistent use of barrier contraception,** and **new** or **multiple sexual partners** put women at risk.

  c. In women, **coinfection** is common.

 2. Clinical features

  a. Infection sites may include the **throat, urethra, cervix,** and **anus**.

  b. **Mucopurulent endocervical discharge** may be accompanied by abnormal bleeding and cramping.

 3. Laboratory studies

  a. Culture for *Neisseria gonorrhoeae* on **Thayer-Martin agar** in CO_2-rich environment is 80%–95% specific.

  b. **Immunoassay or monoclonal antibody tests** are useful for *C. trachomatis*.

 4. **Treatment** is outlined in Tables 7-2 and 7-3.

Table 7-2.

Treatment Regimens for Gonococcal Infections

One of the following:

Ceftriaxone, 125 mg IM in a single dose

or

Cefixime, 400 mg orally in a single dose

or

Ciprofloxacin, 500 mg orally in a single dose

or

Ofloxacin, 400 mg orally in a single dose

PLUS

A regimen effective against possible coinfection with *Chlamydia trachomatis,* such as doxycycline, 100 mg orally twice a day for 7 days or azithromycin 1 g orally in a single dose

IM = intramuscularly.
Centers for Disease Control and Prevention: 1998 Guidelines for Treatment of Sexually Transmitted Diseases. MMWR 1998;47, No. RR-1:60–61.

Table 7-3.

Treatment Regimens for Chlamydial Infections

Doxycycline, 100 mg orally 2 times a day for 7 days

or

Azithromycin, 1 gm orally in a single dose

Alternative regimens:
Ofloxacin, 300 mg orally 2 times a day for 7 days

or

Erythromycin base 500 mg orally 4 times a day for 7 days

or

Erythromycin ethylsuccinate, 800 mg orally 4 times a day for 7 days

Centers for Disease Control and Prevention: 1998 Guidelines for Treatment of Sexually Transmitted Diseases. MMWR 1998;47, No. RR-1:54.

D. HIV/AIDS (see also Chapter 4 IV)

1. General characteristics

a. HIV infection is increasing in women more rapidly than in any other group.

b. Women most commonly acquire HIV infection through **heterosexual contact** and **intravenous drug use.**

c. Infection in a woman **also puts a fetus at risk.**

d. HIV-positive women in the United States are more likely to be **African-American** or **Hispanic.**

2. Clinical features

a. Kaposi's sarcoma is **rare** in women.

b. Herpes simplex virus (HSV) and **cytomegalovirus (CMV) infection, wasting,** and **esophageal candidiasis** are **more common** in women.

c. Refractory *Candida* **vulvovaginitis** is common.

3. Laboratory studies (see Chapter 4 IV C). HIV-infected women should have Pap smears every 6 months.

4. Treatment (see Chapter 4 IV D). Zidovudine therapy during pregnancy decreases mother-to-child transmission.

E. Pelvic inflammatory disease (PID)

1. General characteristics

a. PID is usually polymicrobial.

b. Complications are **infertility** and **ectopic pregnancy.**

Table 7-4.
Treatment Regimens for Pelvic Inflammatory Disease

Outpatient	Inpatient
One of the following:	One of the following:
Cefoxitin, 2 mg IM, plus probenecid, 1 g orally in a single dose,	Cefoxitin, 2 g IV every 6 hours,
or	or
Ceftriaxone, 250 mg IM,	Cefotetan, 2 g IV every 12 hours
or	PLUS
other parenteral 3rd generation cephalosporine	Doxycycline, 100 mg IV or orally every 12 hours
PLUS	
Doxycycline, 100 mg orally 2 times a day for 14 days	
OR	OR
Ofloxacin, 400 mg orally 2 times a day for 14 days	Clindamycin, 900 mg IV every 8 hours
PLUS one of the following:	PLUS
Clindamycin, 450 mg orally 4 times daily,	Gentamicin, loading dose IV or IM (2 mg/kg), followed by a maintenance dose (1.5 mg/kg) every 8 hours
or	
Metronidazole, 500 mg orally 2 times a day for 14 days	

IM = intramuscularly; IV = intravenously.
Centers for Disease Control and Prevention: 1998 Guidelines for Treatment of Sexually Transmitted Diseases. MMWR 1998;47, No. RR-1:82–84.

   2. Clinical features

   a. Classic symptoms are **fever** and **lower abdominal pain.**

   b. **Leukorrhea, cervical motion tenderness ("chandelier sign"),** and **adnexal tenderness** are common.

   c. An **adnexal mass** may indicate a tubo-ovarian abscess.

   3. Laboratory studies

   a. Tests for **gonorrhea** and **chlamydia** should be performed.

   b. **Ultrasound** should be used for diagnosing adnexal masses.

   c. **Diagnostic laparoscopy** may be required.

   4. Treatment (Table 7-4)

   a. Women with mild disease should be treated as outpatients.

   b. **Women with severe disease should be hospitalized** for intravenous antibiotic therapy and possible surgery.

   c. **Sex partners** should be evaluated and treated.

   d. **Pregnant women should not take doxycycline.**

VII. BREAST DISORDERS

   A. Benign breast disorders

   1. General characteristics

   a. **Mastodynia (mastalgia)** or **breast tenderness,** is common, often cyclical, and increases in women with contraceptive pills or HRT.

   b. **Mastitis,** or **breast infection,** is most often due to *Staphylococcus* or *Streptococcus* and occurs primarily in lactating women.

   c. **Fibrocystic breast changes** are caused by cysts, fibroadenomas, and sclerosing adenomas.

2. **Clinical features**

   a. Persistent, noncyclic breast pain suggests underlying cancer; cyclic pain suggests luteal phase tenderness.

   b. **Mastitis** presents with tenderness, heat, fever, chills, and other flu-like symptoms.

   c. **Fibroadenomas** are typically round, firm, smooth, discrete, mobile, and nontender.

3. **Laboratory studies**

   a. **Mammography, ultrasound,** and **biopsy** may be indicated.

   b. In suspected mastitis, **purulent material** or **milk may be cultured** or milk examined for **white blood cells.**

   c. **In suspected cysts, fine needle aspiration is** both **diagnostic** and **therapeutic;** cysts usually contain straw-colored fluid.

   d. **Ultrasound differentiates between** a **solid** and a **cystic mass.**

   e. In a woman over 25 years of age, a **fibroadenomatous mass should be biopsied.**

4. **Treatment**

   a. Treat **mastodynia** with reassurance, vitamin B_6, bromocriptine (a prolactin suppressor), tamoxifen (anti-estrogen), or danazol (attenuated androgen).

   b. Treat **mastitis** with **amoxicillin-clavulanate** or a first-generation **cephalosporin,** and hot compresses.

   c. **Surgical treatment** may be required for abscesses or duct ectasia.

   d. Many types of fibrocystic breast problems need no treatment; aspirate cysts and excise fibroadenomas.

B. **Breast neoplasms**

1. **General characteristics**

   a. Most women with breast cancer have **no identifiable risk factors** other than female sex and increasing age; 5% have genetic susceptibility.

   b. Associated factors include **nulliparity, early menarche, late menopause, long-term estrogen exposure, delayed childbearing,** and **radiation exposure.**

   c. **Ductal carcinomas** comprise 85% of breast cancers; the remainder are **lobular.**

   d. **Lobular carcinoma in situ (LCIS)** and **atypical ductal hyperplasia** predispose to breast cancer.

   e. **Paget's disease** is a ductal carcinoma presenting as an eczematous lesion of the nipple.

   f. **All invasive lobular carcinomas and two thirds of ductal carcinomas are estrogen receptor positive.**

   g. Breast cancer is the **most common female malignancy** and the **second leading cause of cancer death** in women.

2. **Clinical features**

   a. Breast cancer most often presents as a **single, nontender, firm, immobile mass.**

   b. Rarer presentations include **bloody nipple discharge, dimpling, skin thickening,** and **eczematous changes.**

3. **Laboratory studies**

   a. A combination of **physical examination, mammography,** and **fine-needle biopsy** are highly accurate in establishing the diagnosis.

   b. **Ultrasound** and **excisional biopsy** may be indicated.

   c. Biopsy specimen should undergo estrogen and progesterone receptor analysis.

4. **Treatment**

   a. **Modified radical mastectomy** and **partial mastectomy followed by radiation** have equivalent survival rates.

   b. **Adjuvant chemotherapy** benefits some women.

   c. **Tamoxifen** is used to treat women with estrogen receptor-positive disease and postmenopausal women.

   d. **Autologous bone-marrow transplantation** may be helpful in young women with limited metastases.

8

Obstetrics

Jo Hanna Friend D'Epiro

I. ROUTINE PRECONCEPTION AND PRENATAL CARE

A. Preconception care

1. General characteristics

a. Because 40% of pregnancies in the United States are unplanned, **every woman of childbearing age should be considered a candidate for preconception counseling.**

b. **A detailed obstetric and medical history should be taken,** including family history, nutritional habits, drug and environmental exposures, social issues (e.g., marital status, living situation, insurance information), and illicit substance use.

c. **Concerns about fertility can often be aired** during the preconception counseling session. **Infertility** is defined as **failure to conceive after one calendar year of unprotected intercourse.**

2. Clinical features

a. On **pelvic examination, obvious barriers to conception,** such as congenital malformations of the reproductive tract or overt infections, **should be excluded.**

b. **Appropriate weight** for height should be checked.

c. Physical manifestations of **poorly controlled medical disorders** should be identified.

3. Laboratory studies

a. **Rubella titer** should be determined to ascertain immunity to rubella.

b. Laboratory studies pertaining to **chronic medical disorders** should be ordered [e.g., thyroid-stimulating hormone (TSH) for patients with hypothyroidism].

c. **If the patient is at risk** for such infectious diseases as hepatitis B, toxoplasmosis, varicella, or HIV, **titers could be considered.**

d. **Cultures for sexually transmitted diseases** should be offered as needed.

4. Treatment

a. After careful review of history, **the patient should be counseled in regard to risks; any chronic medications should be changed to the safest possible choice for pregnancy;** and **the patient should be referred** to specialists as needed for treatment of **medical disorders** (Table 8-1) and referred for **genetic counseling** as needed.

b. **Dietary supplementation** should be begun with 0.4 mg of **folic acid,** which appears to reduce the risk of neural tube defects.

c. The patient should **take appropriate action if weight loss is necessary** because this may also decrease the incidence of neural tube defects.

d. Appropriate **immunizations** such as hepatitis B vaccine or measles-mumps-rubella (MMR) vaccine should be offered on an as-needed basis.

e. Ask the patient to **keep a menstrual calendar.**

f. If the patient has met the definition of infertility (see I A 1 c), **institute measures to begin evaluation** if desired.

Table 8-1.
Conditions Requiring Perinatology Consultation

Asthma
  Severe (requiring multiple hospitalizations)

Blood group isomimmunization
  CDE (Rh)
  [Exclude ABO or Lewis]

Cardiac disease
  Cyanotic, prior myocardial infarct, aortic stenosis, primary pulmonary hypertension, Marfan syndrome, prosthetic valve, American Heart Association Class II or greater
Diabetes mellitus
  Class D or greater

Family history of genetic problems (e.g., Down syndrome, Tay-Sachs disease)

Hemoglobinopathy
  Sickle cell disease, sickle cell trait, or β-thalassemia

HIV
  Symptomatic or low CD4 count

Hypertension
  Chronic, with renal or heart disease

Pulmonary disease
  Severe obstructive or restrictive

Renal disease
  Chronic, creatinine > 3 without hypertension

At the time of consultation, continued patient care should be determined by collaboration with the referring care provider or by transfer of care. ABO = blood group system consisting of groups A, AB, B, and O; CDE = antigens, also known as Rhesus blood group system or Rh; HIV = human immunodeficiency virus. Modified from March of Dimes Birth Defects Foundation, Committee on Perinatal Health. Toward improving the outcome of pregnancy: the 90s and beyond. White Plains, New York: March of Dimes Birth Defects Foundation, 1993.

B. **Routine prenatal care and prenatal diagnostic testing**

1. **General characteristics**

   a. An initial obstetric history includes **subjective symptoms of pregnancy** such as amenorrhea, breast tenderness, nausea, and fatigue as well as the **patient's general medical, obstetric,** and **family history** (see Table 8-1).

   b. The due date or **expected date of confinement** (EDC) can be calculated using Nägele's or McDonald's rule: First day of last menstrual period (LMP) + 7 days − 3 months = EDC.

   c. The patient's obstetric history can be expressed as **gravida** (number of total pregnancies), **parity** (number of deliveries), and **abortions** (number of miscarriages or abortions) as follows: G_P_Ab_ ; or denoted as a sequence of 4 digits signifying **term infants, premature deliveries, abortions,** and **living children** (i.e., P_ _ _ _).

   d. The **initial visit should take place 6 weeks after the last menstrual period.** Subsequent prenatal visits are to be scheduled **every 4 weeks until the 28th week** of gestation; **every 2–3 weeks up to 36 weeks** of gestation; and **weekly thereafter.**

   e. After the initial visit, each subsequent prenatal visit will include a focused **history and examination regarding fetal movement, blood pressure, check of fundal height, fetal heart tones,** and a **urinalysis** for glucosuria and proteinuria and **vaginal examination as indicated.**

2. **Clinical features**

   a. At 6 weeks from the LMP, the uterine fundus will be enlarged and may have positive **Hegar's** sign (softening of the uterine isthmus).

   b. At 12 weeks, the **uterus is 4 times normal** and can be palpated at the symphysis.

   c. **Fetal heart tones** can be appreciated beginning at 10–12 weeks using Doppler stethoscope and range from **120–180 beats per minute** (i.e., approximately twice the maternal heart rate).

d. At 16 weeks' gestation, the uterus is midway between the symphysis and umbilicus; at 20 weeks the fundus is at the umbilicus, and from 21 weeks on, the height in centimeters of the uterine fundus should correlate roughly ($+/-$ 2 cm) to the number of weeks' gestation (Figure 8-1).

e. Quickening, the first awareness of fetal movements, usually occurs at 20 weeks in a primigravida and as early as 16–18 weeks in a multigravida.

f. Because of the expanding uterus and the dramatically altered hormonal environment, **common complaints,** such as backache, increasing varicosities, heartburn, hemorrhoids, and fatigue, **can be associated with an otherwise healthy pregnancy.**

3. Laboratory and prenatal diagnostic testing (Table 8-2)

    a. Ultrasound

        (1) Obstetrical ultrasound uses sound waves emitted and reflected back to a transducer applied to the abdominal wall. The reflected energy generates a small electrical voltage displayed on a screen that correlates to the difference in densities of the underlying anatomy.

        (2) Transvaginal ultrasound, performed by placing a pencil thin transducer into the vagina, **is sometimes used in the first trimester of pregnancy if an abdominal scan cannot identify structures clearly.**

        (3) Uses in early pregnancy. Ultrasound can **detect fetal heart activity** as soon as 1–2 weeks after the first missed menstrual period. It is an accurate modality to detect **multiple gestations;** to **establish or confirm EDC;** to check for **fetal viability;** to correlate **appropriate growth in relation to gestational age** (large or small for gestational age); to help **check for placental status and location;** to evaluate **vaginal bleeding;**

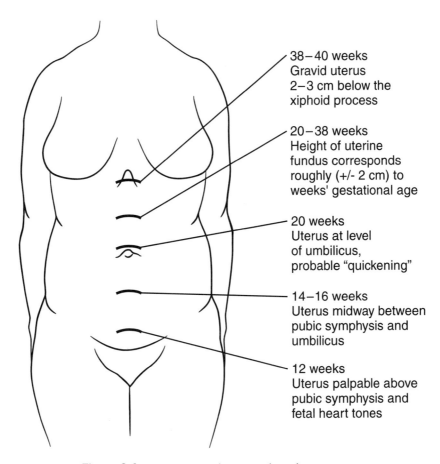

Figure 8-1. Uterine size and position throughout gestation.

Table 8-2.
Prenatal Laboratories and Screening Tests

Early

CBC

Blood type and Rh

Rubella titer

Hepatitis B serum antigen

Cultures for chlamydia, gonorrhea as needed

Offer all women HIV testing

Urinalysis

Coombs' test (irregular antibody screen)

Serologic testing for syphilis

Papanicolaou test

10–12 weeks

Chorionic villus sampling (CVS)

11–14 weeks

Early amniocentesis

15–18 weeks

Alpha-fetoprotein 3 (AFP 3)

Routine amniocentesis

28 weeks

In unsensitized Rh patients, repeat antibody titers (followed by Rh immune globulin)

Screen for gestational diabetes as desired

Hemoglobin and hematocrit

35 weeks

Vaginal–rectal culture for β-streptococcus

Hemoglobin and hematocrit

CBC = complete blood cell count.

to detect **multiple gestation;** and to check **amniotic fluid levels.** It can also be used to help **detect lethal malformations** and as a **follow-up to abnormal alpha-fetoprotein (AFP) testing.**

(4) **Uses in late pregnancy.** Combined with a nonstress test, ultrasound is used late in pregnancy to **monitor fetal well-being** in the form of a scored examination known as a **biophysical profile.** Scaled on a 10-point system, this test includes **fetal motion** and **breathing.**

b. Chorionic villus sampling (CVS) is a diagnostic procedure performed between 10–12 weeks using a catheter or needle to biopsy placental cells (chorionic villi).

(1) CVS is **useful in diagnosing Down syndrome** and several **mendelian conditions** such as cystic fibrosis, hemophilia, muscular dystrophy, and hemoglobinopathies.

(2) Unlike amniocentesis, CVS specimens **cannot** be used for AFP testing for neural tube defects.

(3) The **risk of spontaneous abortion** after CVS is slightly higher than for amniocentesis at 0.5%–1% (versus 0.25%–0.5% for amniocentesis), although the results are available earlier in the pregnancy.

(4) One potentially serious complication after CVS is **limb defects** (0.07%–0.2% risk).

c. Alpha-fetoprotein 3 (AFP 3) test is a multiple marker serum screening test offered to all women between 15–18 weeks' gestation (see Table 8-2).

(1) The AFP 3 test **checks levels of alpha-fetoprotein,** a major circulating protein of the early fetus; **human chorionic gonadotropin (hCG);** and **unconjugated estriol.**

(2) AFP 3 is useful in detecting up to 75% of open **neural tube defects** such as spina bifida and anencephaly and 70%–90% of cases of **Trisomy 18 and 21.**

(3) If an AFP 3 is abnormal, follow-up tests entail either a comprehensive ultrasound with a thorough, detailed examination of fetal anatomy, or amniocentesis, or both.

d. Amniocentesis involves the withdrawal of amniotic fluid via needle under ultrasound guidance for prenatal diagnosis and is usually performed between 15–18 weeks' gestation. Early amniocentesis is performed between 11–14 weeks' gestation. Although early amniocentesis allows for earlier diagnosis, it is considered experimental and has a 2.5-fold increase in pregnancy loss compared with mid-trimester amniocentesis.

   (1) **Indications** for amniocentesis include a mother over 35 years of age, a history of a previously affected fetus, and those at high risk for known genetic diseases such as Tay-Sachs and sickle cell disease.

   (2) The risk of spontaneous abortion following mid-trimester amniocentesis is .25%–0.5%.

e. Fetal monitoring, using Doppler ultrasound for heart tones and an external stress gauge for uterine contractions, **is used near term to monitor fetal well-being.**

   (1) **Baseline fetal heart rate (FHR) tones during labor are 120–169 beats per minute.** Increases in FHR are known as **elevations** and decreases are known as **decelerations.**

   (2) A normal result for a **nonstress test** involves evidence of **3 fetal movements in 10 minutes** and **15 beats per minute acceleration of fetal heart tones** for a duration of 15 seconds.

   (3) **Contractions usually decrease the blood flow to the placenta.** This is poorly tolerated by the stressed or abnormal fetus and leads to hypoxia and concomitant relative bradycardia.

   (4) **Decelerations** have been defined as a **decline in FHR of 15 beats per minute** or lasting more than 15 seconds.

II. COMPLICATIONS OF PREGNANCY

A. Ectopic pregnancy

1. General characteristics

   a. Ectopic pregnancy is the implantation of a pregnancy anywhere but the endometrium.

   b. It is the **second most frequent cause of maternal death** in the United States.

   c. Ectopic pregnancy occurs in **more than 1:100 pregnancies** and has increased in incidence over the past 25 years.

   d. Risk factors for ectopic pregnancy include a **history of a previous ectopic pregnancy, previous infection, abdominal or tubal surgery, more than 2 therapeutic abortions, intrauterine device (IUD) use, assisted reproduction, diethylstilbestrol (DES) exposure,** and **progestin-only contraception.**

   e. Differential diagnosis includes ruptured corpus luteum, appendicitis, renal calculi, pelvic inflammatory disease, torsion of an ovarian cyst, mesenteric adenitis, and gastroenteritis.

2. Clinical features

   a. Presentation of ectopic pregnancy is **widely variable** and may depend on the site of implantation.

   b. The classic presentation includes **abdominal pain, amenorrhea or spotting,** and **tenderness** or **a mass** on pelvic examination (Table 8-3).

   c. Signs and symptoms associated with a ruptured ectopic pregnancy are **severe abdominal or shoulder pain associated with peritonitis, syncope,** and **orthostatic hypotension.**

3. Laboratory studies

   a. Serum levels of hCG less than normal or with an inappropriate serial increase (i.e., less than a 66%–100% increase over 48 hours) should be considered consistent with an ectopic gestation until the diagnosis has been definitively excluded.

   b. Transvaginal ultrasound is diagnostic in 90% of cases of ectopic gestation.

   c. An **hCG titer of greater than or equal to 1500 mIU/ml** should show evidence of a **developing intrauterine gestation** on a transvaginal ultrasound.

Table 8-3.

Signs and Symptoms Associated with Ectopic Pregnancy

Pain	95%
Gastrointestinal symptoms	80%
Amenorrhea with abnormal bleeding	60%–80%
Dizziness or syncope	58%

From: Dorfman SF, Grimes DA, Cates WFr, Binkin NJ, Kafrissen ME, O'Reilly DR: Ectopic pregnancy mortality, United States, 1979 to 1980: Clinical Aspects. *Obstet Gynecol* 64:386, 1984.

Table 8-4.

Definitions

Threatened abortion	The clinical presentation of bleeding, spotting, or cramping, which may be associated with a later spontaneous abortion
Inevitable abortion	This is evidenced by obvious ruptured membranes in the first trimester or cervical dilatation, which will probably lead to expulsion of the pregnancy or infection
Incomplete abortion	Term used to imply that products of conception remain in the uterus after either a spontaneous abortion or a D&C
Missed abortion	Retention of dead products of conception for several weeks
Recurrent spontaneous abortion	Three or more consecutive spontaneous abortions
Elective abortion	Abortion initiated by human intervention at the request of the mother
Septic or infected abortion	Associated with bleeding and sepsis; treatment of infection includes evacuation of the products of conception with appropriate antibiotic therapy

D&C = dilation and curettage.

    4. Treatment

        a. Surgical treatment involves removal of the ectopic gestation, using laparoscopy or laporotomy. The least invasive procedure should be used, depending on the site of gestation and the stability of the patient.

        b. Medical treatment with methotrexate, a folate acid analog, has been used successfully to treat ectopic gestation when it is diagnosed early and the patient is hemodynamically stable.

        c. Follow-up testing using serum hCG levels or pelvic examination is crucial to exclude any remaining evidence of pregnancy.

  B. Spontaneous abortion

    1. General characteristics

        a. Abortion is the **termination of pregnancy,** by any means, **before the fetus is sufficiently developed to survive.**

        b. Spontaneous abortion is the spontaneous premature expulsion of the products of conception, and it **occurs in up to 10% of pregnancies** (Table 8-4).

        c. Of the 80% of spontaneous abortions which occur in the first trimester of pregnancy, **up to 50% are caused by chromosomal abnormalities.**

        d. Possible maternal causes of spontaneous abortion include infection, medical illnesses, immunologic factors, drug use (e.g., tobacco, cocaine, alcohol), and environmental factors (e.g., lead, formaldehyde).

        e. Complications of an improperly treated spontaneous abortion are Rh sensitization, infection, hemorrhage requiring blood transfusion, and potential blood coagulopathies, such as disseminated intravascular coagulation (DIC) from retained tissue or sepsis.

2. Clinical features

    a. **Bleeding** is variable on examination.

    b. The **uterine size often does not correlate appropriately to the last menstrual period,** and the **fundus of the uterus may be boggy or tender.**

    c. A **septic** or **infected abortion** may present with fever, pain, and bleeding.

3. Laboratory studies

    a. **Serial hCG titers, serum progesterone,** or **serial ultrasounds** may be required to confirm a viable pregnancy.

    b. **Ultrasound findings in a nonviable pregnancy** may include **inappropriate development** or **interval growth, poorly formed or unformed fetal pole,** and **fetal demise.**

    c. **Blood type** and **Rh status** are necessary tests to preclude Rh sensitization.

4. Treatment

    a. If the pregnancy has been definitively determined to be no longer viable, the **uterus must be emptied.**

    b. If the pregnancy is early and the patient is managed expectantly, careful follow-up with **pelvic examinations, serial hCG titers,** and **transvaginal ultrasound** can be used to determine whether the abortion is complete.

    c. **Dilation and curettage (D&C)** may also be necessary to ensure complete emptying of the uterus or as one form of induced abortion. Morbidity is caused by uterine perforation or cervical laceration.

    d. **Effective contraception** should be employed after a spontaneous abortion before conception is attempted again.

    e. **Immunoglobulin should be administered to Rh negative women** in the event of either a threatened or spontaneous abortion.

    f. **Septic** or **infected abortion** requires **complete evacuation of the uterine contents, medical support,** and **antibiotics.**

C. Multiple gestation

    1. General characteristics

        a. The overall **incidence of multiple birth in the United States is 1.5%** and has been increasing over the past 30 years, probably secondary to the use of assisted reproductive techniques and ovulation induction. Twins occur in 1:94 births.

        b. **Perinatal morbidity** and **mortality** are **significantly increased** (approximately 2–5 times greater) in multiple birth.

        c. Types

            (1) Two thirds of twins are **dizygotic** or **fraternal** (i.e., formed by the fertilization of 2 ova). The incidence of dizygotic twins is increased in those with a family history of twins, those taking fertility drugs, mothers with above average weight and height, and African American women.

            (2) **Monozygotic** twins, those formed from the fertilization of 1 ovum, occur randomly and are associated with fetal transfusion syndrome and discordant fetal growth.

        d. **Complications.** The most common complication of multiple gestation is **preterm birth.** Other problems that occur with greater frequency are **pregnancy-induced hypertension, fetal growth restriction, cord accidents, congenital anomalies,** and **placenta abruptio** or **previa.**

    2. Clinical features

        a. Size-for-date discrepancies in uterine growth are not usually evident until the second trimester.

        b. Clinical detection by size-for-dates disparity or demonstration of 2 fetal heart tones is unreliable in diagnosing multiple gestation.

    3. Laboratory studies

        a. **Serum AFP is increased** in multiple gestation.

        b. **Ultrasound can detect multiple gestation early in the first trimester** and is very accurate in detecting multiple gestation.

    c. Ultrasound throughout the gestation is used to follow **appropriate growth** for twins and is **used to obtain a biophysical profile at the end of pregnancy** to monitor continued health and to check the position of the twins.

  4. Treatment

    a. Proper prenatal management includes **frequent visits** in which the patient is counseled about **good nutrition**, encouraged to **limit her activity** as the pregnancy progresses, and liberally **tested with ultrasound and nonstress tests** to check fetal growth and well-being.

    b. **Amniocentesis** can be used to assess lung maturity, using the lecithin–sphingomyelin ratio, to help determine the timing of delivery.

    c. **Fetal presentation** is crucial in deciding the route of delivery.

D. Gestational diabetes

  1. General characteristics

    a. In addition to mothers with known diabetes, **approximately one in every 20–30** previously healthy pregnant women is found to have gestational diabetes mellitus.

    b. Poorly controlled gestational diabetes has been associated with increased risk of **macrosomic** infants and consequent difficult deliveries.

    c. The **lifetime risk** of developing diabetes after pregnancy in women who have had gestational diabetes is **increased** to greater than or equal to 50% versus less than 5% in the general population.

    d. **Recurrence** of gestational diabetes is common, occurring in 20%–30% of subsequent pregnancies.

  2. Clinical features

    a. Patients with gestational diabetes are usually **asymptomatic.**

    b. Risk factors for the development of gestational diabetes include a **history of previous large birth weight infant, obesity, age greater than 30 years, glucosuria,** and a **family history of diabetes.**

  3. Laboratory studies

    a. **Screening** of high risk or all pregnant patients with a 50 gram glucola challenge is done at **24–28 weeks' gestation.**

    b. If the **1-hour blood sugar value after 50 grams of glucola is greater than 130–140 mg/dl,** a 3-hour glucose tolerance test should be performed. If **2 or more of the 3-hour values are increased,** the patient is considered to be a gestational diabetic.

    c. **Antepartum testing,** using biophysical profiles and nonstress tests, **is sometimes used in gestational diabetes** beginning at 34 weeks' gestation.

  4. Treatment

    a. **Careful management of gestational diabetes with diet and exercise** is accomplished by performing fasting or 2-hour postprandial blood sugar measurements at each office visit.

    b. Patients with gestational diabetes who have **fasting blood sugar measurements greater than 105 mg/dl** or whose **2-hour postprandial blood sugar measurements are greater than 120 mg/dl require insulin,** according to criteria established by the American College of Obstetricians and Gynecologists (ACOG). Those individuals who maintain their blood sugars below these parameters can be managed with diet and excercise alone.

    c. To help avoid the development of diabetes later in life, the patient should be advised to **obtain and maintain ideal body weight after delivery** and to have **annual evaluations** of fasting glucose concentrations.

E. Preterm labor and delivery

  1. General characteristics

    a. **Preterm delivery** is the delivery of an infant **before 37 weeks' gestation** and occurs in 8%–10% of births.

    b. Preterm delivery **accounts for 75% of neonatal deaths** not due to congenital malformations.

    c. Low birth weight infants born prematurely often have **significant visual or hearing impairment, developmental delays, cerebral palsy,** and **lung disease.**

    d. Multiple gestations account for 10% of all preterm births. Recurrences of preterm labor are common (approximately 17%–37% of patients).

    e. The **etiology** of preterm labor is **poorly understood.** Smoking, cocaine use, lack of prenatal care, uterine malformations, cervical incompetence, and infection are felt to be possible causes of preterm labor. Complications of maternal or fetal health, such as hypertension, diabetes mellitus, or abruptio placentae, are known to be associated with preterm delivery.

2. Clinical features

    a. Preterm labor is defined as **regular uterine contractions between 20–37 weeks' gestation,** which are **5–8 minutes apart or less** with one or more of the following:

        (1) Change in cervix

        (2) Cervical dilatation greater than or equal to 2 cm

        (3) Cervical effacement greater than or equal to 80%

    b. Late symptoms of preterm labor include painful or painless contractions, pressure, menstrual-like cramps, watery or bloody discharge, and low back pain.

3. Laboratory studies. Ultrasound is sometimes used to examine the **length of the cervix.** Examination of the cervicovaginal secretions for **fetal fibronectin,** a glycoprotein, has been used as a **possible marker for preterm labor.**

4. Treatment

    a. Treatments for preterm labor are **unsatisfactory** and **controversial.**

    b. Management techniques include the use of **bed rest, home monitoring, parenteral** and **oral tocolytics,** and, if delivery is imminent, **steroids** administered to the mother prior to delivery to enhance fetal lung maturity.

    c. The goal in managing these patients is to **identify those at risk** and to diagnose this condition before labor is irreversibly established.

F. Hypertension

1. General characteristics

    a. The continuum of hypertension in pregnancy ranges from **pregnancy-induced hypertension** (PIH; isolated hypertension) to **preeclampsia** (hypertension accompanied by proteinuria and edema) to **eclampsia** (the preceding symptoms plus seizures).

    b. The basic underlying pathophysiology of PIH is felt to be **vasospasm** or **arteriolar constriction.**

    c. The **definition of abnormal blood pressure increase** is a blood pressure of **greater than 140/90,** or **an increase of 30 mm systolic** or **15 mm diastolic,** or both.

    d. PIH is **more common among nulliparous** women, mothers in **teenaged** or **advanced years** (i.e., over 35 years of age), those with a **family history of eclampsia, those of low socioeconomic status,** those with **pre-existing hypertension, cases of multiple gestation,** and mothers with **medical disorders** (e.g., diabetes, renal disease).

    e. Complications of PIH, preeclampsia, and eclampsia are **serious.**

        (1) Maternal complications include abruptio placentae, renal failure, cerebral hemorrhage, pulmonary edema, HELLP (*h*emolysis, *e*levated *l*iver enzymes, and *l*ow *p*latelet count) syndrome, and DIC.

        (2) Fetal complications include hypoxia, low birth weight, preterm delivery, or perinatal death.

2. Clinical features

    a. Although generalized edema in pregnancy is common, **swelling of the face or hands** is of greater significance than swelling in the lower extremities in regard to preeclampsia.

    b. Headaches, visual changes, and **epigastric or abdominal pain** often **precede frank seizures.** Epigastric pain can be indicative of hepatocellular necrosis. Reflexes are brisk. Oliguria is an ominous sign in predicting the course of PIH.

    c. Rapid weight gain (e.g., more than 2 pounds per week or 6 pounds per month) may accompany hypertensive disorders.

3. Laboratory studies

a. Proteinuria may be intermittent in PIH and a solitary urinalysis for protein is of limited value. **Twenty-four hour urine protein** test results should remain less than 300 mg/24 hours. Rising urinary protein is often an indication for delivery as it indicates renal tubular necrosis.

b. If the patient can be diagnosed clinically as having preeclampsia, then 24-hour urine, liver function tests, platelet count, creatinine clearance, electrolytes, blood type and crossmatch, and a complete blood cell count (CBC) with a differential should be ordered to facilitate decisions about delivery and to exclude the possibility of HELLP syndrome.

4. Treatment

a. Delivery of the infant is the ultimate treatment for hypertensive disorders of pregnancy.

b. If the patient is not at term and does not have marked preeclampsia, **watchful waiting** is often used with the patient at rest. Hospitalized patients are monitored with frequent blood pressure readings, biophysical profiles, nonstress tests, and maternal laboratory studies.

c. Severe PIH or **eclampsia** are indications for **prompt delivery regardless of gestational age.**

d. Magnesium sulfate, administered by intravenous (IV) drip, is the first line medication for **inpatient management of moderate preeclampsia and eclampsia.**

e. Hydralazine is sometimes given for the acute management of hypertension in a hospital setting.

G. Rh incompatibility

1. General characteristics

a. If the infant's blood type is not identical to the mother's blood type, the mother may develop antibodies against the infant's blood (i.e., Rh sensitization).

b. The most common problem of mismatched blood involves the rhesus D factor (Rh factor). Approximately 15% of the population is Rh-negative. Although 98% of isoimmunizations are secondary to the Rh factor, 43 other antigens exist.

c. Immunoglobulin (Rhogam) administered routinely at 28 weeks' gestation in an Rh-negative patient and after delivery of an Rh-positive infant **helps prevent development of these antibodies to the infant's blood 99% of the time.**

d. Any event that may allow fetal cells to enter maternal circulation such as trauma, spontaneous abortion, therapeutic abortion, ectopic pregnancy, or amniocentesis can sensitize maternal circulation.

e. If antibodies develop, they will attack subsequent Rh-incompatible infants and can lead to severe fetal anemia and death (fetal hydrops).

2. Laboratory studies

a. Routine prenatal blood work should include blood type, Rh factor, and Coombs' test for antibodies.

b. Antibody titers of less than 1:16 will probably not adversely affect the pregnancy.

c. In a sensitized pregnancy, a combination of Coombs' titer, amniocentesis, and ultrasound are used to follow the developing fetus for evidence of distress or fetal hydrops.

3. Treatment

a. 300 micrograms of **D immunoglobulin** (Rho immunoglobulin) are to be **given routinely** to Rh(D-) nonimmunized women at 28 weeks' gestation and within 72 hours of delivering an Rh-positive infant.

b. Rho immunoglobulin is also to be administered at amniocentesis and other instances of uterine bleeding as noted previously.

c. Massive fetal–maternal hemorrhage may require larger doses of immunoglobulin.

H. Abruptio placentae

1. General characteristics

a. Abruptio placentae is the **premature separation of a normally implanted placenta after the 20th week of gestation** and before birth.

b. Abruptio placentae can represent **a true obstetric emergency** as fetal death is as high as 50%–80% and maternal morbidity is as high as 1%. The incidence of abruptio placentae ranges from 0.2%–2.4%.

c. The **etiology** of abruptio placentae is **poorly understood.** However, several **risk factors** are known for the development of abruptio placentae: trauma, smoking, hypertension, decreased folic acid, cocaine use, alcohol (more than 14 drinks per week), uterine anomalies, high parity, previous abruption (the recurrence rate is 10%–17%), and advanced maternal age.

d. Types of abruption include **external,** or revealed, abruption (when blood escapes from the uterus) or **concealed** abruption (when blood is retained between the detached placenta and the uterus). The degree of separation ranges from partial to complete separation of the placenta from its site of implantation (Figure 8-2).

e. Abruption can lead to liberation of tissue thromboplastin or consumption of fibrinogen, thereby activating the extrinsic clotting mechanism. This could eventually lead to **DIC.**

2. Clinical features

a. Vaginal bleeding occurs in the majority of cases (85%) of abruptio placentae.

b. Uterine, abdominal, or **back** pain are also frequent symptoms of abruptio placentae and may be the only symptom if bleeding is concealed.

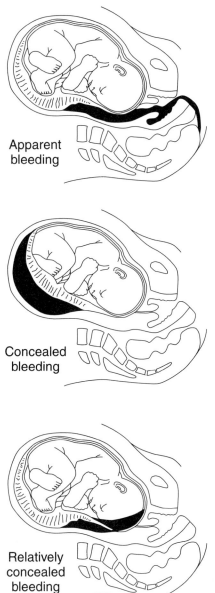

Apparent bleeding

Concealed bleeding

Relatively concealed bleeding

Figure 8-2. Types of abruptio placentae. (Redrawn and reproduced, with permission, from Pernoll M: *CURRENT Obstetric & Gynecologic Diagnosis & Treatment,* 7th ed. Lange, 1991.)

    c. The **uterus becomes hypertonic, irritable, or tender** when the placenta has abrupted and may be enlarged. The uterus may be beyond the expected size because of progressive hemorrhage behind the placenta. Bleeding can also occur within the wall of the myometrium or uterine musculature. That condition is known as a **Couvelaire uterus,** or **uteroplacental apoplexy.**

    d. **Evidence of fetal distress** may or may not be present, depending on the degree of separation.

    e. **Complications** of abruptio placentae that occur in addition to the obvious compromise of placental blood flow to the fetus and hemorrhage are **renal failure, coagulation failure,** and **Couvelaire uterus.**

  3. **Laboratory studies.** Diagnosis is clinical. Ultrasound is usually not helpful in diagnosing this problem.

  4. Treatment

    a. **Delivery of the fetus and placenta** are the definitive treatment of abruptio placentae. **However, management is dependent on the degree of separation and the age of the fetus.**

    b. **Blood type, crossmatch,** and **coagulation studies** are indicated in an unstable patient, as well as **placement of a large-bore IV line.**

    c. **Cesarean section** is often the preferred route for delivering the infant in cases of abruptio placentae.

I. Placenta previa

  1. General characteristics

    a. Placenta previa occurs when **the placenta partially or completely covers the cervical os.**

    b. **Performing a digital examination in a patient with placenta previa can incite severe bleeding.**

    c. Placenta previa occurs in 0.3%–0.5% of pregnancies and is **associated with** advanced age, smoking, high parity, and any process that could have caused scarring of the lower uterine segment (e.g., cesarean section, induced abortion).

  2. Clinical features

    a. **Painless bleeding** is the hallmark of placenta previa.

    b. **Bleeding may continue** from the placenta's implantation site **after delivery** because the **lower uterus contracts poorly.**

  3. Laboratory studies

    a. **Ultrasound is 93%–98% accurate in diagnosing placenta previa.**

    b. When the patient is hemodynamically unstable, **studies for blood type, crossmatch,** and **coagulation** should be ordered as well as **gaining venous access with a large-bore IV line.**

  4. Treatment

    a. Prior to term, if the patient is stable, **watchful waiting** is warranted. Blood transfusion may be necessary during the period of waiting for fetal maturity. Previa found before 20 weeks' gestation often "migrates" and is not present at term.

    b. **Cesarean section** is usually the preferred method of delivering the infant in cases of placenta previa.

III. LABOR AND DELIVERY

  A. Routine vaginal labor and delivery

    1. General characteristics

      a. Twenty percent of perinatal morbidity and mortality occurs during the intrapartum period in otherwise healthy pregnancies.

      b. **Braxton Hicks** contractions, described as weak, slow, and usually painless, accompany the increasing uterine irritability of the last 6 weeks of pregnancy.

      c. Most infants will present in the **vertex** position. However, other possibilities include breech, face, transverse, and compound (arm or leg).

2. Clinical features

    a. Stages of labor

        (1) The **first stage** of labor begins at the onset of true, regular contractions and ends at full dilatation Figure 8-3.

        (2) The **second stage** of labor begins at full dilatation and ends with the delivery of the infant.

        (3) The **third stage** of labor begins after the delivery and entails separation and expulsion of the placenta.

        (4) The **hour following delivery** is sometimes called the **fourth stage** and is critical in assessing and treating tears, lacerations, and hemorrhage.

    b. **"Bloody show,"** which is the passage of a small amount of blood-tinged mucus that has been plugging the cervical os, **often precedes true labor.**

    c. **Amniotic fluid rupture** can occur prior to or during the first stage of labor. Rupture of membranes can be confirmed with the use of Nitrazine Paper.

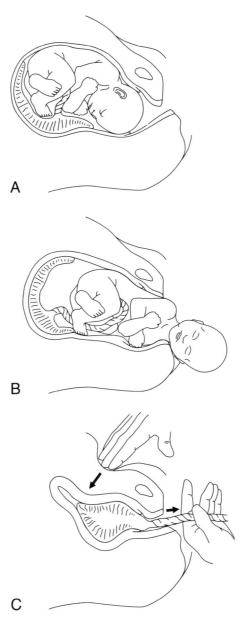

A

B

C

Figure 8-3. Stages of labor. (A) The first stage of labor begins at the onset of true, regular contractions and ends at full dilatation. (B) The second stage of labor begins at full dilatation and ends with the delivery of the infant. (C) The third stage of labor begins after the delivery and entails separation and expulsion of the placenta.

d. Cervical changes are measured in centimeters **(dilatation 1–10 centimeters)** and by percentage of change of thickness **(effacement 0%–100%).**

e. The **descent of the fetus in the pelvis** is denoted in **stations.** The station is the relation of the presenting part to the ischial spines. Stations above the spines are expressed in negative numbers (e.g., −1 cm, −2 cm) and stations below the spine, in positive numbers (e.g., +1 cm, +2 cm).

3. Laboratory studies

a. On admission, a **urinalysis** for protein, glucose, and hematocrit should be obtained.

b. Fetal monitoring is used in labor to assess the fetus's response to labor.

4. Treatment

a. Regular cervical examinations for dilatation, station, and effacement are necessary to check the progress of labor.

b. Continued blood pressure, temperature, and **pulse readings** are critical to exclude late PIH, toxemia, and infection.

c. Analgesia is essential to provide comfort and prevent fatigue. It may take the form of breathing and visualization techniques; intramuscular medications (e.g., meperidine, fentanyl); epidural anesthesia during the second and third stages of delivery; and local infiltration, pudendal block, or spinal block.

d. Amniotomy (deliberate rupture of the fetal membranes to induce labor) can sometimes cause labor to progress more rapidly but increases the likelihood of the risk of a prolapsed cord if the head is not fully engaged.

e. After **crowning** of the presenting part, **pressure** applied from the coccygeal region upward will extend the head at the proper time and help protect the perineal musculature. When the head has been delivered, the **baby can be suctioned** with a rubber suction bulb. The **cord may need to be gently slipped over the head.** The **shoulders are eased carefully through the perineum.** After the rest of the body passes through, **the cord is clamped and cut.**

f. Episiotomy (surgical incision to prevent traumatic tearing) is sometimes used to protect the perineum as the head crowns, for such indications as a large baby or a short perineum.

g. Approximately 3–4 minutes after the baby is delivered, the **uterus contracts,** the **umbilical cord lengthens,** and a significant **increase in postpartum blood flow** signals impending passage of the placenta.

h. The infant is suctioned, kept warm, and assessed for **Apgar** score at 1 and 5 minutes after delivery (Table 8-5).

i. The **placenta** and **umbilical cord should be examined** to ensure that the entire placenta and membranes are passed and that the cord contains 3 vessels (i.e., 2 arteries and 1 vein).

j. Oxytocin, ergotrate, and **methylergonovine maleate** are sometimes used in the third stage of labor to reduce blood loss by stimulating contractions.

Table 8-5.
Apgar Scoring for Newborns

A score is given for each sign at 1 minute and 5 minutes after the birth. If there are problems with the baby, an additional score is given at 10 minutes. A score of 7–10 is considered normal, while 4–7 might require some resuscitative measures, and a baby with Apgar scores of 3 and below requires immediate resuscitation.

	Sign	0 Points	1 Point	2 Points
A	Activity (muscle tone)	Absent	Arms and legs flexed	Active movement
P	Pulse	Absent	Below 100 BPM	Above 100 BPM
G	Grimace (reflex irritability)	No response	Grimace	Sneeze, cough, pulls away
A	Appearance (skin color)	Blue-gray pale all over,	Pink, except extremities	Pink, entirely
R	Respiration	Absent	Slow, irregular	Good, crying

BPM = beats per minute.
Used by permission: APGAR. 1996. [1 screen]. Available from: http://www.childbirth.org/articles/apgar.html.

B. Abnormal labor and delivery

    1. General characteristics

        a. Abnormal labor, or **dystocia,** occurs **when the cervix fails to dilate progressively over time** and the **fetus fails to descend.**

        b. **Macrosomia** (fetal weight more than 4500 grams), **abnormal presentation,** or **fetal anomalies** increase the likelihood of abnormal labor.

        c. **Cord prolapse should be considered** with premature rupture of membranes, particularly with breech or transverse presentation.

        d. If **delivery is delayed more than 24 hours after rupture** of membranes, there is **increased risk for serious intrauterine infection.**

    2. Clinical features

        a. **Inability to deliver vaginally after full cervical dilatation** is a good marker of true dystocia.

        b. **Macrosomia** and **nonvertex presentation can be suspected** on clinical examination prior to the onset of labor.

        c. **Digital examination of the pelvis for its diameters** helps determine the adequacy of the pelvis to deliver the fetus.

        d. **Cord prolapse** is identified with a ropelike, soft, elongated mass on speculum or bimanual examination.

    3. **Imaging studies.** Ultrasound may show evidence of a large baby or gross anatomic defects.

    4. Treatment

        a. Inadequate uterine contractions can be augmented with **oxytocin.**

        b. If maternal pushing is inadequate, **rest or assisted delivery with vacuum extraction** or **forceps** may be used. Forceps or vacuum extractors are used to shorten the second stage of labor and **may be indicated** for fetal distress or maternal indications **only if the head is engaged and the cervix fully dilated.**

        c. The diagnosis of dystocia is a leading indication for **cesarean section.**

        d. If the umbilical cord has obviously prolapsed, **manual elevation** of the presenting part in the knee–chest position is necessary **for temporary reduction of the cord** while administering a tocolytic agent. Emergent delivery is required.

        e. If the baby is in a non-vertex presentation, **external version with ultrasound guidance** can be attempted after 37 weeks' gestation. Tocolysis is used during this procedure.

C. Cesarean delivery and vaginal birth after cesarean delivery (VBAC)

    1. General characteristics

        a. Cesarean section is defined as **the birth of the fetus through an incision in the abdominal and uterine walls** and **constitutes approximately 21%–25%** of deliveries in the United States.

        b. The most frequent **indications** for cesarean section are **repeat cesarean, dystocia, or failure to progress, breech presentation,** and **for fetal well-being.**

        c. The success rate of VBAC depends on the indication for the previous cesarean section.

            (1) When dystocia was the indicator for a previous cesarean delivery, the rate of failure of VBAC is highest. Consequently, many of these patients must have repeat cesarean section deliveries. Conversely, women laboring following a previous cesarean for other indications have no greater risk of a cesarean than the general population.

            (2) The overall success rate of VBAC is 60%–80%.

            (3) Although the incidence of uterine dehiscence in a VBAC following the use of a low transverse incision is relatively low (approximately 1:200), its result can lead to death of the fetus and significantly increased morbidity and mortality to the mother as well.

        d. **Risks** of cesarean section include a greater likelihood of **thromboembolic events, increased bleeding,** and development of **infection.** These all have a lower incidence in women who choose vaginal birth after a cesarean.

2. Treatment

    a. **Prophylactic antibiotics** are often used after a cesarean section to prevent infection.

    b. A **low transverse uterine incision** (versus a classical vertical incision) is usually used in a non-emergent cesarean section because of the decreased blood loss associated with its use, the ease of repair, and because it is **much less likely to rupture than a classical incision.** The incidence of rupture with a classical incision is 12%.

    c. A **trial of closely monitored labor is indicated** in eligible VBAC patients.

IV. PUERPERIUM. The 6-week period following delivery is known as the **puerperium,** or postpartum period.

A. Normal puerperium

    1. General characteristics

        a. Immediately following delivery, the uterus is below the umbilicus. After 2 days, it shrinks or **involutes,** and, after 2 weeks, it descends into the pelvic cavity. It is back to its antenatal size in approximately 4 weeks.

        b. **Lochia,** bleeding that occurs after delivery, represents the sloughing off of decidual tissue. It can last for 4–5 weeks postpartum and may change in color over time from bright red to pale red to white or yellow-white.

        c. In a non-nursing mother, **menses resume 6–8 weeks postpartum.** In contrast, **nursing mothers are usually anovulatory** and may remain amenorrheic throughout the duration of lactation.

        d. The breast produces **colostrum** immediately postpartum. This deep yellow liquid has high levels of maternal antibodies, all vitamins except K, and less sugar and fat than regular breast milk. Over 4–5 days, the increased mineral and protein containing colostrum is replaced by breast milk. The sudden engorgement of the breasts with milk may be accompanied by a transient fever of up to 24 hours.

    2. Clinical features

        a. The **first postpartum visit should be made 4–6 weeks after delivery.** This should include a thorough history with attention to bleeding, pelvic pain, sexual and contraceptive history, future sexual and contraceptive plans, and bowel and bladder function.

        b. **At 6 weeks,** on pelvic examination, **the perineum should be well healed** and the **uterus back to its pregravid size.**

        c. Occasionally, a **lactating mother** will have **atrophic vaginitis.**

    3. Laboratory studies

        a. During the first postpartum visit, a **hemoglobin** and **hematocrit test** are indicated as needed.

        b. If the patient was a gestational diabetic, a **blood sugar screen** should be ordered.

    4. Treatment

        a. **Contraceptive counseling** is an important point to emphasize at the postpartum examination.

        b. **Continuation of vitamin supplementation** is important for the nursing mother because of the increased nutritional needs of lactation.

        c. **Atrophic vaginitis** should be treated with vaginal estrogen as needed.

B. Abnormal puerperium

    1. Hemorrhage

        a. **General characteristics.** Postpartum hemorrhage is defined as blood loss of greater than 500 ml. It is most often caused by abnormal involution of the placental site, cervical or vaginal lacerations, and retained portions of placenta.

        b. **Clinical features.** Complaints of **increased bleeding after delivery** signal a need for evaluation for hemorrhage.

        c. **Laboratory studies. Hemoglobin** and **hematocrit tests** are necessary to quantify complaints of bleeding.

   d. Treatment. Because a D&C can sometimes make the problem worse, **medical management** using intravenous oxytocin, ergonovine, methylergonovine, or prostaglandins is often first line treatment for postpartum hemorrhage.

2. Infection

   a. General characteristics. The most common site of **infection** is the genital tract. Other potential sites of infection are the breast and the urinary tract.

   b. Clinical features

   (1) **Patients with fever** of greater than 100.4°F on more than one occasion should be investigated for suspected infection. A thorough physical examination with attention to the breasts and genital tract is necessary to exclude acute infection.

   (2) **Endometritis** is marked by exquisite uterine tenderness, bleeding, and foul-smelling lochia.

   (3) On examination, **mastitis** presents with localized erythema, tenderness, and possibly induration.

   c. Laboratory studies. **Cultures** of the uterus, healing perineum, surgical incision sites, urine, and occasionally of breast secretions can be helpful prior to the administration of antibiotics.

   d. Treatment. **Empiric antibiotic treatment,** based on the site of infection, should be initiated.

3. Subinvolution of the uterus

   a. General characteristics. Subinvolution of the uterus can be a result of retained placenta, fibroids, or infection.

   b. Clinical features. A subinvoluted uterus will feel **enlarged** and **soft** on examination and the patient may present with complaints of increased bleeding, pain, fever, and foul-smelling lochia.

   c. Laboratory studies. **Ultrasound** can sometimes detect obvious retained placental fragments.

   d. Treatment. Subinvolution of the uterus often responds to **oral agents that increase uterine contraction** (e.g., methergine, ergotrate). Antibiotic treatment may also be necessary.

4. Thromboembolic events

   a. General characteristics. Thromboembolic events (e.g., deep venous thrombosis) are 5 times more common during pregnancy and in the postpartum period. They are much more likely to occur with increased stasis and often involve the iliac veins.

   b. Clinical features. **Deep venous thrombosis** of the extremities presents with **pain** and **swelling.** Iliac thrombosis may present only as fever.

   c. Laboratory studies. **Venography** remains the gold standard for detection of thrombosis. It is variably helpful for iliac thrombosis. Impedance plethysmography and ultrasound are also employed for this problem.

   d. Treatment. Treatment of deep venous thrombosis includes **heparin, rest,** and **analgesia.**

9

Rheumatology and Orthopedics

Eunice E. Gunneson

I. ARTHRITIS

A. Osteoarthritis (OA)

   1. General characteristics

   a. OA is the **most common form of joint disease.**

   b. It results from **cartilage degeneration.** As the cartilage degenerates, joint stresses are transmitted to the underlying bone.

   2. Clinical features

   a. **Decreased range of motion, joint crepitus,** and **pain** are features of OA.

   b. **Joints can become unstable** during the late stages of OA.

   3. Laboratory studies

   a. Laboratory tests are **nonspecific.**

   b. Radiographs show **asymmetric narrowing, subchondral sclerosis, cysts,** and **marginal osteophytes.**

   4. Treatment

   a. **Weight reduction, exercises, acetaminophen, salicylates,** and **intra-articular steroids** are important in managing OA.

   b. Surgical **arthrodesis, osteotomy,** and **total joint arthroplasty** are indicated in **severe cases.**

B. Rheumatoid arthritis (RA)

   1. General characteristics

   a. RA is a **chronic disease** with synovitis affecting multiple joints and other systemic extra-articular manifestations.

   b. The cascade of events after the precipitating cause leads to **joint destruction** with **pannus ingrowth denuding articular cartilage** and causing **chondrocyte death.**

   2. Clinical features

   a. **Malaise, fatigue,** and **morning stiffness** for **more than 6 weeks** are seen.

   b. Arthritis **affects the hands** (i.e., ulnar deviation and subluxation of the metacarpal phalangeal joints) and the **feet** (i.e., claw toes and hallux valgus). **Knee, elbow, shoulder, ankle,** and **neck involvement** is common.

   c. **Subcutaneous nodules** are present and may be associated with a **positive rheumatoid factor.**

   d. **Systemic involvement** may manifest itself as rheumatoid vasculitis (causing ischemic ulcers and peripheral neuropathy), pericarditis, or pulmonary disease (e.g., pleural effusions, fibrosing alveolitis, and nodules).

   3. Laboratory studies

   a. **Erythrocyte sedimentation rate (ESR)** and **C-reactive protein** are elevated.

   b. **Rheumatoid factor** titer will be **positive.**

   c. **Periarticular erosion** and **osteopenia** are seen on **radiograph.**

4. Treatment

a. **Consultation with a rheumatologist** for initiation of treatment and development of a long-term plan.

b. **Physical therapy** should be implemented.

c. **Pharmacologic management** should be early and aggressive to prevent or delay joint destruction.

(1) **Nonsteroidal anti-inflammatory drugs (NSAIDs)** and **aspirin** may control symptoms.

(2) **Gold, antimalarials, steroids,** and **methotrexate** may provide some benefit in preventing or delaying joint damage.

d. **Reconstructive surgery** is indicated for **severe cases.**

C. Other types of arthritis

1. Infectious (septic) arthritis

a. Pathogenesis. The **hematogenous spread** of **metaphyseal osteomyelitis in children,** infection caused by a diagnostic or therapeutic procedure (i.e., intra-articular injection), or an **infection elsewhere** may lead to infectious arthritis. Sexually active young adults are at risk for *Neisseria gonorrhoeae* infection. Patients usually have a preceding migratory polyarthralgia and small red papules.

b. Treatment

(1) **Aggressive treatment** with **intravenous** (IV) antibiotics is required.

(2) **Arthrotomy** (opening into a joint for infections to be drained) and **arthrocentesis** (puncture of joint space with needle for synovial fluid analysis and culture) are often required. Arthrotomy is usually not required when *N. gonorrhoeae* is the infecting organism.

(3) **Oral antibiotics** should follow the IV antibiotics.

2. Psoriatic arthritis

a. General characteristics

(1) This is an **inflammatory arthritis** with onset in patients 30–50 years of age.

(2) **Skin involvement precedes joint disease** by months to years.

b. Clinical features

(1) The course usually is **mild** and **intermittent,** affecting a few joints.

(2) **Symmetric involvement of the hands and feet, cuticle involvement,** and **irregularity, pitting,** and **splitting of the nails** are seen.

(3) **"Sausage" finger appearance** (caused by arthritis and tenosynovitis of the flexor tendon) is a common feature.

(4) **Asymmetric oligoarticular arthritis involving 2–3 joints at a time** occurs.

(5) **Symmetric arthritis** occurs similar to that of RA.

c. Laboratory studies

(1) **ESR** is **elevated; normocytic, normochromic anemia** is seen.

(2) **Hyperuricemia** may occur when skin involvement is severe.

(3) **Rheumatoid factor** is normal.

(4) **"Cup and saucer" appearance** of the proximal phalanx is demonstrated on radiography.

d. Treatment

(1) Psoriatic arthritis drug treatment is **similar to that for RA.**

(2) **Methotrexate** is beneficial for both the skin inflammation and the arthritis.

(3) **Reconstructive surgery** (arthrodesis or joint replacement) is indicated for painful end-stage arthropathy.

3. Reiter's syndrome

a. General characteristics

(1) Reiter's syndrome is a **seronegative arthritis,** predominantly affecting men, with a **triad of urethritis, conjunctivitis,** and **oligoarthritis.**

(2) It is often **secondary to sexually transmitted disease** (chlamydial urethritis) or **gastroenteritis.**

b. Clinical features

(1) Patients have **"sausage toes;"** painful oral ulcers; penile lesions; ulcers on the extremities, palms, and soles; and **plantar heel pain.**

(2) **Patients with human immunodeficiency virus (HIV)** can develop Reiter's syndrome.

c. Laboratory studies

(1) Laboratory studies should include **ESR, alkaline phosphatase, CBC, human leukocyte antigen (HLA)-B27,** and **C-reactive protein**

(2) Evidence of **metatarsal head erosion** appears on **radiograph.**

(3) **Calcaneal periostitis** is present.

d. Treatment

(1) **Physical therapy** and **NSAIDs**

(2) The **underlying condition** [e.g., sexually transmitted disease (STD) or gastroenteritis] must be treated.

D. Gout

1. General characteristics

a. Gout is a **systemic disease of altered purine metabolism** and subsequent **sodium urate crystal precipitation into synovial fluid.**

b. It is **more common in men** than women.

2. Clinical features

a. Most common feature is **initial attack** of the **metatarsal phalangeal (MTP) joint** of the greater toe.

b. Pain, swelling, redness, and **exquisite tenderness develop suddenly at and surrounding the joint.**

3. Laboratory studies

a. **Joint fluid analysis** is diagnostic; or the diagnosis may be **inferred by clinical examination.**

b. **Serum uric acid level** greater than 8 mg/dl is diagnostic.

4. Treatment

a. **Elevation** and **rest** may alleviate symptoms.

b. Pharmacotherapy

(1) **NSAIDs** may be used (i.e., indomethacin 50 mg a day for 2 days, tapered off during the following week).

(2) **Allopurinol** may be used to decrease production of uric acid and prevent further attacks.

(3) **Colchicine** (mechanism of action is unknown) reduces the inflammatory response to deposited crystals, diminishes phagocytosis, and terminates most acute attacks in 6–12 hours.

(4) **Corticosteroids** may be used if other medicines are not tolerated.

E. **Pseudogout** (chondrocalcinosis) results from intra-articular deposition of calcium pyrophosphate.

1. General characteristics

a. Pseudogout affects **peripheral joints,** usually in the lower extremity.

b. It shows marked **similarity to gout,** with **recurrent** and **abrupt** onset of **attacks.**

2. Clinical features

a. Painful inflammation results when crystals are shed into the joint.

b. Most commonly involved joints are the **knee, wrist,** and **elbow** and not the small joints as in gout.

3. Laboratory studies

a. **Calcium pyrophosphate crystals** are found in joint aspiration.

b. **Radiographs** show fine, linear calcifications in cartilage.

4. Treatment

    a. NSAIDs and **intra-articular steroid injections**

    b. Treat **joint destruction** with **surgical procedures** similar to degenerative arthritis.

F. Systemic lupus erythematosus (SLE)

    1. General characteristics

        a. SLE is an autoimmune disorder characterized by **antinuclear antibodies (ANAs)** and **involvement of multiple organs.**

        b. SLE commonly **affects women** of **childbearing age.** Prevalence is also found among certain familial and ethnic groups.

    2. Clinical features

        a. The **diagnosis of SLE** is based on the presence of certain **criteria,** including: malar or discoid rash, photosensitivity, oral ulcers, arthritis, serositis, renal disorder, neurologic disorder, hematologic disorder, immunologic disorder, or antinuclear antibody.

        b. **Common musculoskeletal features**

            (1) Arthralgias and **symmetrical non-erosive arthritis** are found.

            (2) SLE **affects small joints of the hand, wrist, and knees.**

    3. Laboratory studies

        a. **Routine laboratory studies** should include **complete blood cell count (CBC), blood urea nitrogen (BUN), creatinine, urinalysis, ESR,** and **complement** (C3 or C4).

        b. **Antibodies to Smith antigen, double-stranded DNA,** or **depressed levels of serum complement** may be used as markers for the progression of the disease.

        c. **Antibody to nuclear antigens (ANA) is present** 100% of the time but is not specific for SLE.

    4. Treatment

        a. **Mild** or new cases

            (1) **Salicylates** or **NSAIDs** should be administered.

            (2) **Hydroxychloroquine** 200 mg once or twice a day is given.

            (3) **Corticosteroids** are also given, at low doses.

        b. **Acute illness** with renal or central nervous system involvement

            (1) **High-dose steroids** may be used, tapering off as symptoms improve.

            (2) **NSAIDs** may serve as an adjunct therapy.

            (3) **Antimalarial** medications may be helpful, depending on the cause.

            (4) **Pulsed high-dose steroids** or **immunosuppressive medications** can be used in patients with glomerulonephritis or in patients unresponsive to the above treatment.

G. Temporomandibular joint disorder (TMJ)

    1. General characteristics

        a. TMJ, which is the **most common cause of facial pain**, refers to pain affecting the **temporomandibular joint** and **muscles of mastication.**

        b. Causes

            (1) **Neuropsychological** components may play a role.

            (2) **Joint capsulitis from bruxism,** such as grinding of teeth, clenching of teeth, and posturing of the jaw, may cause TMJ.

            (3) **Hypermobility syndrome** and malocclusion may lead to pain in the jaw area.

2. Clinical features

    a. Pain is **aggravated by movement** of the jaw.

    b. There may be **restricted range of motion** and a **click** or **pop** can be felt or heard.

3. Laboratory studies

    a. **Initial** radiographic studies are **normal.**

    b. **Arthritis** is a late finding.

4. Treatment

    a. **Rule out** systemic arthritis such as OA or RA, growth abnormalities, and tumor.

    b. **Most cases resolve** without identification of the cause.

    c. **Refer to a specialist** such as an odontologist or oral and maxillofacial surgeon if the symptoms warrant it.

II. BONE AND CONNECTIVE TISSUE DISORDERS

A. Tendinitis and tenosynovitis

    1. General characteristics

        a. **Tendinitis** refers to **inflammation of the lining** of the tendon sheath. **Tenosynovitis is inflammation of the enclosed tendon sheath.**

        b. Common causes include:

            (1) Overuse injuries

            (2) Systemic disease (e.g., arthritides)

        c. Specific types of tendinitis and tenosynovitis include **stenosing tenosynovitis** of the **wrist** (DeQuervain's), or of the **finger** or **thumb** **(trigger finger).**

    2. Clinical features

        a. Tendinitis and tenosynovitis commonly **appear in the following sites:** rotator cuff, flexor carpi ulnaris, flexor carpi radialis, flexor digitorum, hip, hamstring, quadriceps, patella, Achilles tendon, semimembranous tendon.

        b. Tendinitis and tenosynovitis generally **occur together,** causing **pain with movement, swelling,** and **impaired function.**

        c. The conditions may resolve over several weeks with recurrence common.

    3. Treatment

        a. **Ice, rest,** and **stretching** help relieve inflammation.

        b. **NSAIDs or injection with corticosteroids combined with anesthesia** may be used. Avoid intratendon injection because of risk of rupture.

        c. **Excision of scar tissue** and **necrotic debris** should be performed. The scar tissue is caused by repetitive microtrauma to the tissue, with the most common site being the muscle tendon unit.

B. Bursitis

    1. General characteristics

        a. Bursitis is an **inflammatory periarticular disorder of the bursa** (a thin-walled sac lined with synovial tissue).

        b. The inflammation is caused by **repetitive friction, trauma,** or **systemic disease** (e.g., RA, gout, infection).

    2. Clinical features. The **common sites** of presentation include **subacromial, subdeltoid, trochanteric, olecranon, Achilles bursitis** (pump bump), **ischial bursitis** (Weaver's bottom), and **pre- or suprapatellar** (housemaid's knee) causing pain and tenderness persisting for weeks.

    3. **Treatment** of bursitis includes **prevention of the precipitating factors, rest, NSAIDs,** and **steroid injections.**

C. Fibromyalgia

1. General characteristics

a. The **etiology** and **pathogenesis** are **poorly understood.**

b. It can **occur with RA, SLE,** and **Sjögren's syndrome.**

2. Clinical features

a. Patients have **nonarticular musculoskeletal aches, pains, fatigue, sleep disturbance,** and **multiple tender points** on examination.

b. Anxiety, depression, headaches, irritable bowel syndrome, dysmenorrhea, and **paresthesias** are associated with this condition.

3. Laboratory studies

a. There are **no routine laboratory markers.**

b. **Abnormality of the T-cell sublets** has been described.

4. Treatment

a. **Tricyclic antidepressants** may be prescribed.

b. **Aerobic exercises** improve the functional status by encouraging physical activity rather than avoidance of activity.

c. **Patient education, stress reduction,** and **treatment of psychological problems** may alleviate symptoms.

D. Osteomyelitis

1. General characteristics

a. Osteomyelitis is an **inflammation of the bone** caused by a **pyogenic organism** (most common organism *Staphylococcus aureus*) and can be described by duration (acute, chronic), etiology (hematogenous, exogenous, surgery, true contiguous spread), site (spine, hip), extent (size of defect), and type of patient (infant, child, adult, compromised host).

b. Types

(1) **Acute hematogenous osteomyelitis** most commonly affects the long bones of children.

(2) Osteomyelitis is termed **chronic hematogenous osteomyelitis** when after the original acute infection has had apparently appropriate treatment (antibiotics, surgery), viable colonies of bacteria harbored in necrotic and ischemic tissue cause recurrence of infection.

(3) **Exogenous osteomyelitis** results from open fracture or surgery.

2. Clinical features

a. Acute hematogenous osteomyelitis

(1) **Pain, loss of motion,** and **soft tissue swelling** occur.

(2) Drainage is rare.

b. Chronic hematogenous osteomyelitis

(1) **Recurrent acute flare-ups** of tender, warm, sometimes swollen areas occur at indefinite intervals over months or years.

(2) **Bone necrosis, soft tissue damage,** and **bone instability** can occur.

c. Exogenous osteomyelitis

(1) When **external fixator pin tract** is source of infection, it becomes chronic sinus surrounded by proud flesh.

(2) Clinical findings are similar to chronic osteomyelitis.

3. Laboratory studies

a. **White blood cell count** increases in acute osteomyelitis, and **ESR** is elevated in acute and chronic osteomyelitis.

    b. Identify the organism by **blood culture** or **bone biopsy** (best).

    c. Imaging studies

        (1) Radiographs

            (a) Early—demineralization and soft tissue changes in 10–14 days from the evolution of the infection.

            (b) Late—sequestra (i.e., dead bone surrounding granulation tissue) and involucrum (i.e., periosteal new bone) take several weeks to months to appear.

        (2) Magnetic resonance imaging (MRI) shows the changes before plain films.

        (3) Bone scan shows increased uptake in the area of infection and decreased uptake in the area of sequestra.

  4. Treatment

    a. Six weeks IV antibiotic therapy is recommended, followed by **1–2 weeks of oral antibiotics.**

    b. Immobilization and **surgical drainage** may be indicated.

    c. In **chronic hematogenous osteomyelitis, intermittent long-term antibiotics** will suppress the clinical manifestations. Surgical treatment is required to **remove sequestra, sinus tract** (the abnormal channel permitting escape of exudate to the surface), **infected bone,** and **scar tissue.**

    d. Exogenous osteomyelitis is managed the same as chronic hematogenous osteomyelitis. External or internal fixation devices will need to be removed, if present.

E. Neoplasms

  1. General characteristics

    a. Types

        (1) Common tumors are listed in **Table 9-1**.

        (2) Prostate, breast, lung, kidney, and **thyroid** are the **primary carcinomas** that most commonly **metastasize to the bone.** The **spine** is the common site of metastases.

Table 9-1.
Partial List of Bone Tumors and Tumorlike Conditions

Tissue of Origin	Benign Tumors and Tumorlike Conditions	Malignant Tumors and Tumorlike Conditions

Cartilage	Osteochondroma
	Enchondroma
	Chondroblastoma
	Chondromyxoid fibroma
		Chondrosarcoma
		Variants of chondrosarcoma
		  Dedifferentiated
		  Clear cell
		  Mesenchymal

Bone	Osteoid osteoma
	Osteoblastoma
		Osteosarcoma
		Variants of osteosarcoma
		  Parosteal
		  Periosteal
		  Telangiectatic
		  Postradiation
		  Arising in Paget disease

Marrow elements	Eosinophilic granuloma	Ewing sarcoma Plasmacytoma Multiple myeloma Lymphoma of bone
Fibrous tissue and tissue of uncertain origin	Nonossifying fibroma Aneurysmal bone cyst histiocytoma Simple bone cyst Giant cell tumor Fibrous dysplasia Desmoplastic fibroma	Fibrosarcoma Malignant fibrous histiocytoma

Reprinted with permission from Wilson F, Lins P: General Orthopaedics 12:302, 1997.

b. Incidence

(1) **Benign tumors** of the bone and soft tissue are **more common than malignant. Ecchondroma** (cartilaginous tumor) is the **most common primary benign bone neoplasm of the hand** and is asymptomatic unless complicated by pathologic fracture.

(2) **Lipomas** (soft, nontender, movable mass) and **ganglions** (soft, nontender, transilluminant mass usually on the dorsum of the hand) are common benign soft tissue masses. **Mucous cysts** are ganglia originating from the distal phalangeal joint and often are associated with Heberden's nodules.

(3) **Soft tissue sarcomas occur 3 times more often** than primary bone malignancies.

(4) **Multiple myeloma** is the **most common primary malignant bone tumor.**

c. Age-groups

(1) **Osteogenic sarcomas** are most common in persons **10 to 20 years of age.**

(2) In **adults over the age of 60, metastatic carcinoma** is the most common source of bone lesion.

2. Clinical features

a. Night pain is often associated with malignancy.

b. A **painful mass attached to bone** likely is malignant (some malignant tumors are nonpainful).

c. Severe pain preceded by dull aching pain may indicate **pathological fracture.**

3. Laboratory studies

a. Laboratory studies are of **little value.**

b. Alkaline phosphatase is **elevated** when the bone is broken down and remodeled.

c. Serum and **urine electrophoretic studies** can detect the specific abnormal globulin of multiple myeloma.

d. A **malignant neoplasm is biopsied with an open incision;** then the capsule is closed tightly to prevent bleeding and local spread.

4. Imaging studies

a. Plain radiographs are the **first tool of evaluation.**

b. Computerized tomography (CT) is the best imaging technique if a lesion involves the cortical bones.

c. An **MRI** is most helpful if marrow, soft tissue, or osseous tumors are suspected.

d. Bone scans can evaluate distant osseous metastasis and periosteal involvement of soft tissue masses.

5. Treatment

a. Relieving pain and **maintaining function** are the goals of treatment.

b. For **benign tumors, simple excision** is the treatment.

c. Malignant neoplasms

(1) **Wide surgical resection** is used when feasible.

(2) **Chemotherapy** is used.

(3) **Limb salvage** (using cadaver allograft or endoprosthetic devices) is part of definitive treatment.

(4) **Radiation therapy** followed by **local resection** is the common treatment for **soft tissue sarcomas.**

F. Osteoporosis

1. General characteristics

a. Osteoporosis is a syndrome with **age-related decrease in bone mass** that leads to **fracture of a bone after minor trauma.** In normal bone, the same level of trauma would not cause a fracture.

b. Two types have been characterized.

(1) **Type I (postmenopausal)** occurs **only in women.**

(2) **Type II (age-related)** occurs in **both men** and **women.**

2. Clinical features

   a. Type I is **commonly associated with loss of estrogen** in postmenopausal women.

   (1) The **trabecular bone** is primarily affected.

   (2) The **vertebrae** and **distal radius** are the most common fracture sites.

   b. **Type II.** Patients **older than 75 years of age** with **poor calcium absorption** are at high risk for this type.

   (1) Both **trabecular** and **cortical bone** are affected.

   (2) The **hip and pelvis** are the most common fracture sites.

3. Laboratory studies

   a. **Calcium, hydroxyproline** (index of bone dissolution), and **serum alkaline phosphatase** (index of bone deposition) levels are tested to rule out other abnormalities (e.g., hyperthyroidism, hyperparathyroidism, Cushing's syndrome, hematologic disorders, and malignancy) and will be normal in osteoporosis.

   b. **Dual energy x-ray absorptiometry (DEXA)** is the most helpful way to measure bone density with the least radiation.

   c. **Biopsy** can be used to evaluate the severity.

   d. **Radiographs** will show features of decreased bone density when greater than 30% bone loss is present.

4. Treatment

   a. **Preventative measures** include **physical activity, calcium supplements,** and **estrogen-progesterone therapy.** Conjugated estrogen (0.625 mg daily or the equivalent) will provide effective bone protection.

   b. **Vitamin D** (400 U daily) should be taken by persons over 75 years of age or those who lack sun exposure.

   c. **Intramuscular injections** of **testosterone enanthate,** 150–200 mg every 3–4 weeks, may be considered for men with osteoporosis associated with low testosterone.

   d. **Bisphosphonates** decrease bone formation and resorption.

   (1) **Alendronate,** 10 mg daily, may be taken with a full glass of water on an empty stomach.

   (2) **Recumbency should be avoided** for at least 30 minutes to prevent esophageal irritation.

   e. **Calcitonin** can be used for bone density gain similar to hormonal replacement therapy.

   (1) Calcitonin also has a **modest analgesic effect** after acute fracture.

   (2) It may be given subcutaneously, intramuscularly, or internasally. The **internasal form has fewest side effects; the dose is 200 U daily.**

III. FRACTURES, DISLOCATIONS, SPRAINS, AND STRAINS

A. Classification of fractures

   1. **Location** (e.g., proximal, middle, distal third)

   2. **Direction** [e.g., transverse (at right angle to the axis of the bone), spiral (bone has twisted appearance, also called torsion), oblique (fracture line between horizontal and vertical direction), comminuted (splintered or crushed), segmental (double)]

   3. **Alignment** [e.g., angulation (deviation from straight line), displacement (abnormal position of fracture fragments, such as dorsal displacement of the fracture fragment in a Colles' fracture of the wrist and volar displacement of the fracture fragment in a Smith's fracture of the wrist; both may be complicated by injury to the median nerve or radial artery)]

   4. **Associated factors** [e.g., open fracture (disruption of the skin), closed fracture (skin is intact), dislocation (displacement of bone from a joint)]

B. Imaging studies

   1. **Plain film radiographs** are sufficient to visualize most fractures. Concurrent fractures may also be seen at the joints proximal and distal to the fracture (e.g., distal tibia, proximal fibula, dome of the talus, and lateral malleolus).

2. **Radionucleotide bone scanning** will show increased uptake at the site of the occult fracture or stress fractures (common in athletes and associated with disuse osteopenia when weight bearing started after long periods of immobilization).

3. Although CT has displaced much of its use, tomography allows visualization of the bone's articular surface otherwise obscured by overlying structures (e.g., carpal bones, elbow, and tibial plateau).

4. CT is helpful in diagnosing pelvic, facial, or intra-articular fractures.

5. MRI is **not required.**

C. **Treatment. The following types of fractures** are treated initially with **analgesics, immobilization**, and emergent **referral** to an **orthopedist** after adequate stabilization of the patient.

  1. Open fractures

   a. Ideally, open fractures must be **debrided** and **irrigated** (in operating room) within 4–8 hours of injury.

   b. **IV antibiotics** (first- and second-generation cephalosporins and aminoglycosides) should be administered for **48 hours** after fracture and for 48 hours after surgical procedures.

   c. **Immobilization** and **fixation** should be performed to preserve function.

  2. **Intra-articular fractures** (the fracture line enters a joint cavity)

   a. **Open treatment** may be indicated to restore and maintain articular congruity.

   b. When stable, consider active range of motion.

  3. Femur fractures

   a. Treat neck fractures first with screws, then shaft fractures with intramedullary rods or plates.

   b. There is significant **potential for hemorrhage** with fractures of the femur.

  4. Fractures of both bones of the lower leg in adults

   a. Fractures of the tibia and fibula are associated with ligamental, meniscal, and vascular injuries.

   b. For **simple fractures, reduction** can be **closed** (manipulation or traction) or for more **complicated fractures, open** (usually combined with internal fixation).

D. Fractures in children

  1. **The physis, or growth plate,** is more susceptible to fracture than is injury to attached ligaments.

   a. **Swelling** and **tenderness** are the common findings over the physis when fractured.

   b. **Comparison films** may be helpful.

  2. **Incomplete fractures** (the line of fracture does not include the whole bone)

   a. **Torus fractures** occur when one side of the cortex buckles, due to a compression injury (e.g., falling on an outstretched hand). Treatment is 4–6 weeks in a cast.

   b. **Greenstick fractures** occur in long bones when **bowing causes a break in one side** of the cortex. When the angulation of the fracture is **less than 15°**, a **long arm cast** can be applied for 4–6 weeks. Fractures with angulation **greater than 15°** need **referral** to an orthopedic surgeon.

  3. When **radiographs of a young child** show **fractures in various stages of healing, abuse should be suspected** and the child should be referred to a protective agency.

  4. Growth plate fractures are classified with the **Salter-Harris classification system (Figure 9-1)**

E. Dislocations

  1. General characteristics

   a. **Total loss of congruity** occurs between the articular surfaces of the joint.

   b. Any **less serious** loss of congruity is called **subluxation** (e.g., nursemaids' elbow—subluxation of the head of the radius, occurring when a child, especially 1- to 3-year-olds, are suddenly lifted by the upper limb and the radial head slips anteriorly from the elbow joint out of the annular ligament).

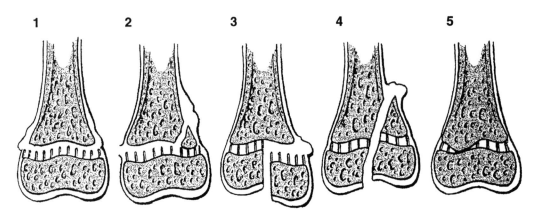

Figure 9-1. The Salter-Harris classification of fractures involving the physis. (1) Fracture through epiphyseal plate. (2) Epiphyseal fracture with associated metaphyseal fragment. (3) Fracture through the epiphysis into the articular surface. (4) Fracture through distal metaphysis, epiphyseal plate, and epiphysis. (5) Impaction of the epiphyseal plate. [From Jarrell BE, Carabasi III RA, *NMS Surgery*, 3rd edition. Baltimore, Williams & Wilkins, 1996, p 533. Redrawn with permission from Salter RB, Harris WR: Injuries involving the epiphyseal plate. *J Bone Joint Surg* 45A:587, 1963.]

  2. Sites of dislocation

      a. Common sites of dislocation are anterior **shoulder,** anterior **hip** (is abducted and radiographs show inferior margin of the acetabulum is overlapped by the femoral head) and posterior **hip** (is abducted and radiographs show the femoral head posterior to the acetabular rim; a common complication of a posterior dislocation is osteonecrosis of the femoral head), and posterior dislocations of the **elbow.**

      b. Less commonly, dislocations may be found in **navicular, subtalar,** and **as part of a combination Lisfranc fracture** and **dislocation involving the second metatarsal,** which will often be fractured at the base with the other metatarsals dislocated.

  3. Treatment

      a. Most dislocations, after assessment of the neurovascular status, are treated with **closed reduction.**

      b. Dislocations that reduce spontaneously require **immobilization 2–4 weeks** followed by range of motion activity and return to normal activity.

      c. If **associated fractures** or **interposed soft tissues** are present, the patient will need to undergo **open reduction** and **internal fixation.**

      d. It is imperative to **assess** the **neurovascular status** after reduction.

F. Strains and sprains

  1. A **strain** is an injury to the **bone-tendon unit** at the **myotendinous junction** or the **muscle** itself.

  2. A **sprain** involves **collagenous tissue** such as ligaments or tendons.

  3. Strain or sprain injury often **follows a sudden stretch.** It can lead to avulsion of tendon (e.g., mallet finger-avulsion or stretch of the terminal extensor tendon; treated with extensor splinting for 6 weeks) and to ligamentous sprain (e.g., stretch of the anterior talofibular ligament causing the common ankle sprain).

  4. Treatment for both requires **supportive therapy.**

IV. DISORDERS OF THE NECK, SHOULDER, AND UPPER EXTREMITY

A. Neck pain

  1. General characteristics

      a. **Spondylosis** is the **most common condition** affecting the cervical spine.

          (1) Degenerative changes occur in the disk, most frequently in C5-C6 with osteophytes and disk narrowing.

          (2) Later, **facet joints** and the **joints of Luschka** are affected.

          (3) Paresthesias and numbness into the fingers, and pain increased with extension and decreased with flexion of the neck may be present.

b. Compression by central disk protrusion or **osteophytes** causes long-tract signs (e.g., clonus, Babinski's sign) and gait disturbance.

2. Treatment

   a. Conservative treatment involves the use of a **cervical collar, traction, exercise,** and **analgesics.**

   b. In advanced disease, **cervical fusion** or **diskectomy** may be necessary.

B. Other conditions of the neck

   1. **Whiplash** and **extension injury are common causes of pain** lasting 18 months or longer.

   a. This may occur as a result of rear impact with rapid extension of the cervical spine followed by flexion.

   b. **Treatment** includes soft cervical collar (short term), local ice or heat, analgesics, and gentle active range of motion.

   2. **Rheumatoid spondylitis** is found in most of the patients with adult RA.

   a. **Ligamentous stretching** causes progressive atlanto-axial and midcervical subluxation.

   b. **Surgical stabilization** is used to treat RA of the cervical spine.

C. Shoulder pain

   1. Shoulder pain can be **referred** pain caused by **cervical spondylosis.**

   2. Pain if **localized** to a **particular area of the shoulder may be the site of pathology** as compared with the diffuse nature of referred pain that cannot be well localized.

D. Rotator cuff syndrome

   1. General characteristics

   a. This syndrome **occurs with eccentric overload** (e.g., a throwing athlete), **underlying glenohumeral instability, poor muscle strength,** and **training errors.**

   b. Adults over the age of 40 commonly have **impingement of the supraspinatus tendon** as it **passes beneath the subacromial arch** as a cause.

   2. Clinical features

   a. **Dull aching in the shoulder** is the main clinical feature. The pain is caused by **inflammation, fibrosis,** and **tears.**

   b. The pain **may interfere with sleep,** and is **exacerbated by abduction** of the arm.

   3. Laboratory studies

   a. **Radiographs** are helpful in ruling out calcific tendinitis, glenohumeral or acromioclavicular arthrosis, and bone tumors.

   b. **Arthrography** or **MRI** can be used to diagnose tears.

   4. Treatment

   a. **Aggravating factors** such as repetitive throwing, other overhead activities, or improper mechanics **must be avoided.**

   b. **NSAIDs** may help alleviate inflammation and pain.

   c. **Local steroid injections** may be considered.

   d. **Physical therapy** may provide relief. Begin nonoperative management of the cuff tears with a **range of motion** and **strengthening program.**

   e. **Arthroscopic subacromial decompression** should be considered for adults with **persistent impingement.**

   f. If the patient is still symptomatic after 1 month, **surgical repair** must be done to avoid progression of the tear.

E. Other conditions of the shoulder

   1. **Adhesive capsulitis (frozen shoulder)** is an inflammatory process that may follow injury to the shoulder or arise on its own (common in diabetes).

   a. It is characterized by **pain** and **restricted glenohumeral movement.**

   b. **Arthrography** may demonstrate **synovitis, capsular contraction,** and **fibrinous adhesions.**

   c. Treatment includes NSAIDs, passive range of motion, and occasionally manipulation under anesthesia.

2. **OA of the humeral head** is usually secondary to osteonecrosis.

   a. **Pain, stiffness,** and **limited range of motion** are features of the condition.

   b. **Radiographs** show osteophytes and joint space narrowing.

   c. Treatment includes NSAIDs, cortisone injections, activity modification, and debridement or total joint replacement in severe cases.

3. **Rupture** of the long **head of the biceps tendons**

   a. This rupture can occur as a **result of spontaneous** or **forced overload.**

   b. In the elderly, this rupture may be caused by **degeneration** or **attritional changes.**

   c. Treatment is by surgical tenodesis to humerus if less than 5–10 days have elapsed since the injury.

F. **Hand and wrist pain**

   1. **OA** and **RA** are the most common conditions of the hand and wrist (see I A, B).

     a. **OA** commonly affects the **carpometacarpal joint of the thumb and distal interphalangeal (DIP) joints.**

     b. OA of the wrist is **post-traumatic** or **follows osteonecrosis of the lunate (Kienböck's disease).**

   2. **Clinical features**

     a. **OA** presents with **Heberden's nodes** and **mucous cysts** in distal joints and **Bouchard's nodes** in proximal interphalangeal joint.

     b. **RA** causes **rupture of extensor tendons, erosion subluxation,** or **dislocation of joints.**

   3. **Dupuytren's disease** affects the palmar aponeurosis, ring, little, and middle fingers, and thumb with painful nodules, pitting, and contractures.

     a. There is **no nonsurgical treatment** for this condition.

     b. Surgical release of the contractures is indicated for contractures of the metacarpal phalangeal joint of greater then 30° and proximal phalangeal contractures of any degree, pain (rare), or nerve compression (digital).

G. **Carpal tunnel syndrome**

   1. General characteristics

     a. The **most common neuropathy,** it involves **compression of the median nerve under the transverse carpal ligament.**

     b. Can be precipitated by premenstrual fluid retention, early rheumatoid arthritis with synovial tendon sheath thickening, acromegaly, pregnancy, repetitive flexion or extension of the wrist (e.g., production line work or keyboard work), and **alcohol abuse.**

   2. Clinical features

     a. Classic findings of **night pain, numbness, paresthesias (sparing the little finger), clumsiness,** and **weakness** are seen.

     b. **Thenar atrophy** may occur.

     c. **Tinel's sign** (tingling with percussion over the volar aspect of the wrist) may be seen.

     d. **Phalen's test** (symptoms with full flexion of the wrist for over a minute) may be seen.

   3. Laboratory studies

     a. Helpful studies include **glucose, thyroid panel, rheumatoid factor, ESR,** and **diagnostic steroid injections.**

     b. Tests of **nerve sensory conduction, if greater than 3.5 milliseconds,** are helpful but not always diagnostic.

   4. Treatment

     a. **Activity modification, volar wrist splint,** and **NSAIDs (except in late pregnancy)** are the first recommended treatment.

b. Steroid injections may be used.

c. Vitamin B_6 taken daily may be helpful.

d. Surgical intervention may be performed to **decompress the nerve.**

V. DISORDERS OF THE BACK AND LOWER EXTREMITY

A. Low back pain (LBP) and sciatica

1. General characteristics

a. The **most common causes** of lower back pain are **prolapsed intervertebral disk** or **low back strain.**

b. When back pain is unrelated to the mechanical use of the back, it can be referred from the intra-abdominal, pelvic, or retroperitoneal areas.

2. Clinical features

a. Pain **originating in the back** and **radiating down the leg** suggests **nerve root irritation.**

b. Pain from **musculoskeletal causes** may be localized to an area of point tenderness.

c. Sciatica (pain in the distributor of the sciatic nerve) is felt in the buttock, posterior thigh, and posterolateral aspect of the leg around the lateral malleolus to the lateral dorsum of the foot and the entire sole.

d. **Unilateral low back** and **buttock pain** that gets worse with standing in one position may have **sacroiliac joint involvement.**

e. Pain in the elderly patient that is **increased by walking** and is **relieved by leaning forward** is suggestive of **spinal stenosis.**

3. Laboratory studies

a. **Radiographs** of the spine in nontraumatic lower back pain are often not required when pertinent directed history and physical examination reveal no sign of a serious condition.

b. **CT scanning** is helpful in demonstrating bony stenosis and identifying lateral nerve root entrapment.

c. **MRI** can be useful in identifying cord pathology, neural tumors, herniated disks, and infections.

d. **Electromyogram (EMG)** is as helpful as physical examination.

4. Treatment

a. **Short-term bed rest** (2 days) with support under the knees and neck, and administration of NSAIDs or analgesics are the first components of treatment.

b. **Progressive ambulation** to normal activities may follow if pain has subsided.

c. A **fitness program,** including postural exercises such as McKenzie exercises for disk derangement, should be implemented for back rehabilitation.

d. If no improvement occurs in 6 weeks, perform further evaluation with bone scan and medical work-up to **rule out spinal tumor** or **infection.**

e. If studies are normal, continue **back rehabilitation.**

f. When conservative treatment fails (CT, possible myelogram, or MRI), **confirm candidates for surgical intervention** (approximately 5% who present with LBP).

B. Scoliosis and kyphosis

1. Scoliosis

a. General characteristics

(1) Scoliosis is defined as **lateral curvature of the spine.**

(2) Some curves are **secondary to underlying causes** (i.e., upper or lower motor neuron disease, myopathies).

(3) **Idiopathic adolescent scoliosis** is the **most common spinal deformity** evaluated by a clinician.

(4) **Girls between onset of puberty growth spurt** and **cessation of spinal growth** are at the greatest risk for idiopathic scoliosis.

(5) The vertebrae at the **apex** of the curve are used for its description. **Right thoracic curves** (i.e., T7 or T8) are the most common, followed by the double major (right thoracic, left lumbar), left lumbar, and the right lumbar.

(6) A **thoracic curve to the left is rare**, and other spinal cord pathology needs to be ruled out before making a diagnosis of scoliosis.

b. Clinical features

(1) **Physical examination** reveals **asymmetry in shoulder, iliac height, asymmetric scapular prominence, flank crease with forward bending showing right thoracic and left lumbar prominence.**

(2) **Gait** and **neurologic examination** are normal.

(3) Curves of less than 20°, 2 years post-menarche, and Risser stage of 2–4 are less likely to progress.

c. Laboratory studies

(1) Single, standing 36″ anteroposterior (AP) **radiographs** should be taken when a patient has scoliometer (device used for measuring curves) readings greater than 5°.

(2) **Vertebral levels** are identified on radiograph with the greatest tilt anterior measured by the Cobb method [measurement perpendicular to the end plate of the most tilted (end) vertebra]. **Curves greater than 15% are significant.**

d. Treatment

(1) **Curves of 10°–15°** are treated by **6-month follow-up of forward bending test,** and **scoliometer test.**

(2) **Curves of 15°–20°** need **serial AP radiograph follow-up every 3–4 months for larger curves** and **6–8 months for smaller curves** or for patients near the end of growth.

(3) **Curves greater than 20° need referral to an orthopedist.**

2. Kyphosis

a. General characteristics

(1) Kyphosis is defined as **increased convex curvature** of the **thoracic spine.**

(2) Scoliosis is also present in **one third of patients** with kyphosis.

(3) **Juvenile kyphosis (Scheuermann's disease)** is idiopathic osteochondrosis of thoracic spine.

(4) **Tuberculosis of the spine** (the most common extrapulmonary location) **causes progressive kyphosis.**

b. Clinical features

(1) A **round back appearance** with a smooth curve when several vertebrae are involved or angular curve when one vertebra is involved is characteristic.

(2) If the curve is a result of faulty posture, it will disappear with spinal flexion.

(3) Excessive **lumbar lordosis** is common.

c. Laboratory studies for kyphosis are the radiographs—standing lateral scoliosis films.

d. Treatment

(1) **Curves of 45°–60°** should be **observed every 3–4 months** and **exercises prescribed for lumbar lordosis** and the thoracic spine.

(2) Curves **greater than 60°** or with persistent pain can be treated with a Milwaukee brace.

(3) **Surgery** is indicated when curvature is unresponsive to above treatment.

C. Spinal stenosis

1. General characteristics

a. Spinal stenosis is **nerve compression** caused by the **narrowing of the spinal canal** or **neural foramina.**

b. Types

(1) **Central stenosis** (compression of the thecal sac) can be **idiopathic** or **developmental.**

(2) **Lateral stenosis** (impingement of the nerve root lateral to the thecal sac) often **accompanies central stenosis** or is an **isolated entity in young adults and the middle-aged.**

c. Spinal stenosis is usually **symptomatic in late middle age,** and is **more common in men** than in women.

2. Clinical features

   a. **Neural claudication** and **exacerbation of pain with walking** that is relieved by leaning forward is associated with this condition.

   b. **Variable back** and **leg pain** may occur.

3. Laboratory studies

   a. **Radiographs** show **soft tissue** and **thecal narrowing.**

   b. **Plain CT, post-myelographic CT**, and **MRI** are standard imaging modalities.

4. Treatment

   a. Conservative management includes **rest, isometric abdominal exercises, pelvic tilt, Williams' flexion exercises, NSAIDs,** and **weight reduction.**

   b. **Decompression** and **fusion** are indicated when studies are positive for neural compressive pathology and quality of life is unacceptable to the patient.

D. Ankylosing spondylitis

1. General characteristics

   a. Ankylosing spondylitis is **inflammation and progressive fusion of the vertebrae.**

   b. This condition involves **back pain, stiffness,** and **hip pain** with **onset during the third and fourth decades** of life, and is seen **more commonly in men** than in women.

   c. This disorder **affects the sacroiliac joint symmetrically** and the spine in a **progressively ascending** manner.

2. Clinical features

   a. **Lumbar motion is restricted.**

   b. **Limited motion in the shoulders and hips, synovitis of the knees, plantar fasciitis, supraspinatus,** and **Achilles tendinitis** are seen.

   c. Patients also have **hip contractures, fixed cervical, thoracic,** and **lumbar hyperkyphosis.**

   d. **Fracture of fused osteopenic spine** may occur (commonly cervical), as well as **sciatica.**

   e. **Extra-articular manifestations** may occur, **including uveitis, cardiac abnormalities,** and **interstitial lung disease.**

   f. Noninvasive tests for spine and thoracic mobility include the **Schober test, thoracolumbar rotation and flexion, finger-to-floor distance, cervical rotation, occiput–wall distance,** and **chest expansion.**

3. Laboratory studies

   a. Evaluation of **ESR** and **HLA-B27** are indicated.

   b. The **"bamboo appearance"** on **radiography** will occur because of **radiographic obliteration** and **marginal syndesmophyte ossification** of the **paraspinal ligaments.**

   c. **Generalized osteopenia of the spine** may be seen.

4. Treatment

   a. **Underlying conditions** must be treated.

   b. Spine **fractures need intervention** and **stabilization.**

10

Endocrinology

Rebecca Lovell Scott

I. THYROID DISORDERS

A. Hyperthyroidism (thyrotoxicosis)

1. General characteristics

   a. This is a condition involving **elevated thyroid hormone concentrations,** and may be caused by **excess production, leakage,** or **exogenous hormones.**

   b. The most common cause (90% of hyperthyroidism) is **Graves' disease,** an autoimmune disorder most often found in women 20–40 years of age. Evidence exists for a genetic predisposition. Graves' disease may also be found in persons with other autoimmune disorders.

   c. Other common causes are toxic nodular goiter, subacute and postpartum thyroiditis, and overdosage of thyroid medication.

   d. **Thyroid storm** is the abrupt onset of more florid symptoms of thyrotoxicosis.

2. Clinical features

   a. Findings include heat intolerance, sweating, weight loss, increased appetite, nervousness, loose stools, frequent urination, irritability, fatigue, weakness, dyspnea on exertion, and menstrual abnormalities.

   b. Patients may also have tachycardia, palpitations, precordial chest pain, warm moist skin, stare, tremor anxiety, and muscle weakness.

   c. In hyperthyroidism caused by Graves' disease, patients will have a goiter, frequently with a bruit; 5% will have ophthalmopathy. Pretibial myxedema occurs in 1% of patients.

   d. Men with hyperthyroidism may develop gynecomastia and impotence.

   e. Findings may be limited to one organ system, and may include isolated atrial fibrillation, psychosis, or myopathies.

   f. Elderly patients are likely to present atypically.

   g. Thyroid storm presents as fever, marked weakness, and muscle wasting; extreme restlessness, confusion, and emotional lability may also occur.

3. Laboratory studies

   a. Laboratory studies are based on levels of thyroid hormones; thyroid-stimulating hormone (TSH) is secreted by the pituitary gland and stimulates thyroid hormone production.

   b. In primary hyperthyroidism, **TSH is low.**

   c. Thyroxine (T_4), triiodothyronine (T_3), free T_4, and free T_4 index will be elevated.

   d. Thyroid function studies are affected by severe illness, cirrhosis, nephrotic syndrome, a variety of drugs, high estrogen states, and acute psychiatric illness.

4. Treatment

   a. *β*-blockers control tachycardia, tremor, and palpitations.

   b. **Methimazole** or **propylthiouracil (PTU)** control hyperthyroidism within several weeks.

  c. Radioactive iodine ablation is preferred to surgery for permanent control.

  d. Thyroid storm is a **life-threatening emergency** requiring prompt and specific treatment. The treatment for thyroid storm includes administration of β-blockers, supportive therapy, and attempts to control hyperthyroidism.

B. Hypothyroidism and myxedema

 1. General characteristics

  a. Hypothyroidism almost always **results from autoimmune thyroiditis, previous thyroid surgery,** or **radiation therapy.**

  b. Hashimoto's thyroiditis (autoimmune thyroiditis) is most common in women; it tends to be familial, and is often associated with other autoimmune disorders (see also I D).

 2. Clinical features

  a. Signs and symptoms tend to be vague and nonspecific.

  b. Common complaints include fatigue, lethargy, anorexia, constipation, menstrual abnormalities, muscle stiffness, memory impairment, depression, cold intolerance, and dry skin.

  c. Signs include weight gain, bradycardia, edema, weakness, hyporeflexia, dementia, and psychosis.

 3. Laboratory studies

  a. TSH will be elevated in primary disease.

  b. Low total T_4 and free T_4 are likely; T_3 may be normal.

  c. Presence of antithyroid peroxidase and antithyroglobulin antibodies in the serum confirm autoimmune disease.

 4. Treatment with synthetic T_4 is best monitored by serial TSH levels.

C. Thyroid cancer

 1. General characteristics

  a. The most common form (70%) is **papillary carcinoma;** women are affected 2–3 times more often than men.

  b. Only 5% of all palpable thyroid nodules are malignant.

  c. Cancer risk is associated with childhood neck irradiation and **family history of multiple endocrine neoplasia II (MEN II) syndrome.**

 2. Clinical features

  a. Patients most often present with **painless neck swelling.** Pain, hoarseness, and hemoptysis may also occur.

  b. The nodule may enlarge over a short period.

  c. Patients may have evidence of metastatic disease.

  d. The gland often has a **stony, hard consistency.**

 3. Laboratory studies

  a. Thyroid function tests are often normal.

  b. TSH should be measured to exclude primary thyroid disease.

  c. Fine-needle biopsy is essential.

  d. Hot nodules on radionuclide scanning are benign.

 4. Treatment

  a. Surgical resection and **partial thyroidectomy** are indicated.

  b. T_4 therapy prevents hypothyroidism and reduces the risk of recurrence.

  c. Radioactive iodine ablation is used for residual disease or to prevent recurrence.

D. Thyroiditis

1. General characteristics

a. **Hashimoto's (chronic lymphocytic)** thyroiditis is the most common thyroid disorder in the United States.

b. **Subacute (granulomatous)** thyroiditis may present with acute symptoms or silently.

(1) It is most common in young or middle-aged women.

(2) **Viral etiology is suspected.**

2. Clinical features

a. In Hashimoto's thyroiditis, the thyroid is usually **diffusely enlarged and firm.**

(1) Signs and symptoms are usually of **hypothyroidism,** but **transient thyrotoxicosis** occurs.

(2) In elderly women (10% of cases) the gland is atrophic.

b. Subacute thyroiditis usually presents as an acute, painful glandular enlargement with dysphagia.

(1) Patients may have thyrotoxicosis and malaise.

(2) Manifestations last from weeks to months.

3. Laboratory studies

a. Testing for Hashimoto's disease involves screening for serum **antithyroid peroxidase** and **antithyroglobulin antibodies,** which will confirm autoimmune disease.

b. **Erythrocyte sedimentation rate (ESR)** is high and antithyroid antibodies are low in subacute disease.

4. **Treatment** is based on specific manifestations.

a. Hashimoto's thyroiditis requires **lifelong replacement with thyroid hormone.**

b. Subacute thyroiditis is treated with **aspirin** and, only as a last resort, **glucocorticoids.**

II. PARATHYROID DISORDERS

A. Hypoparathyroidism and pseudohypoparathyroidism

1. General characteristics

a. Hypoparathyroidism is **most commonly found following thyroidectomy,** but rarely is autoimmune.

b. **Magnesium deficiency** results in functional disease.

c. Pseudohypoparathyroidism results from a **genetic defect.**

2. Clinical features

a. Hypoparathyroidism causes hypocalcemia.

b. Acute disease causes **tetany, carpopedal spasm, cramping, convulsions, oral** and **distal extremity tingling, and irritability.**

c. Positive **Chvostek's sign** and **Trousseau's phenomenon, cataracts,** and **teeth and nail defects** indicate associated hypocalcemia.

d. Findings in patients with chronic disease include lethargy, mental retardation, personality changes, and blurred vision.

3. Laboratory studies

a. Corrected serum calcium, urinary calcium, and parathyroid hormone levels are low.

b. Serum magnesium may be low.

c. Serum phosphate will be high; alkaline phosphatase will be normal.

d. Computed tomography (CT) scan of the skull may show dense bones and basal ganglia calcifications.

e. Electrocardiogram (ECG) findings include prolonged QT intervals and T wave abnormalities.

4. Treatment

   a. Emergency treatment for tetany includes **airway maintenance** and **intravenous calcium gluconate.**

   b. Maintenance therapy includes **oral calcium** and **vitamin D preparations** to keep serum calcium 8–8.6 mg/dl.

   c. Magnesium supplementation may be required.

B. Hyperparathyroidism

   1. General characteristics

   a. This condition is **more common in women** than in men and occurs most often in those **over 50 years of age.**

   b. Causes include parathyroid adenoma and, less commonly, hyperplasia or carcinoma.

   c. Many malignancies also cause hypercalcemia and have clinical findings similar to hyperparathyroidism. Malignancy and hyperparathyroidism may coexist.

   2. Clinical features

   a. Patients may have **polydipsia** and **polyuria;** excessive **calcium** and **phosphate excretion** may lead to renal stones.

   b. Bone pain and arthralgias are common; cortical bone or diffuse bone demineralization, pathologic fractures, and cystic bone lesions may occur.

   c. Mild hypercalcemia is likely to be asymptomatic; if the hypercalcemia is more severe, it may cause anorexia, nausea, vomiting, constipation, anemia, weight loss, and hypertension. Depressed deep tendon reflexes are associated with hypercalcemia.

   d. Depression, muscle weakness, fatigability, paresthesias, pruritus, psychosis, and coma occur in severe disease.

   3. Laboratory studies

   a. **Hypercalcemia** (more than 10.5 mg/dl) is the hallmark; serum phosphate is often less than 2.5 mg/dl.

   b. Urine calcium excretion is low for the degree of hypercalcemia.

   c. **Elevated parathyroid hormone levels** are essential for diagnosis.

   4. Treatment

   a. **Surgical treatment** is recommended for symptomatic and certain asymptomatic patients.

   b. Medical treatment includes **hydration, inhibitors of bone resorption, avoidance of immobility, diuretics,** and **dioxin; postmenopausal estrogen supplementation** and **propranolol** may be helpful.

III. DIABETES MELLITUS

A. General medical problems

   1. Diabetic retinopathy is the leading cause of blindness in people in the United States under 60 years of age. Each year, approximately 5000 patients with diabetes become blind.

   2. Diabetic nephropathy causes approximately one third of end-stage renal disease in the United States.

   3. Diabetic patients have accelerated large-vessel atherosclerosis, putting them at increased risk for stroke and coronary artery disease (CAD). Large-vessel atherosclerosis in diabetic patients is also the cause of at least half of nontraumatic lower extremity amputations in the United States.

   4. Diabetes mellitus causes a characteristic peripheral symmetric polyneuropathy. Nerve damage also causes autonomic dysfunction, leading to impotence, atonic bladder, and delayed gastric emptying.

   5. Skin changes associated with diabetes mellitus include slow wound healing, necrobiosis lipoidica diabeticorum, and acanthosis nigricans.

B. **Insulin-dependent diabetes mellitus (IDDM, type I diabetes)**

1. **General characteristics**

    a. IDDM occurs most often in **young people** of **normal or low weight.**

    b. These persons have **little or no endogenous insulin secretion.**

    c. IDDM is an **autoimmune disease;** a few forms have a genetic component.

2. **Clinical features**

    a. The most common findings include **polydipsia, polyuria,** and **rapid weight loss.**

    b. Untreated IDDM results in diabetic ketoacidosis.

3. **Laboratory studies**

    a. A random plasma glucose more than 200 mg/dl with classic symptoms or 2 fasting levels more than 140 mg/dl are diagnostic.

    b. A plasma glucose more than 200 mg/dl 2 hours after 75 g of oral glucose [oral glucose tolerance test (OGTT)] and more than 200 mg/dl between 0 and 2 hours after oral glucose also meet diagnostic criteria.

    c. Patients may have ketonemia or ketonuria, or both.

4. **Treatment**

    a. **Diet is central to management.**

    (1) Diet must be individualized according to the patient's activity level, food preferences, and need to attain and maintain ideal weight.

    (2) Current recommendations include 55%–60% of calories from carbohydrate, 30% from fat, and 10%–15% from protein.

    (3) Patients should eat at regular intervals.

    b. **Insulin** may be delivered by subcutaneous injection or insulin pump. Glycemic response depends on depth of injection, exercise of injection site, and temperature.

    (1) **Human insulin** causes less antibody response than beef, pork, or combined beef–pork insulin.

    (2) Regular insulin is short-acting and is used before meals.

    (3) Neutral protamine Hagedorn (NPH) insulin and lente insulin are intermediate-acting forms; ultralente insulin is long-acting.

C. **Non–insulin-dependent diabetes mellitus (NIDDM, type II)**

1. **General characteristics**

    a. NIDDM occurs most often in **middle-aged or older people** who are **overweight.**

    b. In NIDDM, **insulin levels are normal or high, but tissues are resistant;** delayed insulin secretion from the pancreas is also often present.

    c. In the United States, NIDDM accounts for 90% of diabetes and is found most often in African-Americans, Hispanics, and Pima Indians.

    d. NIDDM has a strong genetic component.

    e. Exercise and weight loss decrease the risk of NIDDM.

    f. Untreated NIDDM can lead to hyperosmolar nonketotic states.

2. **Clinical features**

    a. Patients usually have **polyuria** and **polydipsia;** ketonuria and weight loss are rare.

    b. Patients may also present with **fatigue, candidal vaginitis, blurred vision,** or **poor wound healing.**

    c. Many patients have few symptoms.

3. **Laboratory studies**

    a. The diagnostic criteria for type II include the same criteria as for type I diabetes mellitus (see III B 3 a, b).

    b. Glycosylated hemoglobin (Hb A_{1C}) and fructosamine are used to monitor chronic control.

4. Treatment

   a. Diet must be individualized, but should include 55%–60% carbohydrate, 30% fat, and 10%–15% protein.

   b. Weight loss may restore insulin responsiveness.

   c. Daily **self-monitoring** is essential to treatment.

   d. Oral hypoglycemic agents (sulfonylureas) potentiate insulin secretion; of these, glyburide and glipizide are second-generation agents with few drug interactions.

   e. Metformin, which reduces hepatic glucose uptake, may be added as a second agent.

   f. Approximately one third of NIDDM patients require **insulin.**

IV. ADRENAL DISORDERS

A. Chronic adrenocortical insufficiency (Addison's disease)

   1. General characteristics

   a. The most common cause is **autoimmune inflammation of the adrenal cortex;** other causes include abrupt cessation of glucocorticoid therapy, destruction of the adrenal gland, tuberculosis, fungal infection, and metastatic disease.

   b. Women are most often affected.

   2. Clinical features

   a. Addison's disease begins insidiously with nonspecific problems such as **fatigue and weakness. Weight loss** is usually present.

   b. Most patients have myalgias and arthritis; many have gastrointestinal symptoms.

   c. Many patients develop sensory hypersensitivities.

   d. Some patients crave salt.

   e. Orthostatic hypotension is common.

   f. Delayed deep tendon reflexes are found.

   g. Hyperpigmentation is found only in primary disease.

   3. Laboratory studies

   a. Laboratory findings include **hyperkalemia (found only in primary disease), hyponatremia, hypoglycemia, anemia, hypercalcemia,** and **eosinophilia.**

   b. A **1-hour adrenocorticotropic hormone (ACTH) stimulation test** is the best screening test. A 1-hour serum cortisol less than 20 μg/dl with a rise less than 7 μg/dl from baseline suggests deficiency.

   c. A 3-day ACTH stimulation test confirms the diagnosis and differentiates primary from secondary causes.

   4. Treatment

   a. Primary disease is treated with **oral cortisone acetate** or **hydrocortisone.**

   b. Addisonian crisis requires **intravenous saline, glucose,** and **glucocorticoids.**

B. Cushing's disease and Cushing's syndrome (hypercortisolism)

   1. General characteristics

   a. Cushing's syndrome may be exogenous or endogenous. The exogenous form is caused by **chronic excess glucocorticoid,** most commonly from corticosteroid drugs used to treat other diseases.

   b. Cushing's disease is caused **by excess secretion of ACTH by the pituitary.**

   (1) Cushing's disease is the **major cause of endogenous Cushing's syndrome.**

   (2) The disease is **most common in premenopausal women.**

   c. Adrenocortical tumors and nonpituitary ACTH-producing tumors (most often small cell lung carcinoma) may also cause Cushing's syndrome.

2. Clinical features

    a. Hypercortisolism may present as **obesity, hypertension,** and **diabetes mellitus.**

        (1) Obesity is centripetal; extremities may appear wasted.

        (2) Fat also causes the buffalo hump and moon facies characteristic of hypercortisolism.

    b. The most specific signs are **proximal muscle weakness** and **pigmented striae** more than 1 cm wide.

    c. Disorders of calcium metabolism may cause **vertebral fractures, hypercalciuria,** and **kidney stones.**

    d. Psychiatric symptoms range from emotional lability to psychosis.

3. Laboratory studies

    a. Excretion of free cortisol in the urine more than 125 μg/dl in 24 hours is diagnostic.

    b. In Cushing's disease the overnight dexamethasone suppression test will result in a plasma cortisol more than 10 μg/dl.

    c. The cortisol excretion test and plasma cortisol test should be confirmed with a low-dose dexamethasone suppression test.

    d. CT scanning [or, for a pituitary tumor, preferably magnetic resonance imaging (MRI)] may show adrenocortical or other tumors.

    e. Hyperglycemia and hypokalemia are not unusual.

4. Treatment

    a. Treatment of Cushing's disease is **transsphenoidal resection** and **hydrocortisol replacement.**

    b. Surgical removal of tumors is the treatment of choice for Cushing's syndrome.

    c. Radiation and chemotherapy may be used for nonresectable tumors.

    d. Adrenal inhibitors can also be used.

        (1) Metyrapone can be combined with aminoglutethimide.

        (2) Mitotane in increasing doses will usually control metabolic disturbances.

        (3) Ketoconazole can also be used to block steroid synthesis.

V. OTHER ENDOCRINE DISORDERS

A. Metabolic bone disease

    1. Osteoporosis (see Chapter 9)

    2. Osteomalacia and rickets

        a. General characteristics

            (1) Osteomalacia and rickets are diseases of defective mineralization.

            (2) Osteomalacia is found in adults; rickets in children.

            (3) Both are most often caused by a **deficiency of vitamin D, calcium, or phosphate.**

            (4) Osteomalacia **may be induced by phenytoin use.**

        b. Clinical features

            (1) Osteomalacia patients present with diffuse muscle weakness and bone pain.

            (2) Children develop skeletal deformities.

        c. Laboratory studies

            (1) In osteomalacia, radiographs show **generalized decrease in bone density;** "Milkman's lines" or "Looser's zones" (pseudofractures) are diagnostic.

            (2) Both may be diagnosed by bone biopsy.

            (3) Hypocalcemia, hypocalciuria, hypophosphatemia, secondary hyperparathyroidism, and decreased 25-hydroxyvitamin D may be present.

   d. Treatment

      (1) **Ergocalciferol** (50,000 units by mouth twice a week for 6–12 months, followed by 400 units daily) treats **vitamin D deficiency.**

      (2) **Phosphate supplementation** and vitamin D are required for renal phosphate wasting.

      (3) **Oral calcium** should be given to treat nutritional calcium deficiency.

3. Paget's disease of bone (osteitis deformans)

   a. General characteristics

      (1) Paget's disease of bone involves localized dysplastic bone formation.

      (2) Paget's disease of bone affects 3% of adults, and 5%–11% of those in their eighties.

      (3) Patients often have a family history of Paget's disease of bone.

      (4) Long-standing lesions in 1%–3% of patients transform into osteosarcoma.

   b. Clinical features

      (1) Most patients are **asymptomatic.**

      (2) **Bone pain** is often the first symptom, with accompanying **joint pain.** Common sites of involvement include spine, pelvis, femur, and skull; patients may present with pathologic fractures or other symptoms related to the site.

      (3) Patients may also have **bowed tibias** and **kyphosis.**

      (4) **Deafness** is the most common neurologic finding.

      (5) **Cardiac output may increase** and progress to failure.

   c. Laboratory studies

      (1) Serum calcium and phosphorus are normal; **alkaline phosphatase is high**.

      (2) Hypercalciuria is common.

      (3) Hypercalcemia occurs in patients on bed rest.

      (4) The extent of the disease should be determined by skeletal radiographs and bone scanning.

   d. Treatment

      (1) Patients with mild disease require only **nonsteroidal anti-inflammatory drugs NSAIDs or acetaminophen.**

      (2) **Calcitonin** restores normal bone remodeling.

      (3) **Alendronate, tiludronate, etidronate,** or **pamidronate** also slow bone turnover.

B. Dyslipidemia

  1. General characteristics

   a. Approximately 20% of American adults have hyperlipidemia.

   b. Dyslipidemias are **highly associated with atherosclerosis,** especially CAD.

   c. Reducing total cholesterol is associated with a lower incidence of myocardial infarction, slowing of disease progression, and regression of lesions.

   d. Low-density lipoprotein (LDL) cholesterol is **associated with increased risk of heart disease,** and **high-density lipoprotein (HDL) cholesterol** with **decreased risk.**

   e. Hypertriglyceridemia is a risk factor for CAD in women and diabetics.

   f. Severe hypertriglyceridemia can cause pancreatitis.

   g. Genetic forms of dyslipidemia are rare but patients with a history of familial hypercholesterolemia, familial hyperchylomicronemia, dysbetalipoproteinemia, or familial combined hyperlipidemia must be screened.

   h. Secondary hyperlipidemia has many possible causes, including diabetes, hypothyroidism, hypercortisolism, acromegaly, obesity, renal and liver problems, estrogens, thiazide diuretics, β-blockers, and alcohol.

2. Clinical features

  a. Xanthomas are pathognomonic for hyperlipidemia.

  b. Nearly two thirds of all persons with xanthelasmas (the commonest form of xanthomas, affecting the eyelids) have normal lipid profiles.

  c. Patients with severe hypercholesterolemia may develop early arcus senilis.

3. Laboratory studies

  a. Patients with any evidence of cardiovascular disease should be screened with a fasting complete lipid profile.

  b. Screening for patients with no evidence of cardiovascular disease and no other risk factors should begin at 35 years of age for men and 45 years of age for women.

  c. Risk factors for cardiovascular disease include family history, hypertension, cigarette smoking, diabetes mellitus, and low HDL cholesterol.

  d. Screening may include total cholesterol alone, total and HDL cholesterol, or LDL and HDL cholesterol levels only.

4. Treatment

  a. Nonpharmacologic therapy

  (1) Dietary changes should include reducing total dietary fat to 30% and saturated fat to 10% of calories; some diets reduce fat even further.

  (2) Soluble fiber, garlic, soy, and vitamin C may also reduce LDL cholesterol.

  (3) The diet should be high in antioxidant-containing fruits and vegetables.

  (4) Patients should be encouraged to increase aerobic exercise to increase levels of HDL.

  b. Pharmacologic treatment

  (1) Patients with high LDL cholesterol and a significant risk of CAD should take **325 mg aspirin every other day** unless contraindicated.

  (2) Postmenopausal estrogen replacement increases HDL and reduces LDL cholesterol.

  (3) Niacin is associated with reduced long-term mortality and has an optimal effect on lipids, but is poorly tolerated at full doses.

  (4) Resins that bind bile acids include **cholestyramine** and **colestipol.** They reduce the incidence of coronary events, but have no effect on mortality. Their mechanism of action is binding bile acids in the intestine.

  (5) 3-Hydroxy-3-methylglutaryl coenzyme A (HMG-CoA) reductase inhibitors, which include **lovastatin, pravastatin, simvastatin, fluvastatin,** and **atorvastatin,** inhibit the rate-limiting enzyme in formation of cholesterol. They also reduce CAD and total mortality. Myositis is a common side effect.

  (6) Fibric acid derivatives include **gemfibrozil** and **clofibrate;** they reduce synthesis and increase breakdown of very low-density lipoprotein (VLDL). Their side effects include cholelithiasis, hepatitis, and myositis. Clofibrate is associated with a statistically significant increase in cancer mortality.

  (7) Probucol should be reserved for patients with genetic disorders who have failed other treatments.

VI. NUTRITIONAL PROBLEMS

  A. Protein-energy (protein-calorie) malnutrition (PEM)

  1. General characteristics

  a. PEM results from **inadequate food intake; secondary PEM** is **related to other illness**.

  (1) Marasmus (wasting of subcutaneous fat and muscle) is the predominant form of PEM and is associated with early abandonment or failure of breastfeeding.

  (2) Kwashiorkor (generalized edema, enlarged fatty liver, apathy) is seen in children living in areas where staple and weaning foods are deficient in protein and are excessively starchy.

(3) In the United States approximately 20% of hospitalized patients have PEM caused by decreased intake, increased losses, or increased nutritional requirements related to underlying disease.

   b. PEM affects all body systems; losses of 35%–40% of body weight result in death.

2. Clinical features

   a. Findings range from **weight loss** and **mild growth failure** to classic marasmus and kwashiorkor.

   b. Patients may have **dry skin** and **thin hair** or **edema.**

3. Laboratory studies

   a. **Serum albumin** may be low.

   b. Other tests are indicated for underlying conditions.

4. Treatment

   a. **Fluid and electrolyte abnormalities** should be **corrected.**

   b. **Acute infection** should be treated.

   c. **Protein, calorie, vitamin,** and **mineral depletion** should be **corrected slowly** to prevent complications (e.g., refeeding edema, congestive heart failure).

B. Vitamin deficiencies

1. General characteristics

   a. Single vitamin deficiencies are rare.

   b. Multiple vitamin deficiencies are associated with protein–calorie undernutrition, malabsorption syndromes, alcoholism, hemodialysis, various medications, total parenteral nutrition, certain restrictive diets, and genetic metabolic disorders.

   (1) The **most common cause of thiamine deficiency** in the United States is **alcoholism.**

   (2) **B_6 deficiency** is found in patients taking isoniazid, cycloserine, penicillamine, and oral contraceptives; patients who are alcoholic; and those who have genetic errors of metabolism.

   (3) **Vitamin C deficiency** is most often found in the urban poor, the elderly, chronic alcoholics, patients with cancer or chronic renal failure, smokers, and infants with poor dietary intake.

   (4) **Vitamin A deficiency** in the United States is usually due to fat malabsorption syndromes, alcoholism, laxative abuse, or inadequate intake.

   (5) **Vitamin E deficiency** is seen in patients with severe malabsorption problems and in children with chronic liver disease, biliary atresia, or cystic fibrosis.

2. Clinical features

   a. Symptoms are **nonspecific;** physical examination is normal in early deficiency states.

   b. Glossitis, cheilosis, and sore mouth are seen with various vitamin B deficiencies.

   c. **Thiamine (B_1) deficiency** is associated with anorexia, muscle cramps, paresthesias, irritability, high output cardiac failure, symmetrical motor and sensory neuropathy, and Wernicke-Korsakoff syndrome.

   d. Advanced niacin deficiency **(pellagra)** includes a classic triad of dermatitis, dementia, and diarrhea.

   e. **B_6 deficiency** leads to mouth problems, irritability, and weakness; severe deficiency is associated with anemia, peripheral neuropathy, and seizures.

   f. Advanced vitamin C deficiency **(scurvy)** causes bleeding problems, anemia, and impaired wound healing.

   g. For B_{12} and folate deficiency, see Chapter 4; for vitamin D deficiency, see V A 2 d; for vitamin K deficiency, also see Chapter 4.

   h. The earliest symptom of vitamin A deficiency is night blindness; xerosis and Bitot's spots (superficial, foamy patches on the exposed bulbar conjunctiva) are other early signs.

   i. Vitamin E deficiency leads to areflexia, gait problems, and decreased proprioception and vibratory sense.

3. Laboratory studies include obtaining serum levels for levels of the suspected vitamin.

4. Treatment is aimed at the specific cause and is often empiric.

C. Vitamin toxicities

1. **General characteristics.** In the United States, vitamin excess, especially of A, D, and B_6, is more common than vitamin deficiency.

2. **Clinical features**

a. **Niacin excess** is characterized by flushing and gastric irritation; sustained release preparations are associated with fulminant hepatitis.

b. **B_6 excess** can cause an irreversible sensory neuropathy at doses as little as 200 mg/day.

c. **Vitamin C excess** can cause gastric irritation, flatulence, and diarrhea. It can cause a false positive fecal occult blood test and errors in urine glucose tests.

d. **Excess β-carotene** causes yellow staining of the palms and soles, but spares the sclera.

e. **Chronic excess vitamin A** causes dry skin, hair loss, mouth sores, anorexia, and vomiting; acute toxicity causes nausea, vomiting, abdominal pain, headache, papilledema, and lethargy.

3. **Laboratory studies** include serum levels of the vitamin in question.

4. **Treatment** consists of elimination of the offending agent.

D. Obesity

1. **General characteristics**

a. Obesity is one of the most common disorders seen in medical practice and is **associated with increases in morbidity and mortality.**

b. African-American women and persons of lower socioeconomic status are more likely to be obese.

c. Disorders most commonly associated with obesity include **hypertension, type II diabetes, hyperlipidemia, cardiovascular disease,** and **degenerative joint disease.**

d. Obese and overweight people are subject to social disapprobation and discrimination.

2. **Clinical features**

a. Obesity is defined as a **body weight in excess of 120% of expected weight.**

b. It can be classified as **mild** (20%–40% overweight), **moderate** (41%–100% overweight), or **severe** (more than 100% overweight).

c. Weight due to excess fat tissue is more of a problem than weight due to muscular tissue.

d. Fat distribution primarily in the upper body poses a greater health risk than fat in the thighs and buttocks.

3. **Laboratory studies**

a. Relative weight (RW) is computed by the body weight divided by "desirable weight" times 100; controversy surrounds the definition of "desirable weight."

b. Body mass index (BMI) is computed by dividing the weight in kilograms by the height in meters squared.

(1) Normal BMI is 20–25 kg/m^2.

(2) BMI more accurately reflects adipose versus lean tissue.

c. Less than 1% of patients have secondary obesity; testing for hypothyroidism and Cushing's syndrome may be needed.

d. For all obese patients, fasting levels of glucose, cholesterol, and triglycerides should be measured.

4. **Treatment**

a. **Multidisciplinary modalities** include **hypocaloric diet, behavior modification, aerobic exercise,** and **social support.**

b. **Maintenance of weight loss** is important.

c. Medications to treat obesity are controversial and associated with potentially serious health consequences.

d. Gastric surgery is considered the treatment of last resort.

11

Neurology

William H. Marquardt

I. CEREBROVASCULAR DISEASE

A. Stroke

1. General characteristics

    a. Stroke is the **third most common cause of death** in the United States and the **most disabling neurologic disorder.**

    b. The incidence of stroke **increases with age,** is **higher in men** than in women, and is **higher in blacks** than in whites.

    c. The major risk factors for stroke include hypertension, hypercholesterolemia, cigarette smoking, and heavy alcohol use.

    d. Ischemic strokes account for 80% of all strokes. Two thirds of ischemic strokes are **thrombotic** and one third are **embolic.**

    e. Hemorrhagic strokes, which are usually secondary to hypertension, account for 20% of strokes.

2. Clinical features

    a. Signs and symptoms of stroke **correlate with the area of the brain supplied by the affected vessel,** especially with ischemic events.

    b. Hemiparesis or hemisensory deficit is revealed in most cases on history and physical examination. One can **localize the lesion to one side, contralateral** to these deficits.

    c. Strokes involving the **anterior circulation,** which supplies the cortex, subcortical white matter, basal ganglia, and the internal capsule, are commonly associated with **hemispheric signs and symptoms** (i.e., aphasia, apraxia, hemiparesis, hemisensory losses, and visual field defects).

    d. Strokes involving the **posterior circulation,** which supplies the brain stem, cerebellum, thalamus, and portions of the temporal and occipital lobes, are commonly associated with **evidence of brain stem dysfunction** (i.e., coma, drop attacks, vertigo, nausea, vomiting, and ataxia).

3. Laboratory studies

    a. Routine blood tests include complete blood cell count, erythrocyte sedimentation rate, platelet count, prothrombin time, partial thromboblastin time, and blood glucose level.

    b. Additional blood tests should include Venereal Disease Research Laboratory (VDRL) for syphilis, antinuclear antibodies (ANA), and serum lipids.

    c. Routine imaging studies in suspected stroke include a chest radiograph, computed tomography (CT) scan (in emergencies), and magnetic resonance imaging (MRI).

    d. Additional imaging tests to evaluate stroke patients include carotid ultrasound, echocardiography, and angiography.

4. Treatment

    a. Antiplatelet therapy is initiated for ischemic stroke and transient ischemic attack, whereas **anticoagulant therapy** is indicated in the setting of cardiac embolus.

    b. Endarterectomy may be indicated if 70%–99% stenosis of the common or internal carotid artery is present.

c. Hemorrhagic stroke is treated with conservative and supportive measures, including **management of hypertension.**

B. Subarachnoid hemorrhage (SAH)

1. General characteristics

a. SAH refers to **spontaneous (nontraumatic) bleeding into the subarachnoid space.** It is usually the result of a ruptured cerebral arterial aneurysm or an arteriovenous malformation (AVM).

b. Ruptured saccular ("berry") aneurysm accounts for approximately 75% of cases of SAH. It occurs most often during the fifth and sixth decades with an approximately equal sex distribution.

c. Intracranial AVM accounts for approximately 10% of SAH. It occurs twice as often in men and typically occurs during the second to fourth decades.

2. Clinical features

a. The classic SAH presents as sudden onset of an **unusually severe generalized headache,** which patients may describe as "the worst headache I've had in my life."

b. The headache may remain unchanged for several days and subside only slowly over 1–2 weeks.

c. **Frequently, blood pressure rises precipitously** as a result of the hemorrhage.

d. Patients with an SAH may develop a **temperature** of up to 102°F, and frequently display **confusion, stupor, coma,** and **nuchal rigidity** or other signs of meningeal irritation.

3. Laboratory studies

a. **CT scan** is the initial investigation modality for suspected SAH; more than 90% of patients with aneurysmal rupture will be identified this way.

b. **Evaluation of cerebrospinal fluid (CSF)** reveals markedly elevated opening pressures and grossly bloody fluid.

c. An **echocardiogram** may reveal several abnormalities including peaked or deeply inverted T waves, a short PR interval, or tall U waves.

4. Treatment

a. **Supportive medical treatment** involves prevention of elevated arterial or intracranial pressures that might lead to rerupture of the affected vessel. It also may include strict bed rest, mild sedation, or administration of stool softeners to prevent straining.

b. **Hypertension management** is important, but care must be taken to prevent hypotension and inadequate cerebral perfusion.

c. **Surgical management** includes the clipping or wrapping of aneurysms depending on the clinical state of the patient, and either removal or embolization of an arteriovenous malformation by intra-arterial catheter.

II. SEIZURE DISORDERS

A. General characteristics

1. Seizures are **transient disturbances of cerebral function** due to abnormal, paroxysmal neuronal discharges in the brain.

2. Seizures are characterized as either **generalized** or **partial** depending on whether the disturbance affects the entire brain, or only a portion.

B. Clinical features

1. **Generalized seizures** are characterized by a sudden loss of consciousness and are either **convulsive (grand mal or tonic-clonic) seizures** or **nonconvulsive (absence) seizures.**

a. **Generalized convulsive seizures** are associated with a postictal obtundation and confusion lasting from minutes to hours.

b. **Generalized nonconvulsive seizures** are associated with only minor motor activity such as blinking.

2. Partial seizures

   a. **Simple partial seizures** are not accompanied by an impairment of consciousness. In **simple partial seizures** there may be isolated tonic or clonic activity of a limb or transient altered sensory perception. This may spread to include the entire side of the body in a "jacksonian march."

   b. **Complex partial (temporal lobe) seizures** are often characterized by an aura (transient abnormalities in sensation, perception, emotion, or memory), followed by impaired consciousness lasting seconds to minutes. Nausea or vomiting, focal sensory perceptions, and focal tonic or clonic activity may accompany a **complex seizure.**

C. Laboratory studies

   1. In **generalized seizures,** the electroencephalograph (EEG) typically shows generalized spikes and associated slow waves.

   2. In **simple partial seizures** the EEG may show a focal rhythmic discharge at the onset of the seizure, but occasionally no ictal activity will be seen.

   3. The EEG in **complex partial seizures** often reveals interictal spikes or spikes associated with slow waves in the temporal or frontotemporal areas.

   4. Other laboratory studies are indicated to evaluate **potential metabolic** or **toxic causes.**

D. Treatment

   1. **Correction of hyponatremia, hypoglycemia, or drug intoxication** may be all that is necessary to control seizures.

   2. **Anticonvulsant therapy is typically not indicated** in the setting of a single, unprovoked seizure in a patient with a normal neurologic examination and normal brain imaging and EEG.

   3. The goal of medical therapy is to **prevent seizures with a single agent in progressive doses** until seizures are controlled or until toxicity occurs.

   a. Generalized convulsive, simple partial, and complex partial seizures are typically treated with **carbamazepine, phenytoin, valproic acid, phenobarbital,** and **primidone.**

   b. **Valproic acid** or **ethosuximide** is used for generalized, nonconvulsive (absence) seizures.

III. MULTIPLE SCLEROSIS (MS)

A. General characteristics

   1. MS is characterized by inflammation associated with **multiple foci of demyelination** in the **central nervous system (CNS) white matter.**

   2. Patients with MS typically follow either a **relapsing-remitting pattern** of episodes, or a **chronic progressive course.**

   3. MS is **thought to be an immunologic disorder** associated with CNS immunoglobulin production and alteration of T lymphocytes.

B. Clinical features

   1. Patients may initially present with **any of an array of symptoms,** including **focal weakness, numbness or tingling, optic neuritis, diplopia, balance problems,** or **urinary symptoms.**

   2. The diagnosis must be questioned if signs and symptoms are not **related to multiple areas of the CNS over time.**

C. Laboratory studies

   1. An **MRI done with gadolinium** is very effective in visualizing white matter lesions in the CNS.

   2. **CSF examination** can reveal a sterile inflammation with a mild protein elevation, an elevated immunoglobulin G (IgG) index, oligoclonal bands, and increased myelin basic protein.

   3. **Visual, auditory,** and **somatosensory evoked potentials** are helpful in assessing nerve transmissions.

D. Treatment

1. **Corticosteroids** may hasten maximal recovery from acute exacerbations. High-dose intravenous corticosteroids are often used in the setting of optic neuritis.

2. **Interferon-β** decreases the frequency of relapses, especially moderate and severe attacks.

3. **Copolymer** also decreases the frequency of relapses, especially in mild disease.

4. Otherwise, therapy is **symptomatic.**

   a. Amantadine and pemoline can improve fatigue.

   b. Baclofen and diazepam improve spasticity.

   c. Several agents may relieve urologic dysfunction.

IV. DEMENTIA is characterized by **a progressive impairment of intellectual functioning** with compromise in at least 2 of the following spheres of mental activity: language, memory, visuospatial skills, emotional behavior, or personality and cognition. Alzheimer's disease is the most common form of dementia; other forms are referred to as "senile dementia."

A. Alzheimer's disease

1. **General characteristics**

   a. Alzheimer's is the **most common cause of chronic dementia,** representing 60%–80% of demented patients.

   b. The disease is characterized by **steadily progressive memory loss** and other **cognitive deficits** and typically begins in the sixth or seventh decades.

   c. **Genetic factors** in Alzheimer's have been identified, and familial cases have been mapped to chromosomes 1, 14, 19, and 21.

   d. Alzheimer's disease has a characteristic pathology consisting of **intracellular neurofibrillar tangles** and **extracellular neuritic plaques.**

2. **Clinical features**

   a. The diagnosis of Alzheimer's can be made when an **otherwise alert patient exhibits progressive memory loss and other cognitive deficits,** such as disorientation, language difficulties, inability to perform complex motor activities, inattention, visual misperception, poor problem-solving abilities, inappropriate social behavior, or hallucinations.

   b. Intellectual decline should be present in 2 or more areas of cognition and documented by a mini-mental status examination or similar scale.

   c. Formal neuropsychological testing can confirm the diagnosis and document disease progression.

3. **Laboratory studies.** Laboratory testing, including serum electrolytes, calcium, glucose, thyroid-stimulating hormone, vitamin B_{12}, renal and liver function tests, drug and alcohol levels, and MRI or CT, is only helpful in ruling out other treatable causes of dementia.

4. **Treatment**

   a. **Standard medical therapy,** initially in low doses, is useful in treating insomnia, agitation, and depression (see also Chapter 12).

   b. **Cholinesterase inhibitors,** such as tetrahydroaminoacridine, may improve memory function.

   c. The patient will require vigilant family supervision. **Day care centers** and **respite care** are adjuncts to family supervision.

B. Senile dementia

1. **General characteristics**

   a. Fifteen percent to twenty percent of patients with a chronic dementia have a **vascular dementia,** usually referred to as **multi-infarct dementia,** which includes lacunar and multiple cortical infarcts. Multi-infarct dementia is **more common in men** and is associated with hypertension with or without history of transient ischemic attack (TIA) or stroke.

   b. A similar percentage of patients (15%–20%) have evidence of both vascular and Alzheimer's-type dementia; the correct diagnosis for the large majority of these patients is Alzheimer's-type.

2. Clinical features

    a. Senile dementia is usually manifested as **forgetfulness in the absence of depression and inattentiveness.**

    b. Social graces may be well maintained, so mental status testing is important to establish the diagnosis.

    c. Progression of the disease leads to **loss of computational ability, word-finding** and **concentration problems, difficulty with routine daily activities,** and, ultimately, **complete disorientation** and **social withdrawal.**

3. Laboratory studies. Laboratory testing and imaging are only useful in establishing other, treatable, causes of dementia.

4. Treatment

    a. As in Alzheimer's, standard medical regimens can be used to treat insomnia, agitation, or depression.

    b. Caregivers should identify and reduce home hazards and arrange, as necessary, community services or preparation of an advance directive.

V. PRIMARY HEADACHE

A. Tension headache

    1. General characteristics

        a. Tension headaches are **caused by muscle contraction.** They are typified by **"band-like" pain** around the head or generalized pain.

        b. There may be an associated history of **significant stress** or **minor trauma** to the head or neck.

    2. Clinical features

        a. Discomfort is usually reported as **steady** or **aching** and is not associated with focal neurologic symptoms.

        b. Posterior cervical and occipital muscles, or the scalp, may be tender.

    3. Laboratory studies

        a. Routine laboratory tests are helpful only in ruling out concurrent illness or an underlying rheumatologic condition.

        b. Imaging studies are done only if there is a high index of suspicion for structural lesion.

        c. Lumbar puncture or electroencephalography is similarly done only for selected patients with specific clinical findings.

    4. Treatment

        a. Medical treatment is generally with **simple analgesics** such as aspirin, acetaminophen, or nonsteroidal anti-inflammatory drugs (NSAIDs).

        b. When appropriate, **local heat** and **muscle relaxants** may be employed for muscle-tension discomfort.

        c. If in the setting of depression or significant stress, **antidepressants** or **psychotherapy** may be indicated.

B. Migraine headache

    1. General characteristics

        a. Migraine headaches more typically present **unilaterally,** with **throbbing or pulsating discomfort.**

        b. Migraine patients often relate a **family history** of migraine disease.

        c. The pathophysiology of migraines has been classically attributed to intracranial vasospasm followed by extracranial vasodilatation. More current theories relate to dysfunction of the trigeminovascular system resulting in the perivascular release of substance P.

    2. Clinical features

        a. Migraine with aura (formerly called classic migraine) presents with an aura, commonly involving visual changes, field cuts, or flashing lights affecting one visual hemifield.

            (1) The throbbing pain is often contralateral to the visual aura and associated with the other symptoms seen in migraine without aura.

            (2) Migraine with aura can also be associated with transient neurologic deficits and hemisensory loss.

b. **Migraine without aura** (formerly called common migraine) is frequently accompanied by nausea, vomiting, photophobia, sonophobia, and anorexia.

c. Migraine patients often retreat to **quiet, dark rooms** and prefer to lie quietly.

3. Laboratory studies

a. Routine laboratory tests are done only to help rule out other concurrent disorders.

b. Imaging studies or lumbar puncture is done only in select clinical settings and then only to rule out causes of acute secondary headache.

4. Treatment

a. **Mild to moderate migraine headache**

(1) **Abortive therapy** may include aspirin, NSAIDs, or isometheptene.

(2) Subsequent abortive measures for migraine might include **serotonin-receptor agonists** such as sumatriptan and various forms of ergotamine.

b. In the setting of frequent migraine headache, **prophylactic measures** may be employed.

(1) **Medical prophylaxis for migraine** might include β-blockers, tricyclic antidepressants, calcium channel blockers, NSAIDs, or valproic acid.

(2) **Biofeedback therapy** is often employed in migraine patients in the hope of reducing the number of headaches by helping patients deal more effectively with stress.

C. Cluster headache

1. General characteristics

a. Cluster headaches are **severe, unilateral, periorbital headaches** that last 30–90 minutes and **occur several times a day over a period of weeks to months.**

b. Typical cluster headache patients are **middle-aged men.**

2. Clinical features

a. The unilateral pain of cluster headache is often accompanied by ipsilateral lacrimation, conjunctival injection, nasal congestion, and Horner's syndrome.

b. Patients with cluster headache often pace incessantly around the room because the pain is severe and is not relieved by rest.

3. Laboratory studies

a. As in other headache syndromes, laboratory studies only help to identify other concurrent conditions and rule out other causes of acute head and facial pain.

b. Imaging studies or lumbar puncture is only accomplished in specific clinical settings and to rule out other causes of acute cephalgia.

4. Treatment

a. **Abortive and symptomatic therapy** for cluster includes administration of 100% oxygen, ergotamines, sumatriptan, and analgesics as indicated.

b. **Prophylactic therapy** for cluster includes lithium, calcium channel blockers, and oral corticosteroids.

VI. MOVEMENT DISORDERS

A. Benign essential (familial) tremor

1. General characteristics

a. The **cause** of benign essential tremor **is unknown.** It is sometimes inherited in an autosomal dominant manner, and thus may be called familial tremor.

b. Tremor **may begin at any age.**

c. It is **enhanced by emotional stress.**

   d. Small quantities of alcohol commonly provide dramatic, temporary relief from the tremor.

   e. Although the tremor **may interfere with manual skills,** it causes only minimal disability.

2. Clinical features

   a. Patients with benign essential tremor display a **rhythmic 6- to 8-hertz to-and-fro movement,** usually of the **upper extremities** but sometimes of the **head** (titubation).

   b. Speech may also be affected if the laryngeal muscles are affected.

3. Laboratory studies. No laboratory testing is needed or warranted.

4. Treatment

   a. Low doses of β-blockers, usually propranolol, may be useful in controlling tremor but will have to be used indefinitely unless tremor is associated only with certain circumstances and intermittent dosing is helpful.

   b. Primidone may be useful in controlling tremor if propranolol fails.

B. Parkinson's disease

1. General characteristics

   a. Idiopathic Parkinson's **occurs in all ethnic groups,** with an approximately **equal sex distribution,** and begins most often between 45 and 65 years of age.

   b. Parkinson's disease is characterized by a degeneration of cells in the substantia nigra, causing a **deficiency of the neurotransmitter dopamine** and an **imbalance of dopamine and acetylcholine.**

   c. Patients with Parkinson's generally complain of problems related to their slowed movements, difficulty arising from a seated position, difficulty ascending and descending stairs, trouble getting dressed, and difficulty with handwriting.

2. Clinical features

   a. The essential features that are **diagnostic** in Parkinson's include: **resting tremor, bradykinesia, rigidity,** and **postural instability.**

   b. The **tremor is most noticeable at rest,** at about 4–6 cycles per second, and may be only very slight with voluntary effort.

   c. Initially the tremor is **confined to one limb or the limbs on one side,** but may eventually be present in all limbs, and the lips and mouth.

   d. Bradykinesia, or a **generalized slowness of voluntary movements,** is evident in the slow, shuffling gait, the reduced arm swing, slowed rapid alternating movements, infrequent blinking, and masklike facies.

   e. Rigidity is noted with passive range of motion testing and **cogwheel rigidity** may be noted.

   f. Postural instability is noted, including difficulty in standing from a seated position, unsteadiness on turning, difficulty in stopping, and a tendency to fall.

   g. Cognitive impairment develops in over 50% of patients over time.

3. Laboratory studies. Generally, no laboratory testing is needed or warranted.

4. Treatment

   a. Treatment is designed to best **restore the balance between dopamine and acetylcholine** either by blocking the effect of acetylcholine with anticholinergic drugs, or by administering levodopa (the precursor of dopamine) or a combination of both.

   b. Amantadine, a mild anticholinergic, is often helpful for patients with mild symptoms but no disability.

   c. Benztropine and other anticholinergic drugs are particularly helpful in treating the tremor of Parkinson's.

   d. Levodopa is converted to dopamine in the body and improves all symptoms of Parkinson's. **Carbidopa,** when added to levodopa in various combinations, allows for lower doses of levodopa and reduced side effects.

   e. Dopamine agonists, such as bromocriptine, act directly on dopamine receptors and are often reserved for patients who become refractory to levodopa therapy.

   f. Physical therapy may help some patients, and quality of life may be improved with **household modifications** or the **availability of special utensils.**

C. Huntington's disease

1. General characteristics

a. Huntington's disease is an **inherited autosomal dominant disorder** and occurs throughout the world in all ethnic groups, with a prevalence of approximately **5 per 100,000.**

b. The gene responsible for Huntington's disease is on **chromosome 4.**

c. Symptoms of the disease usually **do not develop until after 30 years of age.** By this time, those who are affected have often already had children who may be similarly affected.

2. Clinical features

a. The disease is characterized by **progressive chorea** and **dementia,** which usually is fatal within 15–20 years.

b. The **earliest mental changes are often behavioral,** with irritability, moodiness, and antisocial behavior that generally progress to an obvious dementia.

c. The **earliest physical signs may be a mere restlessness** or fidgetiness but eventually severe choreiform movements and dystonic posturing occur.

3. Laboratory studies. **CT scanning** usually demonstrates cerebral atrophy and atrophy of the caudate nucleus.

4. Treatment

a. Huntington's disease has **no cure** and **progression of the disease cannot be halted.**

b. **Symptomatic treatment** for the disease may include phenothiazines to control dyskinesia, and haloperidol or clozapine to control any behavioral disturbances.

c. Offspring of Huntington's patients should receive **genetic counseling** in conjunction with genetic testing, which is now available for making a definitive diagnosis even in the presymptomatic state.

D. Tourette's syndrome

1. General characteristics

a. Tourette's syndrome is characterized by **multiple motor and phonic tics,** with the **onset of symptoms occurring in childhood** between the ages of 2 and 25 years.

b. For a diagnosis of Tourette's syndrome the **tics must occur frequently for at least a year** and vary in number, frequency, and nature.

2. Clinical features

a. **Motor tics involving the face, head, and shoulders** (e.g., sniffing, blinking, frowning, shoulder shrugging, and head thrusting) occur initially in 80% of patients.

b. **Phonic tics,** initially seen in approximately 20% of patients, are characterized as **grunts, barks, hisses, coughing, or verbal utterances.**

c. Some tics are self-mutilating and may include nail-biting, hair-pulling, and biting of the lips or tongue.

3. Laboratory studies. All diagnostic evaluations are normal, with the exception of possible minor, nonspecific EEG changes that have no diagnostic relevance.

4. Treatment

a. **Haloperidol** is generally regarded as the drug of choice for treatment, with doses slowly increased until maximum benefit with minimal side effects.

b. **Clonazepam or clonidine** may also be helpful and can minimize the side effects of long-term haloperidol use.

E. Wilson's disease

1. General characteristics

a. Wilson's disease results from a **deficiency in the copper-binding protein ceruloplasmin** leading to accumulation of copper in the brain, liver, and other tissues.

b. Wilson's disease is an **autosomal recessive disorder localized to chromosome 13** that usually presents between the first and third decades.

2. Clinical features

   a. Slit lamp examination reveals **Kayser-Fleischer rings (representing copper deposition) of the cornea,** the pathognomonic sign of the condition.

   b. Movement disorders seen in Wilson's disease include **rigidity, parkinsonian tremor, masklike facies, dystonia,** and **athetosis.**

3. Laboratory studies

   a. Diagnosis is established by a **low serum ceruloplasmin level** and **increased levels of hepatic copper.**

   b. A **24-hour urine test** will show **increased copper excretion.**

   c. Complete blood count (CBC) may show a hemolytic anemia.

   d. **MRI** can reveal atrophy of the caudate and putamen with increased signal intensity on T-2 weighted images.

4. Treatment

   a. Therapy for Wilson's disease consists of **copper chelation,** with penicillamine being the drug of choice.

   b. **Liver transplantation** is indicated for fulminant hepatitis and end-stage cirrhosis.

VII. PERIPHERAL NEURAL DISORDERS

A. Polyneuropathy

   1. General considerations

   a. Peripheral nerves can be affected by:

   (1) Inherited and immune system-mediated diseases

   (2) Several metabolic or toxic conditions

   (3) Idiopathic inflammatory polyneuropathy (Guillain-Barré syndrome)

   b. The pathologic feature of a polyneuropathy may be:

   (1) **Axonal degeneration** (axonal or neuronal neuropathies)

   (2) **Paranodal** or **segmental demyelination**

   c. Diffuse polyneuropathies produce a **symmetric sensory, motor,** or **mixed deficit,** most often marked distally.

   d. **Diabetes mellitus** may lead to **symmetric motor neuropathy** (diabetic amyotrophy), a thoracoabdominal radiculopathy, autonomic neuropathy, or isolated lesions of individual nerves; these may occur singly or in any combination.

   e. **Uremia** may produce a symmetric sensorimotor polyneuropathy typically affecting the lower extremities more than the upper and more distally than proximally.

   f. **Alcoholics** may have an axonal distal polyneuropathy accompanied by painful cramps, muscle tenderness, and painful paresthesias more marked in the legs than in the arms.

   g. **Infectious** and **inflammatory conditions** associated with neuropathy include leprosy, AIDS, Lyme disease, sarcoidosis, polyarteritis, and rheumatoid arthritis.

   2. Clinical features

   a. Patients with peripheral neuropathy commonly complain of **changes in sensation** (often described as numbness or tingling) or **pain described as aching, burning, or sharp.**

   b. **Disorders affecting large fibers** (the immune-mediated demyelinative neuropathies) often result in a **painless numbness** and **decreased sensation to light touch** and vibration as well as weakness.

   c. **Disorders affecting small fibers** (diabetes, amyloidosis) frequently are **painful** and can cause **decreased sensation** to **touch, pinprick, and temperature.**

   d. Involvement of motor fibers leads to a **flaccid weakness that is most marked distally,** and deep tendon reflexes may be depressed or absent.

    e. **Guillain-Barré syndrome often follows infective illness or inoculations** and is associated with preceding *Campylobacter jejuni* enteritis.

    f. **Weakness is the chief complaint** in Guillain-Barré. The weakness begins in the legs and spreads to the arms, face, and possibly the muscles of respiration or deglutition.

3. Laboratory studies

    a. Conduction velocity in electromyography (EMG)

        (1) In **axonal neuropathies,** conduction velocity is normal or only mildly reduced and needle EMG demonstrates denervation in affected muscles.

        (2) In **demyelinating neuropathies,** conduction may be markedly slowed in affected fibers and, in severe cases, blocked completely.

    b. Cutaneous nerve biopsy may help provide the diagnosis, but, in most cases, no specific etiology is identified.

4. Treatment

    a. Treatment is of the **underlying cause** when it can be established, with symptomatic therapy as needed.

    b. **Physical therapy** helps prevent contractures.

    c. **Splints** and other supports may be utilized for weak limbs.

    d. Anesthetic areas, particularly in the distal extremities, must be protected from injury by heat or pressure.

B. Mononeuropathy

1. General considerations

    a. A nerve may become **injured** or **compressed** by adjacent anatomic structures at any point along its course. This leads to sensory, motor, or a mixed deficit **restricted to the area of the affected nerve.**

    b. The relative contributions of mechanical factors and ischemia to local nerve damage are not clear.

2. Clinical features

    a. With involvement of a sensory or mixed nerve, **pain** is commonly felt **distal to the lesion.**

    b. **Percussion** of the nerve at the site of the compression or injury **may produce distal paresthesias.**

    c. **Ulnar nerve lesions** are likely to occur.

        (1) At the **medial epicondyle** of the elbow, ulnar nerve lesions produce sensory changes in the medial 1½ digits and along the medial border of the hand, with weakness of the associated muscles of the forearm and hand.

        (2) At the **wrist** or in the **palm of the hand,** ulnar nerve lesions may develop secondary to repetitive trauma, ganglia, or benign tremors.

    d. **Radial nerve injuries** commonly occur.

        (1) In the **axilla,** radial nerve injuries produce weakness or paralysis, including the triceps muscle.

        (2) The radial nerve can also be injured at the **spiral groove** during deep sleep or in intoxicated individuals (Saturday night palsy), but the triceps is spared.

        (3) The radial nerve may also be injured at the elbow area by the branch of the nerve supplying the extensors of the wrist and fingers.

        (4) The superficial radial nerve may be compressed by handcuffs or a tight watch band.

    e. **Femoral neuropathy**

        (1) **Weakness** and **wasting of the quadriceps muscle** result from femoral neuropathy, with sensory changes over the anteromedial aspect of the thigh.

        (2) The femoral nerve may also be compressed by the inguinal ligament when the thighs are markedly flexed and abducted, as in the lithotomy position.

        (3) Meralgia paresthetica (compression of the lateral femoral cutaneous nerve) produces pain, paresthesia, or numbness at the lateral aspect of the thigh and is associated with obese and pregnant women.

    f. Injury to the **common peroneal nerve** at the head or neck of the fibula (caused by sitting cross-legged or wearing high boots) may produce weakness of dorsiflexion and eversion of the foot, accompanied by numbness or blunted sensation of the anterolateral aspect of the calf and dorsum of the foot.

    g. **Sciatic nerve** injuries most commonly result from misplaced deep intramuscular injection, but may be caused by trauma to the buttock, hip, or thigh.

    h. Tarsal tunnel syndrome results from compression of the **posterior tibial nerve** as it passes behind and below the medial malleolus causing pain, paresthesia, and numbness over the bottom of the foot, sparing the heel.

    i. **Carpal tunnel syndrome** results from compression of the **median nerve** as it passes through the carpal tunnel causing burning and tingling initially, and then activity-related pain in the distribution of the median nerve. It may be evidenced by a positive **Tinel's sign** (tingling or shock-like pain on volar wrist percussion) or **Phalen's sign** (pain or paresthesias with wrist flexion to 90° of 60 seconds).

3. **Laboratory studies.** Electrodiagnostic studies may be necessary to evaluate and monitor evidence of partial denervation in weak muscles.

4. **Treatment**

    a. No treatment is necessary in most cases of mononeuropathy and **complete recovery occurs within 2 months.**

    b. In chronic compression or nerve entrapment, careful **avoidance of aggravating factors** and **correction of any concurrent systemic condition** are necessary.

    c. Local infiltration with **corticosteroids** may be of value.

    d. **Surgical decompression** may be necessary in the setting of progressive neurologic deficit.

VIII. CENTRAL NERVOUS SYSTEM INFECTION

A. Bacterial meningitis

    1. General characteristics

        a. Typical symptoms of meningitis are based on 3 processes: **inflammation, increased intracranial pressure,** or **tissue necrosis.**

        b. **Causes** of bacterial meningitis tend to **vary with the age of the patient.** *Escherichia coli* is seen frequently in infants, *Haemophilus influenzae* in children up to approximately 6 years, *Neisseria meningitidis* in adolescents and young adults, and *Streptococcus pneumoniae* in adults.

    2. Clinical features

        a. **Fever, headache, vomiting,** and a **stiff neck** are the typical signs and symptoms of meningitis, although all may not be present.

        b. Symptoms are **typically acute,** with patients presenting within hours, or 1–2 days, of infection.

        c. Careful initial examination may reveal evidence of **soft tissue abscess,** otitis, or other **parameningeal infection.**

        d. **Meningeal signs** may be absent or very subtle at the age extremes, or difficult to assess with impaired consciousness.

    3. Laboratory studies

        a. Prompt **lumbar puncture** and **CSF analysis** are essential, following **imaging studies** to rule out evidence of increased intracranial pressure.

        b. The CSF may be slightly turbid to grossly purulent.

        c. CSF pressure is elevated in approximately 90% of cases.

        d. CSF white cell count is elevated, ranging from 1000 to as high as 10,000, with increased neutrophils.

        e. CSF protein concentrations of 100–500 mg/dl are most common.

        f. CSF glucose levels are often decreased, and may be less than 40 mg/dl.

        g. Gram stain and cultures of the CSF are diagnostic in approximately 80% of cases.

4. Treatment

    a. Antibiotic treatment is begun immediately if the CSF is not clear and colorless. The initial choice of antibiotic is **based empirically on the patient's age.**

        (1) Neonates receive ampicillin and gentamicin.

        (2) Infants up to 3 months of age receive the same combination, with higher doses of gentamicin.

        (3) Children and adolescents up to 18 years of age generally receive a third-generation cephalosporin, or ampicillin plus chloramphenicol.

        (4) Adults generally receive penicillin G, IV or ampicillin.

        (5) The elderly are generally treated with ampicillin plus a third-generation cephalosporin.

        (6) If the meningitis is postsurgical or posttraumatic, the patient generally receives a third-generation cephalosporin, with or without nafcillin to cover *Staphylococcus aureus* and gram-negative bacilli.

    b. Repeat lumbar puncture and **CSF analysis** are crucial to assess response to treatment.

        (1) The CSF should be sterile after 24 hours.

        (2) A decrease in pleocytosis and the proportion of neutrophils should be seen within 3 days.

B. Viral (aseptic) meningitis and encephalitis

  1. General considerations

    a. The most frequent causes of these infections are **enteric viruses** in the summer and fall: 50% are **coxsackievirus** A or B, 30% are **echoviruses,** and 10%–15% are **mumps virus.**

    b. Aseptic meningitis may also reflect an inflammatory process in the parameningeal area (i.e., sinusitis, otitis, abscess).

  2. Clinical features

    a. Viral meningitis and encephalitis often present as an **acute confusional state,** especially in children and young adults.

    b. Signs and symptoms are generally not as acute and may have persisted for several days.

    c. Examination may reveal a number of **systemic manifestations** suggesting a particular etiologic agent (e.g., rash, pharyngitis, adenopathy, pleuritis, carditis, jaundice, organomegaly, diarrhea).

    d. In **encephalitis,** because it involves the brain directly, there may be **marked altered consciousness, seizures, or other focal neurologic signs.**

  3. Laboratory studies

    a. As with bacterial meningitis, **prompt lumbar puncture** and **CSF analysis** are crucial, after assessing for evidence of increased intracranial pressure.

    b. The CSF opening pressure is generally normal.

    c. Cells present in the CSF are more likely to be lymphocytes or monocytes, and the count is generally less than 1000.

    d. The CSF protein, glucose, and serum blood counts are more likely to be normal.

  4. Treatment

    a. The course of aseptic meningitis is generally **benign and self-limited,** with no specific therapy required.

    b. Mild headaches can be treated with **acetaminophen.**

    c. Seizures can be suppressed with **anticonvulsants.**

    d. Breathing can be supported, if necessary.

C. Brain abscess

  1. General characteristics

    a. Brain abscess typically results from direct **spread of infection from sinus, ear, or soft tissue infection;** hematogenous spread to the brain is rare.

    b. Abscesses may be localized to the **extradural (epidural) space, subdural spaces,** or in the **brain parenchyma.**

2. Clinical features

    a. Brain abscesses present as a **space-occupying lesion;** symptoms may include **vomiting, fever, altered mental status,** or with **focal neurologic signs.**

    b. These signs and symptoms may have been preceded by **previous evidence of otitis, sinusitis, or pharyngitis.**

3. Laboratory studies

    a. A **lumbar puncture** and **CSF analysis** should be performed, following a CT scan.

    b. The **CT,** or **MRI,** is helpful in establishing the diagnosis, especially if done with a contrast medium.

    c. The bacteriology of brain abscess is usually **polymicrobial** and may include both gram-positive and gram-negative organisms.

4. Treatment

    a. Acute treatment may involve **respiratory and circulatory support, airway management,** and **monitoring of other vital functions.**

    b. Brain abscesses are treated with **appropriate antibiotics that penetrate brain tissues well,** including penicillin, chloramphenicol, and metronidazole.

    c. **Surgical excision or decompression** may be required in cases of very large lesions or a delayed response to therapy.

IX. PAIN SYNDROMES

A. Discogenic low back pain

  1. General characteristics

    a. **Disease of the vertebral discs, including prolapse, nerve pathology, or degenerative disease,** may produce **local pain, root (radicular) pain,** or **pain referred to other parts of the involved dermatomes.**

    b. **Local pain** may result in secondary, reflex muscle spasm causing further pain as well as altered posture and limited movement.

    c. **Radicular pain** arises from compression, stretching, or irritation of nerve roots, being exacerbated by coughing, straining, or movements stretching the nerve fibers.

    d. Root disturbances may produce paresthesias and numbness in a dermatomal distribution and may lead to weakness in segmental distribution.

    e. Reflex changes may accompany involvement of motor or sensory nerve fibers.

  2. Clinical features

    a. Acute intervertebral disc prolapse generally involves the L4-L5 or the L5-S1 disc and leads to back and radicular pain.

    b. An L-5 radiculopathy causes weakness of dorsiflexion in the foot and toes.

    c. An S-1 root lesion produces weakness of eversion and plantar flexion of the foot, and a depressed ankle jerk.

    d. A centrally prolapsed disc may produce bilateral limb disturbances.

    e. Degenerative lumbar disc disease may lead to local pain, stiffness, and restricted activity.

  3. Laboratory studies

    a. **Plain radiographs** help to rule out other disorders such as local primary cancers or metastatic deposits.

    b. **CT myelography** or **MRI** is utilized in the setting of persistent pain and/or increasing neurologic deficit.

    c. **Electromyography** may be helpful in assessing the extent and severity of root involvement.

  4. Treatment

    a. Symptoms are generally relieved with **rest, NSAID analgesics,** and **muscle relaxants.**

    b. Persistent or increasing neurologic compromise requires **surgical treatment.**

    c. Long-term therapy may include **back strengthening exercises** and **weight loss,** if appropriate.

B. Discogenic neck pain

1. General characteristics

   a. A number of **congenital abnormalities** may involve the cervical spine and lead to neck pain; including hemivertebrae, fused vertebrae, basilar impression, and instability of the atlantoaxial joint.

   b. When **rheumatoid arthritis** involves the spine, it tends especially to affect the cervical region.

   c. Neck pain may also be caused by **disc protrusion, herniation,** or **degenerative disease.**

2. Clinical features

   a. Acute **cervical disc protrusion** produces neck pain and **radicular pain in the arm,** made worse by head movement.

   b. With **lateral herniation** (often C6 or C7) motor, sensory, or reflex changes may be seen on the affected side.

   c. With a more **central herniation** the spinal cord may be involved leading to **spastic paraparesis and sensory disturbances in the legs.**

   d. Severe **cervical degenerative disease** may result in compression, stretching, or angulation of one or more nerve roots, producing neck pain, occipital headaches, restricted head movement, or a variety of **radicular symptoms in the upper as well as lower extremities.**

3. Laboratory studies

   a. **MRI** or **CT myelography** will confirm a diagnosis of acute disc protrusion.

   b. **Routine radiographs** may show evidence of cervical spondylosis resulting from chronic cervical disc degeneration.

   c. **Electromyography** may be helpful in determining the extent and severity of root involvement.

4. Treatment

   a. In mild cases of discogenic neck pain, **bed rest** or **intermittent neck traction** may be helpful, followed by **immobilization in a collar** for several weeks.

   b. If conservative measures are unsuccessful or there is an increasing neurologic deficit, **surgical removal of the protrusion** may be necessary.

C. Herpes zoster (shingles)

1. General characteristics

   a. Herpes zoster results from the **spontaneous reactivation of the latent varicella virus.**

   b. Herpes zoster becomes **increasingly common with advancing age** and is common in **patients with lymphoma,** especially following radiotherapy.

2. Clinical features

   a. The initial complaint is of a **burning or shooting pain in the involved dermatome,** followed within 2–5 days by the development of a **vesicular erythematous rash.**

   b. The rash becomes crusted and scaly after a few days and then fades, leaving small anesthetic scars.

   c. Signs are **usually limited to a single dermatome,** most commonly on the thorax.

   d. If the first division of the 5th cranial nerve (CN) is involved, the patient may develop corneal scarring.

   e. The pain and dysesthesias may last for **several weeks,** or may persist for **many months** (postherpetic neuralgia).

   f. The pain of shingles is exacerbated by touching the involved area.

3. **Laboratory studies.** No laboratory testing is needed or warranted.

4. Treatment

   a. **Corticosteroids** may lesson the risk of postherpetic neuralgia if utilized during the acute phase.

   b. Corticosteroids, as well as **acyclovir,** or **famciclovir,** may reduce the duration and severity of the acute eruption.

   c. The chronic pain syndrome can be treated with **tricyclic antidepressants, carbamazepine,** or **phenytoin.**

D. Reflex sympathetic dystrophy (RSD)

    1. General characteristics

        a. RSD is a **chronic, sympathetically mediated pain condition** that can occur idiopathically or develop following **minor soft tissue trauma** to a limb, bone fracture, or myocardial infarction.

        b. The **disparity between the severity of the inciting injury and the degree of pain experienced** is the most characteristic feature.

    2. Clinical features

        a. Early in RSD, the **pain, tenderness,** and **hyperesthesia** may be **strictly localized to the site of the injury** and the extremity may be warm, dry, swollen and red, or slightly cyanotic.

        b. The involved extremity is held in a splinted position, and the nails may become ridged and the hair long.

        c. When advanced, the **pain is more diffuse and worse at night;** the limb becomes cool and clammy and intolerant of temperature changes, with the skin becoming glossy and atrophic.

        d. The **joints of the affected limb become stiff,** generally in a position that renders the extremity useless.

    3. **Laboratory studies. Radiographs** of the affected limb may reveal severe osteopenia, in excess of that anticipated due to simple disuse.

    4. Treatment

        a. It is vital that the condition be **diagnosed** and **treated early,** before major secondary changes develop.

        b. **Physical therapy** combined with **diazepam** or **alprazolam** may relieve symptoms in mild, early cases with minimal skin and joint changes.

        c. **Paravertebral sympathetic ganglion blocks** and **aggressive physical therapy** are typically employed if advanced or severe.

        d. **Medical management** may include tricyclic antidepressants or anticonvulsants.

X. NEUROMUSCULAR DISORDERS

A. Myasthenia gravis

    1. General characteristics

        a. Myasthenia gravis involves **muscle weakness and fatigability, which improves with rest.**

        b. The **onset** of myasthenia gravis is **usually insidious** but the disorder is sometimes made evident by a **coincidental infection** that exacerbates the symptoms.

        c. The disorder may occur at any age, but is **more common in young women** and older men.

        d. Antibodies directed against the acetylcholine receptor on the muscle surface cause an **increased rate of receptor destruction leading to weakness.**

    2. Clinical features

        a. Typical presenting problems include **ptosis, diplopia, difficulty in chewing or swallowing, respiratory difficulties, limb weakness,** or a combination of any of these.

        b. Symptoms may **fluctuate in intensity during the day,** and there is a tendency to longer term spontaneous relapses and remissions that may last for weeks.

        c. Clinical examination confirms the weakness and fatigability of affected muscles, which improve after a short rest.

        d. **Sensation is normal,** and there are **usually no reflex changes.**

        e. The diagnosis may be confirmed if **marked clinical improvement** is achieved by administering a short-acting anticholinesterase, **edrophonium.**

    3. Laboratory studies

        a. **Lateral** and **anteroposterior chest radiographs** should be obtained to rule out a coexisting thymoma.

        b. **Electrophysiologic studies** may show a decrementing muscle response.

  c. Assay of serum **for elevated levels of circulating acetylcholine receptor antibodies** is another way of diagnosing the condition in 80%–90% of patients.

 4. Treatment

  a. The mainstay of therapy is administration of a **cholinesterase inhibitor** such as pyridostigmine. It produces a transient improvement in strength.

  b. **Thymectomy** often leads to improvement of symptoms.

  c. **Corticosteroids, immunosuppressive agents, intravenous immunoglobulin,** or **plasmapheresis** are effective in patients with refractory disease.

B. Amyotrophic lateral sclerosis (ALS)

 1. General characteristics

  a. ALS has a prevalence of approximately 1 in 100,000 with **half of the patients dying within 3 years of the onset** of disease.

  b. The **cause of ALS is unknown,** although the gene for familial ALS has been localized to chromosome 21 and other evidence points toward a possible immunopathogenesis.

 2. Clinical features

  a. Progressive weakness is the hallmark of ALS.

  b. Patients typically exhibit signs of both **upper and lower motor neuron dysfunction.**

  c. Early in the disease, weakness is usually focal and may only affect **speech, swallowing, or the use of a single extremity.**

 3. Laboratory studies

  a. **Electromyography** may show changes of chronic partial denervation, with abnormal spontaneous activity in resting muscle.

  b. **Motor conduction velocity** is usually normal and **sensory conduction studies** are also normal.

  c. **Biopsy** of a wasted muscle shows the histologic changes of denervation.

 4. Treatment

  a. Therapy is **supportive,** as there is **no cure.**

  b. Particular attention is paid to providing **support for breathing and swallowing** functions.

C. Muscular dystrophy

 1. General characteristics

  a. The muscular dystrophies are a group of **inherited myopathic disorders** characterized by **progressive muscle weakness and wasting.**

  b. The various dystrophies are subdivided by mode of inheritance, age of onset, and clinical features.

   (1) **Duchenne's muscular dystrophy** is an X-linked recessive disorder. The onset is in early childhood, and many patients do not become weak until 3–5 years of age.

   (2) **Becker's muscular dystrophy** is an X-linked recessive disorder with a much more benign course than Duchenne's. Patients are often able to walk into their late twenties.

   (3) **Myotonic muscular dystrophy** is an autosomal dominant disorder with the onset of symptoms usually occurring between the ages of 2–25 years.

 2. Clinical features

  a. In **Duchenne's muscular dystrophy,** patients initially have progressive proximal weakness, followed eventually by distal weakness and respiratory distress, and death by the third decade.

  b. In **Becker's muscular dystrophy,** patients follow a more benign course with 50% survival to age 50 with predominantly proximal (pelvic and shoulder girdle) symptoms.

  c. In **myotonic muscular dystrophy,** patients display a characteristic muscle myotonia, distal weakness, cataracts, frontal balding, impaired intellect, hypersomnia, testicular atrophy, cardiomyopathy, mitral valve prolapse, and cardiac conduction defects, with death in the fifth or sixth decade, typically due to respiratory compromise or cardiac arrhythmia.

3. Laboratory studies

    a. Patients typically have an **elevated serum creatine kinase level.**

    b. **Electromyography** demonstrates a myopathic pattern (i.e., brief, small-amplitude muscle potentials).

    c. **Muscle biopsy** is often informative.

4. Treatment

    a. There is **no specific treatment** for the muscular dystrophies.

    b. **Physical therapy** and **orthopedic procedures** can often lessen or prevent deformities and contractures.

    c. **Prolonged bed rest must be avoided,** because inactivity often leads to a worsening of disability.

XI. CENTRAL NERVOUS SYSTEM TRAUMA

A. Brain injury

    1. General characteristics

        a. **Head injury** accounts for nearly half of the trauma-related deaths in young people.

        b. Prognosis is directly related to the site and severity of brain damage.

        c. **Loss of consciousness for greater than 2 minutes implies a worse prognosis.**

        d. The degree of retrograde and post-traumatic amnesia is also directly related to the severity of brain injury.

    2. Clinical features

        a. During the physical examination, special attention must be given to **level of consciousness** and to the extent of any **brain stem dysfunction.**

        b. In **concussion,** there may be a brief loss of consciousness with bradycardia, hypotension, and respiratory arrest for a few seconds.

        c. In the setting of **acute epidural hemorrhage,** signs and symptoms might include headache, confusion, somnolence, seizures, and focal deficits occurring several hours after the injury.

        d. **Bruising** may be on the side of the injury (referred to as a "coup injury") or contralaterally ("contracoup injury").

    3. Laboratory studies

        a. **Skull radiographs** or **CT scans** may detect skull fractures, and further studies of the cervical spine should be done to look for related injuries.

        b. **CT scanning** is also important to demonstrate intracranial hemorrhage, to show evidence of cerebral edema, and to identify displacement of midline structures.

    4. Treatment

        a. **Surgical evacuation** may be necessary following acute epidural, acute subdural, and cerebral hemorrhage.

        b. Increased intracranial pressures may be relieved by **induced hyperventilation, intravenous mannitol infusion,** and **intravenous furosemide.**

B. Spinal cord injury

    1. General characteristics

        a. Whiplash injury may cause spinal cord damage, but severe injury typically relates to fracture or dislocation causing compression or angular deformity of the cord.

        b. Sites of injury may extend from the cervical to the upper lumbar region.

        c. Extreme hypotension following acute injury may result in cord infarction.

2. Clinical features

    a. Total cord transection

        (1) Total cord transection results in **immediate flaccid paralysis** and **loss of sensation** below the level of the lesion.

        (2) **Reflex activity is lost** for a variable time, and there is urinary and fecal retention.

        (3) With the slow return of reflex function, **spastic paraplegia or quadriplegia develops,** with hyperreflexia and extensor plantar responses.

    b. Lesser cord injury

        (1) Patients may be left with mild limb weakness or distal sensory disturbance.

        (2) Sphincter function impairment may lead to urinary urgency and urgency incontinence.

    c. A **unilateral cord lesion** produces an ipsilateral motor disturbance with accompanying impairment of proprioception and contralateral loss of pain and temperature below the lesion (Brown-Séquard's syndrome).

    d. A **central cord syndrome** may lead to a lower motor neuron deficit and loss of pain and temperature, with sparing of posterior column functions.

    e. A **radicular deficit** may occur at the level of the injury; if the cauda equina is involved, there may be dysfunction in several lumbosacral roots.

3. **Laboratory studies.** No laboratory testing is needed or warranted.

4. Treatment

    a. Treatment of spinal cord injury involves **immobilization,** as well as **decompressive laminectomy** and **fusion** if there is cord compression.

    b. **Early treatment with high-dose corticosteroids** has been shown to improve neurologic recovery if commenced within 8 hours of the injury.

    c. **Anatomic realignment of the spinal cord** by traction and other orthopedic procedures is important.

    d. Subsequent care of **residual neurologic deficit** requires therapy for spasticity and care of the skin, bowel, and bladder.

XII. PRIMARY CENTRAL NERVOUS SYSTEM NEOPLASMS

A. General characteristics

    1. Approximately half of all primary intracranial neoplasms are gliomas, and the remainder are meningiomas, pituitary adenomas, neurofibromas, and others.

    2. Approximately 10% of spinal tumors are intramedullary, with ependymoma being the most common.

    3. Certain tumors, especially neurofibromas, hemangioblastomas, and retinoblastomas, may have a familial basis.

    4. The most common source of intracranial metastasis is carcinoma of the lung, breast, kidney, and the gastrointestinal tract.

B. Clinical features

    1. Spinal tumors may lead to spinal cord dysfunction by direct compression, by ischemia secondary to arterial or venous obstruction, or by invasive infiltration.

    2. Intracranial tumors may produce a generalized **disturbance of cerebral function** and lead to evidence of increased intracranial pressure (i.e., personality changes, intellectual decline, emotional lability, seizures, headaches, nausea, and malaise).

    3. Intracranial tumors may also produce **focal deficits** depending on their location.

        a. **Frontal lobe lesions** often produce progressive intellectual decline, slowing of mental activity, personality changes, contralateral grasp reflexes, and possible expressive aphasia.

        b. **Temporal lobe lesions** may lead to seizures, olfactory or gustatory hallucinations, licking or smacking of the lips, depersonalization, emotional and behavioral changes, visual field defects, and auditory illusions.

    c. Parietal lobe lesions typically cause contralateral disturbances of sensation and may cause sensory seizures, a cortical sensory loss (impaired stereognosis) or inattention, or some combination of all these.

    d. Occipital lobe lesions characteristically produce crossed homonymous hemianopia or a partial field defect, visual agnosia for objects and colors, or unformed visual hallucinations.

    e. Brain stem and cerebellar lesions produce cranial nerve palsies, ataxia, incoordination, nystagmus, and pyramidal and sensory deficits in the limbs on one or both sides.

  4. Symptoms of spinal tumors usually develop insidiously, with pain characteristically aggravated by coughing or straining and either localized to the back or felt diffusely in an extremity as motor defects, paresthesias, or numbness, especially in the legs.

  5. Physical examination of patients with spinal tumors may reveal **localized spinal tenderness.**

C. Laboratory studies

  1. CT or MRI with contrast may detect the lesion, define its location and size, evaluate the extent to which normal anatomy is distorted, and the degree of any associated cerebral edema or mass effect.

  2. Arteriography may demonstrate stretching or displacement of normal cerebral vessels, as well as the presence of tumor vascularity.

  3. EEG may demonstrate a focal disturbance due to the neoplasm or a more diffuse change reflecting altered mental status.

  4. CT myelography or **MRI** may be needed to identify and localize the site of spinal cord compression.

  5. CSF removed at myelography is often xanthochromic and contains greatly increased protein concentration, normal cell content, and normal glucose concentration.

D. Treatment

  1. Complete surgical removal of the tumor may be possible if it is extra-axial or is not in a critical or inaccessible region of the brain.

  2. Surgical **shunting** of an obstructive hydrocephalus may dramatically reduce clinical deficits.

  3. Radiation or **chemotherapy,** or both, increases median survival rates regardless of any preceding surgery.

  4. Corticosteroids help reduce cerebral edema and are usually started prior to surgery.

  5. Anticonvulsants are commonly administered in standard doses.

  6. Intramedullary cord lesions are treated by **decompression** and **surgical excision** and by **irradiation.**

  7. Treatment of epidural spinal metastases consists of **irradiation,** irrespective of cell type.

XIII. SLEEP DISORDERS

A. General characteristics

  1. Dyssomnia (insomnia) complaints include difficulty getting to sleep or staying asleep, intermittent wakefulness during the night, early morning awakenings, or combinations of all. Psychiatric disorders, including depression and manic disorders, are often associated with persistent insomnia.

  2. Hypersomnia (excessive daytime sleepiness) is generally a more severe problem and may manifest in patients with sleep apnea, narcolepsy, or those who demonstrate nocturnal myoclonus.

  3. Parasomnias (abnormal behaviors during sleep) include sleep terrors, nightmares, sleepwalking, and enuresis.

B. Clinical features

  1. Taking a **careful history** of those with insomnia may reveal depression, abuse of alcohol, heavy smoking (more than 1 pack a day), inappropriate use of sedatives-hypnotics, or a medical history including uremia, asthma, or hypothyroidism.

  2. Sleep apnea is often seen in obese middle-aged and older men with hypertension and associated congestive heart failure.

3. Patients with **narcolepsy** experience sudden, brief sleep attacks, cataplexy, sleep paralysis, and hypnagogic hallucinations, which may precede sleep.

C. **Laboratory studies**

   1. **Polysomnography (sleep studies)** assesses EEG activity, heart rate, respiratory movement, and oxygen saturation.

   2. **Thyroid studies** may be helpful if hypothyroidism is suggested.

D. **Treatment**

   1. **Insomnia**

      a. In transient insomnia, **de-emphasis** and **reassurance** are sufficient treatment.

      b. A variety of **"sleep hygiene"** rules should be discussed to remove numerous barriers to effective sleep.

      c. Medications should be avoided if possible, but **antihistamines** may be effective for milder problems while **rapidly acting** hypnotics may be used for short periods if necessary.

   2. **Sleep apnea treatment** includes **weight reduction,** if appropriate, and administration of air under continuous pressure through the nasopharynx during sleep, called **continuous positive airway pressure (CPAP).**

   3. Narcolepsy is managed by administration of **stimulants.**

   4. **Nocturnal myoclonus** is typically treated with clonazepam.

   5. **Sleep terror** and **sleep walking** can be treated with benzodiazepines.

12

Psychiatry

Francis J. Winn, Jr.
Charles C. Lewis

I. DIAGNOSIS OF PSYCHIATRIC DISORDERS IN THE UNITED STATES

A. Background

    1. Psychiatric diagnoses conform to the *Diagnostic and Statistical Manual of Mental Disorders,* 4th edition (DSM-IV).

    2. DSM-IV has gained wide acceptance because professionals from a number of specialties outside of psychiatry (e.g., internal medicine, family practice, psychology, social work, clergy, occupational therapy, nursing) have been involved in its conception and development.

B. DSM-IV is a criteria-based diagnostic approach that requires the following three conditions be met prior to one or more diagnoses being made for any given patient.

    1. The condition is not caused by the direct effects of any drug.

    2. The psychiatric disorder is not caused by the effects of a medical condition.

    3. There is significant impairment in social functioning, occupational functioning, or both.

C. If a patient's signs and symptoms result from a medical condition or substance abuse, then the diagnosis should reflect that fact, with the psychiatric symptoms taking a secondary role. This relation holds regardless of the behavior manifested by the patient.

D. The DSM-IV contains a catchall category for each group called "not otherwise specified" (NOS). This catchall diagnosis allows a physician assistant (PA) in general practice to make a diagnosis for patients with atypical symptoms, thus avoiding diagnostic uncertainty by forcing a classification based on incomplete or contradictory symptom pictures. Therefore, a patient can always be assigned to a diagnostic group, even if assignment to one of the formal conditions listed in the DSM-IV is not possible or feasible.

II. SCHIZOPHRENIA AND OTHER PSYCHOTIC DISORDERS

A. Overview

    1. **Brief psychotic disorder, schizophreniform disorder,** and **schizophrenia** are three disorders that present with common symptoms. The primary criteria for differentiating among these disorders are the **severity** and the **duration of the symptoms.**

    2. In all disorders of this group, memory or consciousness is not adversely impacted, but there are severe problems with any or all of the following: social and occupational functioning, affect, motivation, perception, reality orientation, spontaneity, or the ability to communicate appropriately (e.g., disorganized speech).

    3. Subtypes of schizophrenia and other psychotic disorders include:

        a. Paranoid type

        b. Disorganized type

    c. Catatonic type

    d. Undifferentiated type

    e. Residual type

    f. Schizoaffective disorder

    g. Delusional disorder

    h. Shared psychotic disorder (e.g., the folie à deux)

    i. Psychotic disorders caused by alcohol, drugs, or medications

    j. Psychotic disorders caused by general medical conditions

    k. Psychotic disorders NOS

4. Temporal sequencing of symptoms is important for making an appropriate diagnosis in this group.

    a. A diagnosis of **brief psychotic disorder** is made when symptoms are present for at least 1 day but less than 1 month. The patient returns to premorbid levels of functioning after the symptoms abate. The clinician is most likely to see this disorder in a patient following the death of a loved one or similar catastrophic experience.

    b. A patient with **schizophreniform disorder** presents with the same symptoms as those seen in a patient with brief psychotic disorder, but the symptoms have lasted at least 1 month and have not exceeded 6 months.

    c. If symptoms exceed 6 months, then a diagnosis of **schizophrenia** should be made.

B. Clinical features. Certain symptoms must be exhibited by the patient prior to making a diagnosis of schizophrenia. The subtypes of schizophrenia are defined by variations of the presenting symptoms.

  1. At least two of the following symptoms must be present concurrently.

    a. Delusions are erroneous beliefs based on a misinterpretation of reality.

    b. Hallucinations are false perceptions in any of the sensory modalities. In order to qualify for the diagnosis, the hallucination must not occur as an isolated experience, in a clouded sensorium, or as part of a religious experience or in a cultural context.

    c. Disorganized speech is used as a marker for disorganized thought processes. Disorganized speech is exhibited by the patient's inability to stay on a topic (i.e., loose associations), the inability to provide an answer related to a question (i.e., a tangential response), or both. The symptoms need to be severe enough to impair an individual's ability to communicate effectively.

    d. Grossly disorganized behavior may be exhibited as unpredictable agitation, inappropriate sexual behavior, childlike silliness, or catatonic motor behavior. Grossly disorganized behavior may also be manifested as a reduced level of self-care and hygiene.

    e. Negative symptoms are manifested as flat affect, poor eye contact, poor posture, nonproductive speech, or lack of goal-directed activities.

  2. Social functioning, occupational functioning, or both must be impacted.

    a. This impairment may be manifested as an inability to hold a job for an extended period or maintain relationships (e.g., a marriage).

    b. The PA may find that the patient's educational progress is disrupted (if the patient is an adolescent) or uncompleted (if an adult).

    c. Problems with social relationships are not uncommon. For example, the patient may have trouble making friends or may have withdrawn from established friends and social relationships. Such individuals appear to have isolated social contacts.

C. Differential diagnosis. If a major mood disorder has been diagnosed (e.g., a bipolar disorder), then this diagnosis takes precedence over a diagnosis of schizophrenia or psychosis. The proper diagnosis would be the particular mood disorder diagnosed with a note that psychotic features are present.

D. Treatment

    1. Hospitalization

        a. Patients exhibiting suicidal ideation or an inability to care for themselves should be hospitalized.

        b. Most states require hospitalization if a patient is considered a danger to him- or herself or others.

        c. According to the *Tarasoff v. Regents of University of California* ruling, a patient who makes a credible threat of harm toward another in front of a health professional automatically obligates the health care professional to breach practitioner–patient confidentiality guidelines and report the threat to the authorities, the intended victim, or both.

    2. **Pharmacotherapy.** Neuroleptics (e.g., **haloperidol, loxapine, fluphenazine**) are viewed as the preferred treatment, with behavioral-oriented therapy targeted toward social skills training as an adjunct. The health care provider should remember that no therapeutic intervention is totally effective in ameliorating all symptoms encountered with the various schizophrenias and psychoses, and that patients with diagnostic subtypes of these conditions will react differently to the various neuroleptics available.

III. MOOD DISORDERS

A. Overview

    1. **Definition.** Mood disorders are a group of clinically distinct entities, identified by a mood episode (e.g., **depressive, manic,** or **mixed**) that requires a specific treatment regimen. The defining feature is a change in mood from a premorbid state.

    2. **Major categories of mood disorders** include:

        a. **Depressive disorders,** including the **major depressive disorder, dysthymic disorder,** and the **NOS** category

        b. **Bipolar disorders,** including **bipolar I, bipolar II, cyclothymic disorder,** and **bipolar disorder NOS**

        c. **Mood disorders,** such as those caused by a **general medical condition, substance-induced mood disorder,** and **mood disorder NOS**

    3. General considerations for diagnosis

        a. For the three categories of mood episodes, both **social** and **occupational** functioning should be **impaired.**

        b. If **psychotic features** are present, or the patient is viewed as a threat to him- or herself or others, then hospitalization must be recommended.

B. Major depressive episode

    1. In order to make this diagnosis, five or more of the symptoms presented under the "**depression**" heading in Table 12-1 must be present for the better part of a 2-week period.

    2. At least one of the symptoms must be indicative of a depressed mood while a second should be anhedonia.

    3. Symptoms presented by the patient should have resulted in a decreased level of functioning and could be manifested as:

        a. The inability to hold a job for an extended period

        b. The inability to maintain a relationship or marriage

        c. The inability to complete an education

        d. Difficulty making friends, a withdrawal from social relationships, or isolated social contacts

    4. A diagnosis of major depressive episode under this heading should not be made if the patient exhibits symptoms falling under the "**mania**" heading in Table 12-1, or if the mood episode is due to bereavement.

C. **Manic episode** is characterized by an abnormally elevated, expansive, or irritable mood that lasts at least 1 week.

    1. At least three of the symptoms listed under the "**mania**" section of Table 12-1 are present.

    2. The patient does not exhibit symptoms listed under the "**depression**" section of Table 12-1.

Table 12-1.
Symptoms of a Mood Episode

Depression
Depressed mood (reported by either the patient or observed by others)
Anhedonia
Excessive feelings of guilt
Indecisiveness
Lack of self-worth
Sleep problems or terminal insomnia
Cognitive problems (difficulty with memory and concentration)
Psychomotor retardation or agitation
Either a decreased or increased appetite or a 5% or greater change in body weight over a 1-month period
Decreased interest in sex
Either suicidal ideation or thoughts of death without suicidal ideation
Chronic fatigue

Mania
Inflated self-esteem or grandiosity
Irritability
Decreased need for sleep
Pressured speech
Flight of ideas
Distractibility
Impaired judgement resulting in pursuit of pleasurable activities with a high probability of adverse outcomes
Psychomotor agitation

D. Hypomanic episode is characterized by at least 4 continuous days of an abnormally and persistently elevated, expansive, or irritable mood.

   1. In order to diagnose the hypomanic episode, at least 3 of the symptoms listed under **"mania"** in Table 12-1 must be present if the mood is elevated; 4 are required if the mood is irritable.

   2. Psychomotor agitation and anhedonia are usually present.

   3. Although the patient's mood and functioning have changed from premorbid functioning, social and occupational functioning have not been significantly impacted and there are no psychotic features.

E. Mixed episode is characterized by rapidly alternating moods in conjunction with symptoms of both a **manic episode** and a **depressive episode**, which last at least 1 week.

   1. Symptoms are severe enough that there is a marked impairment in occupational or social functioning. Hospitalization is required because patients are usually a threat to themselves or others, or exhibit psychotic symptoms.

   2. The condition is not caused by a general medical condition, or by the direct effect of a prescribed or illegal drug.

F. Major depressive disorder

   1. Diagnostic criteria

      a. The presence of a **major depressive episode** that is not better accounted for by a disorder mentioned in section II

      b. The absence of a **mixed, hypomanic,** or **manic** episode

   2. Diagnostic considerations

      a. Major depressive disorder is **more common in women** than in men.

      b. Core symptoms tend to vary by age cohort but the DSM-IV notes that there tends to be a large proportion of women across age cohorts who report a worsening of symptoms just prior to menses.

      c. There are no laboratory tests diagnostic of the condition.

   3. Clinical course

      a. Major depressive disorder can occur at any age, but the first episode is usually seen in the early 20s.

      b. Premorbid problems tend to be rare and premorbid functioning may return between episodes.

4. Treatment

   a. Monitoring. Patients with a **major depressive disorder** must be monitored closely because they pose a substantial suicide risk. The DSM-IV indicates that the condition is associated with a 15% mortality rate owing to suicide.

   (1) Perhaps the time of greatest risk for the patient is after treatment has been initiated. **Patients who may not have the psychic energy to make a suicide attempt while in the depths of a depressive episode develop that energy as they start to improve.**

   (2) The clinician should remember that the goal of treatment is to **diagnose early** and **prevent relapse.**

   (3) The most important objective in meeting the treatment goal is to reduce and eventually eliminate all signs of the disorder, even if that requires maintaining a patient on medications for an indefinite period.

   (4) It is easier to maintain a patient who has a history of relapse on medication than it is to regain control of the symptoms. By maintaining the patient, the health care provider also reduces the chance of a successful suicide.

   b. Pharmocotherapy. Selective serotonin reuptake inhibitors (SSRIs), heterocyclic antidepressants, tricyclic antidepressants, and monoamine oxidase (MAO) inhibitors have all been proved beneficial.

   (1) SSRIs are usually considered **first-line therapy** because they have minimal adverse effects. Selection of a particular SSRI should be based on side-effect profiles and the problems with which the patient presents.

   (2) MAO inhibitors. The tyramine-free diet required to avoid side effects experienced with the use of MAO inhibitors makes this class of drugs the least likely to be used.

   c. Psychotherapy. Because of the broad range of consequences affecting social and occupational functioning that arise from a major depressive disorder, a comprehensive approach to the condition must include psychosocial intervention. The specific intervention should be based on the responsiveness of the patient.

G. Bipolar disorders

   1. Types

   a. Bipolar I disorder is characterized by the occurrence of one or more **manic** or **mixed episodes.** The patient may have experienced **depressive episodes,** but this is not required for the diagnosis.

   b. Bipolar II disorder is characterized by a history of at least one or more **major depressive episodes** and at least one **hypomanic episode.** The patient has never experienced a **manic episode** or a **mixed episode.**

   c. Cyclothymic disorder is characterized by recurring periods of depression and hypomania over a 2-year period, with symptom-free periods lasting no more than 2 months at any one time. The depressive episodes are not severe enough to be classified as a **major depressive episode,** nor have **manic** or **mixed episodes** occurred.

   2. Treatment

   a. Monitoring. Patients with **bipolar I** or **bipolar II** disorder should be monitored closely because they pose a substantial suicide risk.

   b. Pharmacotherapy

   (1) Lithium is indicated in the treatment of **bipolar I, bipolar II,** and **cyclothymic** disorders.

   (2) Anticonvulsants are usually recommended for patients with **bipolar I** and **bipolar II disorders.**

   (3) Antidepressants may also be used, but caution must be exercised because use of these drugs can result in rapid cycling between mood states.

   c. Electroconvulsive therapy. If psychopharmacology is ineffective or contraindicated, then electroconvulsive therapy should be considered for patients with **bipolar I** and **bipolar II disorders.**

IV. ANXIETY DISORDERS

A. Overview

   1. Definition. Anxiety disorders are characterized by **excessive amounts of anxiety** that **impede performance** and can result in **physiologic symptoms** such as tachycardia, palpitations, a loss of appetite, nausea, and others symptoms that cause the patient distress.

2. Types of anxiety disorders

    a. Generalized anxiety disorder

    b. Panic disorder

    c. Obsessive–compulsive disorder (OCD)

    d. Posttraumatic stress disorder

    e. Acute stress disorder

    f. Phobias

    g. Agoraphobia

    h. Anxiety disorder NOS

B. Generalized anxiety disorder

1. Characteristics

    a. Generalized anxiety disorder is characterized by **excessive anxiety** over **several life events** that lasts 6 months or more. The patient has difficulty coping with the anxiety, usually expressed as worry or apprehension, generated by these events.

    b. The patient with a diagnosis of **generalized anxiety disorder** presents with at least 3 of the following symptoms (only 1 if the patient is a child).

        (1) Restlessness or hypervigilance

        (2) Easy fatigability

        (3) Irritability

        (4) Sleep disturbance

        (5) Muscle tension

        (6) Difficulty concentrating

2. Treatment

    a. **Pharmacotherapy.** SSRIs and buspirone are effective. **Tricyclic antidepressants** have also been used.

    b. A **behaviorally oriented therapy** should also be initiated in addition to pharmacotherapy.

C. Panic disorder

1. Characteristics

    a. Panic disorder is characterized by recurrent unexpected **panic attacks** that abruptly occur in the presence of debilitating fear and that peak within 10 minutes of onset.

    b. Attacks may occur repeatedly and rapidly with severe anxiety lasting several hours after the termination of the attack.

    c. Panic attacks can occur while the patient is sleeping.

    d. A National Institutes of Health (NIH) consensus conference has indicated that the diagnostic criteria for this disorder include a clustering of at least 4 attacks over a 4-week period or 1 or more attacks followed by 1 month of fearful anticipation about experiencing additional attacks.

2. Presenting symptoms. At least 4 of the following symptoms should be present during the attack.

    a. Palpitations or tachycardia

    b. Chest discomfort

    c. Sweating

    d. Trembling or shaking

    e. Shortness of breath

    f. Choking

    g. Nausea or abdominal distress

h. Vertigo, light-headedness

i. Fear of dying

j. Paresthesias

k. Chills or hot flashes

l. Fear of losing control or fear of going crazy

m. Derealization (a defense mechanism in which people, events, and surroundings appear changed or unreal) or depersonalization (a state in which the individual feels estranged from himself and/or the external world)

3. Treatment

    a. Pharmacotherapy

        (1) Alprazolam has historically been the only Food and Drug Administration (FDA)-approved medication for panic disorder.

        (2) MAO inhibitors, benzodiazepines, and **tricyclic antidepressants** have also been used successfully.

    b. Cognitive and behavioral therapies have been shown to be effective in treating panic disorder. The NIH consensus statement has indicated that combined psychotherapeutic approaches that include **cognitive therapy** tend to be the most effective in treating the disorder and in reducing panic attacks. Initial improvement should be noted with most patients within the first 3 to 6 weeks.

D. Obsessive-compulsive disorder (OCD)

  1. Characteristics. OCD has the following two components.

    a. Obsession refers to the cognitive component that causes the patient's anxiety. The anxiety is generated by the persistent thoughts, images, or impulses that are both intrusive and inappropriate. The thoughts are not based on real problems encountered by the patient.

        (1) The patient avoids the anxiety-producing thoughts by attempting to ignore or suppress them or to neutralize them with other thoughts or actions.

        (2) Adult patients are usually aware that they are causing their own distress and that the symptoms are not being imposed by others.

    b. Compulsions are the ritualistic or repetitive behaviors that patients feel **compelled** to engage in to prevent or control the anxiety or distress caused by the obsessions. The behaviors or mental acts are excessive and not realistically connected with the events the patient is trying to avoid.

  2. Treatment

    a. Pharmacotherapy. Clomipramine and certain SSRIs have been found to be effective in the treatment of OCD. Patients who show only a partial remission of symptoms should have their medication augmented with buspirone or a benzodiazepine.

    b. Behaviorally oriented therapies should also be initiated. Traditionally oriented insight therapies, however, have not been found to be helpful.

E. Posttraumatic stress disorder results from exposure to a traumatic event and is manifested in overwhelming sensations of helplessness, fear, and horror. Posttraumatic stress disorder must be differentiated from brief psychotic disorder.

  1. Characteristics. Posttraumatic stress disorder is caused by a physiologic or psychological trauma that is out of the range of normal human experience (e.g., war, natural disaster, catastrophic accident). A patient with the disorder may repeatedly relive the event, have intrusive memories of the event, or experience distress when exposed to stimuli that trigger event review. At least 3 of the following symptoms must be present for more than 1 month after the event and must impair occupational functioning, social functioning, or both.

    a. Patients are unable to recall an important aspect of the event.

    b. Patients make an effort to avoid activities, places, and events that remind them of the event.

    c. Patients attempt to avoid thinking or talking about the event associated with the trauma.

    d. Patients experience anhedonia.

  e. Patients experience restricted affect.

  f. Patients believe their lives have been irrevocably changed for the worse because of the event.

  g. Patients have an increased state of arousal characterized by at least 2 of the following symptoms: insomnia, irritability, poor concentration, hypervigilance, or exaggerated startle response.

 2. Treatment

  a. Pharmacotherapy. SSRIs and buspirone have been reported to be effective for the treatment of posttraumatic stress disorder. Tricyclic antidepressants have also shown modest success in the treatment of this disorder.

  b. Psychotherapy

   (1) Crisis counseling should be initiated as a preventive measure when feasible.

   (2) Membership in a support group and **cognitive** or **behaviorally oriented therapies** should be initiated. The specific modality is less important than the therapist's experience in dealing with the type of trauma encountered.

F. Phobias

 1. Characteristics. This disorder is characterized by **excessive anxiety** when presented with an object or situational event.

  a. Exposure to the object or situational event results in an immediate **increase in anxiety** and can precipitate a **panic attack**. Because of the discomfort caused by the increased anxiety, the panic attack, or both, the situation or object that provokes the event is either feared and avoided or endured with considerable apprehension.

  b. Except for children, patients with this disorder know that their fear is excessive and unreasonable.

 2. Diagnosis of a phobia should be made only if the response to a phobic stimulus interferes with a patient's daily routine or with his or her social or occupational functioning. The DSM-IV recognizes five subtypes of phobias. A patient with a phobic subtype is at greater risk for having an additional phobia within the subtype.

  a. Animal type. Animals or insects are the phobic stimulus. Onset for this type is generally in childhood.

  b. Natural environment type. Natural phenomena (e.g., storms, heights, water, lightning) are the trigger.

  c. Blood-injection injury type. Fear of invasive procedures is paramount and the phobic trigger is the possibility of injury, the sight of blood, or contamination by exposure to bodily fluids.

  d. Situational type. Examples of phobic stimuli include bridges, tall buildings, flying, driving, and confined spaces.

  e. Other type

 3. Treatment

  a. Pharmacotherapy. SSRIs should be tried first. If these are not successful, the practitioner should turn to tricyclics, MAO inhibitors, or low-dose benzodiazepines.

  b. Behaviorally oriented therapies should also be initiated. Desensitization, flooding, and similar procedures have been shown to be powerful techniques for the treatment of this type of disorder.

G. Agoraphobia may occur with or without a history of panic disorder.

 1. Characteristics include an intense anxiety about placing oneself into a situation where an incapacitating problem could occur and no help would be available. The potential occurrence of the incapacitating event is usually viewed by the patient as extremely embarrassing or humiliating. If the feared incapacitating event is a panic attack, then agoraphobia is diagnosed secondary to the panic disorder.

 2. Diagnosis. Any of the 13 symptoms characteristic of a panic attack may be present. In addition, the patient may have a potentially incapacitating or embarrassing medical condition, such as a heart condition or a lack of bowel or bladder control. In extreme cases, symptoms may render the patient unwilling or unable to leave his or her home.

 3. Treatment should be consistent with the recommendations provided for panic disorder.

V. EATING DISORDERS include **anorexia nervosa, bulimia nervosa, eating disorders NOS,** and **eating disorders of childhood** (e.g., pica, rumination disorder).

A. Anorexia nervosa

1. **Definition.** The patient either refuses to maintain a body weight above 85% of what is considered normal for age and height, or fails to make weight gains to maintain a weight that is 85% of what would normally be expected for any increase in height. The percentage noted is somewhat subjective because appropriate body weight is a function of body build as well as height.

2. **Characteristics.** The patient has an inappropriate perception of his or her body shape and size, and denies the seriousness of the low body weight. Postmenarchal women may have amenorrhea.

3. **Treatment**

   a. Hospitalization. Given the high mortality rate associated with this condition (approximately 10%), a patient should be hospitalized if he or she meets any of the following conditions.

   (1) Thirty percent or more weight loss in a 6-month period

   (2) Electrolyte disturbance that cannot be controlled on an outpatient basis

   (3) Diuretic abuse that cannot be controlled on an outpatient basis

   (4) Arrhythmias

   (5) Severe dehydration

   (6) Suicidal ideation

   (7) Uncontrolled binging and purging

   (8) Severe depression

   b. Pharmacotherapy. Both antidepressants (e.g., amitriptyline) and SSRIs (e.g., fluoxetine) can be of use, especially when depression is present. An appetite stimulant may be of use, as might a drug that has weight gain as a side effect. Overall, however, medications do not play a major role in the treatment of this disorder.

   c. Behaviorally oriented therapies. While insight-oriented therapy is usually not of value, family therapy and various behavioral techniques usually are. The behavioral techniques should focus on cognitive restructuring to change the patient's perceptions toward body image and food.

B. Bulimia nervosa

1. **Characteristics.** As with anorexia nervosa, a bulimic's self-image is unduly influenced by body weight and shape.

   a. The patient engages in recurrent episodes of **binge eating** (i.e., consuming excessive amounts of food over a 2-hour period) at least twice a week for 3 months.

   b. Bulimic patients believe that they have no control over their eating behavior and thus use inappropriate measures to prevent weight gain (e.g., **purging** via vomiting, **diuretic use**). The health care practitioner must carefully differentiate between anorexia and bulimia because both entail binging and purging. The binging and purging with bulimia, therefore, should not occur during anorexic episodes.

2. **Treatment.** The prognosis for bulimic patients is better than for anorexic patients because there is less denial concerning their disorder.

   a. Hospitalization is required when the same risk factors noted for anorexics are noted for the bulimic patient.

   b. Pharmacotherapy. Antidepressants are useful for bulimia (e.g., imipramine), as are SSRIs (e.g., fluoxetine) and MAO inhibitors.

   c. Behaviorally oriented psychotherapies should be used in conjunction with family therapy. Group therapy with others suffering from bulimia should also be considered. The broad-based goal of therapy with bulimics is the same as with anorexics.

VI. SUBSTANCE ABUSE DISORDERS

A. **Overview. Substances of abuse** include alcohol, nicotine, and drugs (e.g., opiates, barbiturates, over-the-counter). The number of substances that can be abused is limited only by their availability and the desire of the patient to experiment.

B. Types of Abuse

1. **Addiction** is a nonscientific, nonmedical term denoting psychological and/or physical dependence that results in drug-seeking behavior that may or may not pose risks to the individual.

2. **Physical dependence** is used to refer to the physiologic changes that occur with drug use and result in withdrawal symptoms on termination of use.

3. **Psychological dependence** refers to the craving or desire for the substance independent of the physiologic withdrawal symptoms. Because both physiologic and psychological dependence occur together, a more appropriate term is substance dependence.

4. **Substance dependence.** Substance dependence occurs when substance use results in impairment as manifested by three of the following seven conditions occurring within a 12-month period.

   a. **Tolerance** (either a decreased effect over time when the same amount of substance is used or a need for an increased amount of a substance over time to achieve a baseline effect)

   b. **Withdrawal** (the need to use a substance to relieve or avoid physical symptoms associated with deprivation of the substance)

   c. **Use of increasingly larger amounts of a substance over a longer period than desired**

   d. **Unsuccessful efforts to either stop or decrease** the amount of a substance used

   e. **Significantly larger amounts of time spent** in attempts to acquire or use the substance or to recover from its effects

   f. **Social, occupational, or recreational impairment**

   g. **Continued use of a substance despite the awareness that doing so has adverse consequences**

5. **Substance abuse** is substance use that has not met the criteria for dependence but has resulted in impairment as manifested by at least one of the following criteria within a 12-month period.

   a. Failure to meet home, school, or work obligations

   b. Repeated use of the substance in hazardous situations

   c. Recurrent substance-related legal problems

   d. Continued use of the substance even though the patient is experiencing interpersonal or social problems as a result

6. **Substance intoxication** refers to maladaptive behavioral or psychological changes **attributed to recent ingestion of a substance.** Intoxication is reversible and is **not caused by a mental disorder or medical condition.**

C. Treatment. Substance dependence is viewed as a **chronic, relapsing disease** by the Substance Abuse and Mental Health Services Administration (SAMHSA). Relapses are not considered a failure in treatment but rather a step toward what will hopefully be a complete remission of all symptoms.

1. SAMHSA recognizes that some forms of dependence **require ongoing medication** to keep an individual free of drugs (e.g., daily methadone as therapy for a patient with a dependence on opiates).

2. A popular form of therapy, for a number of different types of substance use, is a **12-step program.** Twelve-step programs are available for both substance users [e.g., Alcoholics Anonymous (AA)], as well for their family members (e.g., ALANON and ALATEEN).

   a. Perhaps the best short-term predictor of abstinence from alcohol is whether an individual is enrolled in AA.

   b. The best predictor of abstinence 1 year from the onset of sobriety is sponsorship of another member in the 12-step program.

3. The best and most cost-effective approach to treating substance abuse is to prevent it. One of the more successful **prevention** approaches uses the risk and protective factor framework of Catalano and Hawkins. Risk factors can be assessed in an office environment through use of the CAGE screening test for alcohol abuse or the Drug Abuse Screening Test (DAST) for drug abuse.

VII. ATTENTION-DEFICIT HYPERACTIVITY DISORDERS (ADHD)

A. Definition. ADHD has been overdiagnosed in recent years. The primary diagnosis is attention deficit disorder (ADD), with some children manifesting hyperactivity and impulsivity, and others manifesting inattentiveness. Most children manifest symptoms that result in a diagnosis emphasizing both attentional deficits and hyperactivity.

B. Diagnosis

   1. The following must be ruled out prior to making a diagnosis.

     a. **Normal childhood behavior.** Parents may have unrealistic expectations concerning age-appropriate behavior or they may have failed to set limits resulting in poor behavior on the part of the child.

     b. **Grief, a change in family status,** or **abuse** can lead to behavioral problems that can be confused with ADHD. The diagnosis of ADHD should not be made if a school official claims that a child's behavior has become unmanageable after having been judged acceptable in previous years.

     c. **Other childhood neuropsychiatric disorders.** The child may have symptoms of another childhood neuropsychiatric disorder (e.g., conduct disorder, oppositional defiant disorder).

   2. With ADHD, initial symptoms of hyperactivity, impulsivity, or inattentiveness resulting in impairment must have been manifest prior to age 7.

   3. A diagnosis of ADHD requires that at least 6 of the following 9 symptoms of inattention are **developmentally inappropriate** and that they have been present for at least 6 months.

     a. Makes careless mistakes and has trouble attending to details

     b. Experiences problems in sustaining attention

     c. Does not appear attentive when directly addressed

     d. Does not follow through or complete assigned work

     e. Forgetful

     f. Easily distracted from activities by other things going on at the same time

     g. Loses items critical to accomplishing assigned activities

     h. Avoids activities requiring sustained mental effort

     i. Has difficulty in organizing tasks

C. **Treatment.** Central nervous system (CNS) stimulants in combination with behavior-oriented therapies are the recommended treatment.

   1. **Pharmacotherapy.** Individual response to this class of drugs is idiosyncratic and needs to be closely monitored. Although **dextroamphetamine** has received FDA approval for children older than 3 years and **methylphenidate** has been approved for those older than 6 years, all drugs in this class are equally effective.

   2. **Behavioral therapy** should include behavior modification, classroom management where appropriate, and family therapy. Multimodality therapy is a crucial component in successfully dealing with these patients.

VIII. ABUSE AND NEGLECT

A. **Child abuse.** In most states, PAs are required to alert the appropriate authorities if abuse or neglect of a child is suspected. When a young patient presents with any condition that appears questionable for abuse, it is best to consult with a mental health professional or family social services so that additional help can be offered to the patient.

   1. A child who has been deliberately **burned, severely beaten,** or **starved** is in obvious need of immediate attention for medical problems. Abuse and neglect can also be manifested in subtle ways, such as **failure to thrive.**

     a. In cases of overt abuse, appropriate authorities need to be contacted immediately so that the child can gain relief from the care giver's actions.

     b. While the PA's responsibility to contact the authorities is real, it must be tempered with a dose of understanding.

   2. **Munchausen by proxy syndrome** is a form of abuse usually perpetrated by the mother. Symptoms are fabricated or clinical signs are induced in a child, resulting in repeated visits to a health care provider for relief. The perpetrator induces the various signs and symptoms in the child in order to receive attention as being either an attentive or a suffering parent. Authors of a recent article in a major journal speculated that a large number of sudden infant death syndrome (SIDS) cases may actually have been examples of Munchausen by proxy syndrome.

   3. **Other types of abuse.** Abuse can be inferred in some cases where there are no obvious physical indications.

     a. Although **corporal punishment** within reason is not normally considered abuse, it **becomes abuse if the parent indicates that he or she received gratification while administering the punishment.**

    b. **Neglect** can be considered when a client allows a minor to engage in potentially harmful behaviors (e.g., alcohol consumption) or remain unattended. In some states, leaving a child younger than 13 years home alone is considered neglect.

B. **Spousal abuse.** When confronted with a patient who is thought to be a victim of spousal abuse, the PA needs to take the following actions:

    1. The PA must provide immediate medical attention to address the physical sequelae.

    2. The PA must recognize suspected abuse and take the initiative to engage the patient in nonthreatening questioning to confirm whether or not abuse has occurred.

        a. If abuse has occurred, the PA must stress to the abused patient that someone does care, and that there are better alternatives than the one he or she has chosen.

        b. Contact numbers for referral agencies should be readily accessible to the practitioner. The following may be sought:

            (1) **Legal recourse,** such as criminal penalties and restraining orders

            (2) Services of a **local emergency shelter**

            (3) Services of **private support groups** (e.g., the House of Ruth) or the **National Coalition Against Domestic Violence**

        c. The decision to accept a referral is ultimately the patient's, but if help is offered and accepted, the **PA must ensure that a referral can be made immediately.** Nothing can be more devastating for an abused woman than to make the decision to leave an abusive spouse and find that she has nowhere to go but back to the environment in which she was abused because referrals could not be made or could not be acted on in a timely manner. This tends to reinforce the patient's poor self-image and results in the patient losing trust in her health care provider.

        d. **Caution** is required in dealing with cases of spouse abuse. Because of the dangers involved, the health care practitioner should present the patient with options and let him or her decide the path to take. There are many reasons for this approach.

            (1) It is not uncommon for a practitioner to stress the importance of leaving an abusive spouse only to find that the abused closes ranks with the abuser, confronting the clinician for attempting to break up a family.

            (2) The Federal government estimates that a woman who leaves an abusive husband has a **70% greater risk of being killed by the batterer** than one who stays.

            (3) Battered spouses have suffered a blow to their ego defenses and may not be assertive enough to believe that their rights have been violated. It is not uncommon to find battered women who believe that they either deserved the beating or must accept the beatings as price for a roof over their head and food on the table.

C. **Elder abuse** has been reported to affect approximately 4% of the population older than 65 years.

    1. Elder abuse can be physical, psychological/emotional, financial, or neglect. Physical abuse may be suspected when the health care provider notices:

        a. Bruises

        b. Puncture wounds

        c. Cuts

        d. Poor hygiene

        e. Hair loss in clumps

        f. Weight loss

        g. Burns

        h. Soiled clothing

2. Because most cases of elder abuse are committed by a caregiver, the health care provider should be alert to the following:

   a. Previous history of abuse by the caregiver

   b. Conflicting accounts of accidents by caregivers

   c. Unwillingness of a caregiver to agree to implementation of treatment plans

   d. Inappropriate defensiveness by the caregiver

   e. A caregiver who will not allow, or limits, the patient's responses to questions

3. Some states have the same reporting requirements for suspected elder abuse as for child abuse. The following web sites provide additional information on this relatively new area of concern.

   a. www.oaktrees.org/elder/

   b. www.txlegal.com/nursing.htm

IX. RAPE CRISES

A. Definitions

   1. Rape is an act of aggression that may be perpetrated on a spouse, a partner of the same sex, or a partner of the opposite sex.

   2. Sodomy. Legally, penetration of the anus or fellatio is considered sodomy and not rape; however, forced participation in these acts can result in psychological sequelae similar to those seen in rape victims, regardless of the sex of the victim.

B. Characteristics. A patient who has been raped or sodomized may experience:

   1. Depression

   2. Lack of appetite

   3. Sleep disturbances

   4. Rage and anger

   5. Feelings of worthlessness

   6. Enduring patterns of sexual dysfunction

   7. Agoraphobia

   8. Fear of future violence, death, or of contracting a sexually transmitted disease (STD)

   9. Feelings of being used or "dirty"

   10. Anxiety attacks

C. Approach to the patient

1. History and physical examination

   a. Because rape constitutes both a psychiatric emergency and legal situation, all procedures should be documented, clothing saved, and samples taken.

   (1) Emergency rooms in most medical centers have a rape kit with instructions on questions to include in the examination, what specimen samples should be collected and under what conditions, and how samples should be handled after collection to ensure that they cannot be tampered with.

   (2) If a rape kit is not available, the health care professional should consult with local or state law enforcement agencies to determine his or her obligations.

   b. It is important to explain to the patient the purpose of all procedures prior to the examination, and to inform the patient of what is being done prior to doing it. This procedure provides the patient with a feeling of control. The health care provider should remember that the patient has already suffered an assault and loss of control and should exhibit as much compassion as possible.

   2. Prevention of STDs and pregnancy. Prophylactic antibiotic therapy should be initiated to reduce the patient's risk of developing certain STDs. The patient should be given the option of taking drugs to prevent or terminate a pregnancy.

   3. Counseling. As soon as possible after the event (i.e., preferably before leaving the emergency department), the patient should talk to a mental health professional and follow-up counseling should be scheduled.

X. UNCOMPLICATED BEREAVEMENT

   A. Definition. Uncomplicated bereavement is defined as a normal response to a major loss. The **length of the grief reaction** and the consequences depend on a number of factors, including the suddenness of the loss, the relationship of the survivor to the deceased, and the age or physical condition of the person who has died (e.g., the death of a 90-year-old relative with Alzheimer's disease may be viewed as expected or a blessing, whereas the death of a 3-year-old child is usually taken much harder, regardless of the child's condition).

   B. Presenting characteristics

   1. Shock can be manifested as confusion (e.g., inability to attend to immediate problems, problems focusing, difficulty in maintaining goal-directed behavior).

   2. Feelings of numbness or **guilt over how the patient treated the deceased** may be noted.

   3. Depression. Symptoms of depression (e.g., weight loss, emotional lability, decreased libido) may be seen.

   C. Treatment. Patients exhibiting uncomplicated grief will not be helped by antidepressive medications, but will respond to social contact and reassurances.

   1. It is important to **document that a grief reaction has occurred** because denial can lead to both psychological as well as medical problems.

   2. Encouraging the patient to talk about feelings allows the clinician to evaluate how well the patient is handling the grief.

13

Dermatology

Edward D. Huechtker
Pamela D. Bailey

I. DIAGNOSIS OF DERMATOLOGIC CONDITIONS. At least 30% of visits to health care providers are for dermatologic conditions, according to some estimates.

A. History and physical examination

    1. **History.** The most important technique in diagnosing a skin disorder is obtaining a thorough history. Important elements of the history include:

        a. Past medical illnesses

        b. Medication history (prescription and nonprescription drugs)

        c. Family history

        d. Psychosocial history

        e. Recreational and employment histories

        f. Diet

        g. Environmental exposures

    2. **Physical examination.** A general examination, paying particular attention to the **skin, hair,** and **mucocutaneous surfaces** should be carried out under **natural** or **bright light.** A **magnifying glass** may be useful. Common skin lesions that may be noted during examination are summarized in Table 13-1.

B. Definitions of significant terms

    1. **Angioma**—a swelling or tumor due to proliferation, with or without dilation of blood vessels

    2. **Bulla**—a vesicle measuring less than 5 mm in diameter

    3. **Crusted**—hard and rough surface formed by dried sebum, exudate, blood, or necrotic skin

    4. **Lichenification**—thickened skin with distinct borders

    5. **Macerated**—swollen and softened by an increase in water content; the appearance skin gets when left in water too long

    6. **Macule**—a flat, nonpalpable lesion measuring less than 10 mm

    7. **Nodule**—same as a papule only larger than 10 mm

    8. **Papule**—a solid, palpable lesion measuring less than 10 mm

    9. **Patch**—same as a macule but larger than 10 mm

   10. **Petechiae**—minute hemorrhagic spots in the skin of pinpoint to pinhead size, which are not blanched by diascopy

   11. **Plaque**—a plateau-like lesion measuring larger than 10 mm; could also be a group of confluent papules

   12. **Scale**—heaped-up particles of horny epithelium with a non-hydrated appearance

   13. **Telangiectasia**—dilated, superficial blood vessels

Table 13–1.
Common Skin Lesions and Their Descriptions

Papule		Solid, palpable lesion measuring less than 10 mm in diameter	Vesicle		Circumscribed, elevated lesion containing serous fluid and measuring less than 5mm in diameter
Nodule		Solid, palpable lesion measuring more than 10mm in diameter	Bulla		Vesicle larger than 5 mm in diameter
Macule		Flat, nonpalpable lesion measuring less than 10mm in diameter	Wheal		Transient, elevated lesion caused by local edema
Patch		Flat, nonpalpable lesion measuring more than 10mm	Petechiae		Minute hemorrhagic spots that cannot be blanched by diascopy
Plaque		Plateau-like lesion measuring more than 10mm in diameter; could also be a group of confluent papules	Crust		Hard, rough surface formed by dried sebum, exudate, blood or necrotic skin
Scale		"Heaped up" piles of horny epithelium with a dry appearance			

14. **Verrucous**—irregular, rough, and convoluted surfaces

15. **Vesicle**—circumscribed, elevated lesion containing serous fluid and measuring less than 5 mm in diameter

C. Diagnostic techniques

1. **Darkfield microscopy** is used in the diagnosis of syphilis. The causative organism, a spirochete, is visible in the serous exudate from the genital lesions.

2. **Diascopy.** A glass slide or diascope is pressed against the skin to reveal changes produced in the underlying skin when the skin is blanched.

3. **Potassium hydroxide (KOH) test.** Microscopic examination of skin scrapings mounted in KOH, which dissolves keratin and cellular material but does not affect fungi, is a fast way of detecting dermatophytes.

4. **Scraping for mites.** Mineral oil is used to help capture and contain mites, eggs, or feces in skin scrapings, which are then examined microscopically.

5. **Tzanck smear.** Cells from the base of a vesicle caused by herpes virus or varicella-zoster virus are stained with Giemsa or Wright stain. The presence of multinucleated giant cells suggests infection.

6. **Wood's light examination** is used to assess pigment changes or to fluoresce infectious lesions.

II. SKIN INFECTIONS

A. Viral infections

1. Pityriasis rosea

a. Etiology. The cause of this condition is unknown, but is thought to be viral.

b. Clinical features. A herald patch precedes a widespread symmetrical papular eruption by approximately 1 week.

(1) The **herald patch** is a solitary, round or oval pink lesion with a raised border and fine, adherent scales in the margin.

(2) The **rash** appears on the trunk and consists of round or oval, salmon-colored, slightly raised papular and macular lesions, usually less than 1 cm in diameter.

(a) A **"Christmas tree" distribution** of lesions results because the long axis of each lesion is usually aligned with the natural skinfolds.

(b) **Fine scale** covers the lesions in the beginning. The lesions then desquamate, leaving a collarette scale around each lesion.

(c) **Resolution.** After 3–8 weeks, the rash disappears spontaneously.

b. Treatment

(1) **Lotions** or **emollients** may be used to treat the scale. No other treatment is usually indicated.

(2) **Ultraviolet B therapy** is thought by some practitioners to be helpful.

(3) **Antipruritics, oral antihistamines,** or **lotions** may help if there is itching.

2. **Molluscum contagiosum** is a fairly common viral infection of the skin and mucous membranes. Children are most often affected, but adults can develop the condition as well. Boys are affected more often than girls. The organism can be sexually transmitted.

a. Clinical features. Discrete, **flesh-colored, umbilicated papules** appear over the face, trunk, and extremities in children. In adults, flesh-colored, often translucent, dome-shaped lesions with a depression in the center appear on the groin and lower abdomen.

(1) Lesions range in size from 3–6 mm in diameter and **appear in groups.** In immunocompromised patients, the lesions can be larger (up to 1.5 cm in diameter) and more widespread.

(2) A **white, curd-like material** can be expressed from under the depression of the lesion.

b. Treatment is usually not necessary because the disease is self-limiting. If therapy is indicated, it consists of local destruction of individual lesions by curettage, cryotherapy, electrodesiccation, or an acid or exfoliative peel.

B. Bacterial infections

1. **Cellulitis** is an acute, spreading inflammation of the dermis and subcutaneous tissue. Bacteria (e.g., *Haemophilus influenzae, Streptococcus, Staphylococcus*) are usually the cause.

a. Clinical features

(1) The involved area is **swollen, red, hot,** and **tender.**

(2) The patient may have **lymphadenopathy, fever, chills**, and **malaise.**

b. Laboratory findings. The causative organism can be identified by culturing any drainage or discharge, or by needle aspiration.

c. Treatment

(1) **Antibiotic therapy** should be initiated immediately to cover *H. influenzae*, streptococci, and staphylococci.

(a) Appropriate agents include a penicillinase-resistant penicillin (e.g., dicloxacillin) or a first-generation cephalosporin. For patients who are allergic to penicillin, erythromycin is used.

(b) Patients started on parenteral therapy may be switched to oral therapy when the fever, chills, and malaise subside.

(2) **Marking the margins of involvement** with a pen may be appropriate in order to follow the progression or regression of the area.

(3) **Surgical intervention** is mandatory if there is poor response to antimicrobial therapy, or if a necrotizing soft tissue infection is suspected.

2. Impetigo is a highly contagious superficial pyoderma caused by *Staphylococcus aureus* or group A *Streptococcus* most often seen in infants and children.

   a. Clinical features. A **superficial, flaccid vesicle** ruptures, forming a **thick, yellowish crust** (often described as "honey-colored").

   b. Laboratory findings. Bacterial culture and Gram stain reveal gram-positive cocci and confirm the diagnosis.

   c. Treatment

      (1) **Antibiotic therapy.** A **topical antibiotic** (e.g., **bacitracin**) should be applied for at least 10 days. In more advanced cases, **oral antibiotics** (e.g., **dicloxacillin, cephalexin, erythromycin**) are appropriate.

      (2) **Gentle débridement** of the scab with warm soaks is appropriate.

C. Fungal infections

1. Candidiasis is caused by *Candida* species, especially *Candida albicans*. This organism, part of the normal flora in humans, becomes pathogenic when there is a disturbance in the balance of normal flora or the host becomes debilitated.

   a. Clinical features

      (1) **Oral candidiasis (thrush)** appears as a **white, curd-like layer** of variable thickness on the oral mucosa and tongue. When the layer is scraped off, it leaves an **erythematous base**.

         (a) An estimated 60% of people older than 60 years who wear dentures have experienced some form of thrush. Infants are also prone to thrush.

         (b) **HIV-infected patients** are one of the groups at highest risk for oral candidiasis. Ninety percent of these patients become infected, and the infection is very difficult to treat.

      (2) **Genital candidiasis** is common; it is estimated that 75% of all women have been affected by at least one episode of vaginal candidiasis during their lifetime. **Patients with diabetes, uncircumcised males,** and **pregnant women** are predisposed.

         (a) **Vaginal candidiasis** is associated with a **"cottage cheese" discharge**.

         (b) **Candidal balanitis** is characterized by erythema and tenderness, sometimes accompanied by papulo-pustular lesions.

         (c) **Diaper rash** is another form of genital candidiasis.

      (3) **Cutaneous candidiasis** typically presents with a **bright red-orange rash,** which may be surrounded by papules and pustules. Other forms of candidiasis can include **nail infections, paronychia,** and **candidal folliculitis.**

         (a) Areas most often affected include the axillae, the region under the breasts, and the inguinal and perianal regions (in obese patients).

         (b) People exposed to water in their occupations (e.g., bartenders, housekeeping staff, waiters) may present with candidiasis between their fingers.

      (4) **Systemic candidiasis.** *Candida* can cause life-threatening systemic illnesses, including **meningitis, endocarditis,** and **bronchopulmonary infections.**

   b. Laboratory findings. A **KOH preparation** can assist in diagnosing candidiasis.

   c. Treatment depends on the location of the infection, the duration of the symptoms, and the immune status of the patient. Therapy is usually 7–14 days, but now there are single-dose therapies available that enhance compliance and may actually be more cost-effective than a 2-week regimen.

      (1) **Topical medications** are effective for oral and genital candidiasis. **Imidazoles, azoles,** and **polyenes** all work well and come in a variety of formulations (e.g., creams, oral suspensions, ointments, powders, troches, lozenges, suppositories).

       (2) Oral ketoconazole, fluconazole, and **itraconazole** are usually effective for treating resistant mucocutaneous infections.

  2. Dermatophytoses, superficial fungal infections that affect the hair, nails, and skin, are most often caused by **Microsporum, Trichophyton,** or **Epidermophyton.**

    a. Types

      (1) Tinea pedis (infection of the foot)

      (2) Tinea cruris (infection of the groin)

      (3) Tinea corporis (infection of the chest, back, neck, or shoulders)

      (4) Tinea capitis (infection of the scalp)

      (5) Tinea barbae (infection of the lower jaw in bearded men)

      (6) Tinea unguium (infection of the nails)

      (7) Tinea manus (infection of the hand)

    b. Clinical features

      (1) Most forms of tinea. An **erythematous, annular patch** with **distinct borders** and a **central clearing** is seen. The patch is usually covered with a fine scale. The affected region may itch, sting, or burn.

      (2) Tinea unguium presents as thickening, discoloration, and onycholysis of the nail bed and plate.

      (3) Tinea capitus. A kerion (i.e., a granulomatous, secondarily infected, raised, boggy lesion) can appear with any form of tinea, but is most commonly found with tinea capitis.

    c. Treatment

      (1) Topical antifungal creams, ointments, lotions, powders, or **sprays** are applied twice daily for 4 weeks. Tolnaftate 1% or ketoconazole 2% is recommended. If there are vesicles, powders help to dry the area and prevent maceration.

      (2) Oral fungicidal agents (e.g., griseofulvin, itraconazole, tolnaftate, first-generation azoles, terbinafine, naftifine) are required for patients with chronic or resistant infections. Some infections, such as tinea unguium, require therapy for several months.

        (a) Kerions. Oral **fluconazole** (50 mg daily for 20 days) should be used if there is a kerion.

        (b) Monitoring for hepatotoxicity. Antifungal agents can be hepatotoxic. Baseline hepatic enzyme values should be obtained, and the patient should be monitored closely throughout the course of therapy.

  3. Tinea versicolor is caused by **Malassezia furfur,** a yeast found in the skin of humans. This yeast, for reasons not understood, **manifests in the spore and hyphal form** in some patients, causing tinea versicolor.

    a. Clinical features. Patients develop **pale macules that will not tan.** Most patients are **asymptomatic** and only notice that they have the infection during the summer months, when the skin around the lesions tans.

    b. Laboratory findings. A **KOH preparation** shows **hyphae** and **spores** under the microscope.

    c. Treatment

      (1) Selenium sulfide lotion is applied daily from the neck to the waist and left on for up to 15 minutes for 7 days. This treatment can be repeated monthly for maintenance therapy as necessary.

      (2) Oral ketoconazole (200 mg daily for 1 week or 400 mg as a single oral dose) in association with topical treatment is an alternate therapy, although this approach is less popular than selenium sulfide treatment. Patients using ketoconazole should be advised not to shower for 18 hours because the drug is delivered to the skin surface through the patient's sweat glands.

      (3) Topical imidazole. The new creams, lotions, and solutions are effective, but their cost is often prohibitive.

D. Other skin infections

  1. Abscess. An abscess is **a localized infection** characterized by a **collection of purulent material in a cavity** formed by necrosis or disintegration of tissue.

    a. Clinical features

      (1) The abscess is **tender, erythematous,** and **often fluctuant,** indicating the formation of pus.

      (2) The **axilla, buttocks, perirectal region,** and **head and neck** are the most common locations.

b. **Laboratory findings.** Discharge or drainage can be cultured, but there is **usually more than one causative organism.**

c. **Treatment**

   (1) **Hot soaks** may be used to treat an abscess in the early stages. The area should be soaked for 20 minutes, 4 times daily, until the abscess "reaches a head." When the lesion is fluctuant, it is **incised and drained,** and an iodoform gauze wick is placed in the wound to allow drainage. Alternatively, a **drawing salve** (e.g., **ichthammol**) may be used instead of surgery.

   (2) **Oral antibiotics** (e.g., dicloxacillin, cephalosporins, erythromycin) must be administered if the patient has a fever or cellulitis surrounding the abscess. Most practitioners feel that antibiotics are not indicated for mild abscesses.

2. **Injection site abscesses** may occur in patients who regularly inject therapeutic or illicit drugs. *S. aureus,* streptococci, and oral anaerobes are the most common infecting organisms. The abscesses should be **incised and drained,** and **antibiotic therapy** (e.g., with a first-generation cephalosporin) should be initiated.

3. **Infected epidermal cysts.** The initial injury is usually a result of trauma; secondary infection then develops. Aggressive treatment is needed for any infected lesions on the face, especially in the "dangerous triangle" (i.e., the bridge of the nose to the corners of the mouth).

   a. **Surgery.** The cysts **should be drained with a 16- or 14-gauge needle** or **lanced with a number-11 blade.** If the cyst is not infected, it can be surgically removed with an elliptical incision.

   b. **Antibiotic therapy** is necessary if there is cellulitis.

4. **Furuncles and carbuncles** are **infections of the hair follicles.** They may be referred to colloquially as "boils" or "risens." A furuncle is an infection of a single hair follicle, while a carbuncle involves more than one hair follicle.

   a. **Clinical features.** These lesions present as **red, hard, tender lesions** and progress to become **fluctuant or pus-filled.**

   b. **Treatment.** Initial treatment is with **warm, moist compresses.** Cloths used for warm compresses or towels used to dry the lesions should be handled with care to avoid spreading infection to others. **Antibiotic therapy** and **incision and drainage** may be appropriate.

5. **Acne vulgaris** is an inflammatory follicular, papular, and pustular eruption involving the pilosebaceous apparatus. Acne vulgaris is probably the most common skin disorder, and can affect all age-groups, from neonates to postmenopausal adults. It is so **prevalent in adolescents** that it is considered physiologic in that age-group.

   a. **Clinical features**

   (1) Acne lesions can be **open comedones ("blackheads,"** melanin depositions on a keratinous plug) or **closed, noninflammatory comedones ("whiteheads,"** flesh-colored papules approximately 1 mm in diameter). Open or closed comedones can become **erythematous papules, pustules,** or even **cysts** ranging in size from 1 mm to 5 mm. Inflammatory lesions can lead to hyperpigmentation and scarring.

   (2) Acne is seen most commonly on the **face, neck, back,** and **shoulders.**

   b. **Treatment**

   (1) **Mild acne.** The affected areas should be kept clean. **Retinoids, azelaic acid,** or **salicylic acid** can be applied topically. If there are inflammatory lesions, **benzoyl peroxide, tretinoin, topical erythromycin, clindamycin,** or **sodium sulfacetamide** can be used.

   (2) **Cystic acne**

      (a) **Oral antibiotics** (e.g., **tetracycline**) should be used in conjunction with the topical preparations.

      (b) **Isotretinoin (Accutane)** is hepatotoxic and teratogenic and therefore should be used only as a last resort and in consultation with a dermatologist.

      (c) **Dermabrasion.** Once severe acne is under control, dermabrasion can be used for scarring.

III. NEOPLASMS OF THE SKIN

A. Benign neoplasms

1. **Keratoderma.** A keratoderma is a **generalized thickening of the horny layer of the epidermis.**

   a. Types of keratoderma

   (1) **Punctate keratodermas** (found on the palms of the hands and the soles of the feet) and **keratodermas on the digits** are more prevalent in **African-American patients.**

   (2) **Senile keratoderma (actinic keratosis)** is a premalignant condition brought on by cumulative exposure to the sun, and it is **more prevalent in fair-skinned people.**

   (3) **Actinic cheilitis** is actinic keratosis of the lip.

   b. Clinical features

   (1) **Punctate keratoderma** and **keratoderma of the digits.** The lesions develop central plugs.

   (2) **Actinic keratosis.** The thickened lesions progress very slowly to squamous cell carcinomas. They can also progress to a cutaneous horn (i.e., a white, compact, protuberant growth seen in elderly patients).

   c. Treatment

   (1) **Liquid nitrogen** can be used to successfully treat keratodermas.

   (2) **Electrodesiccation** and **curettage** are used by some practitioners.

   (3) **Mild acid treatments** or the application of **Monsel's solution** has also been used.

   (4) **5-Fluorouracil** (applied topically twice daily for 2–4 weeks) is effective, but patients must be warned that their lesions will look worse before they look better.

2. **Lipomas (adipose tumors)** are **benign neoplasms of mature fat cells.** These neoplasms pose no harm to the patient. Surgical excision may be appropriate for cosmetic reasons, or if the lipoma is located where it is constantly irritated (e.g., a belt line, under the edge of a brassiere).

3. **Pyogenic granulomas (capillary hemangiomas).** Pyogenic granuloma is a misnomer because the lesion does not have an infectious etiology.

   a. **Clinical features.** These **bright red, raspberry-like growths** usually **present on exposed parts of the body** such as the arms, hands, fingers, or legs. They often appear following an injury or surgery, but can also appear spontaneously.

   b. **Treatment** consists of **electrodesiccation and curettage** or **excision.** Cauterization with silver nitrate and cryosurgery has not proved to be curative.

4. **Warts** are caused by **papillomavirus.**

   a. Types of warts

   (1) **Verruca vulgaris (common wart)** is common in children.

   (2) **Condylomata acuminata (genital warts)** are usually found in adult patients and are **sexually transmitted.**

   b. **Clinical features.** Warts are **raised, rough-surfaced lesions** that range in size. The warts may be **flesh-colored** and **slightly erythematous** to **pigmented** or **dark.**

   c. **Treatment.** Warts usually **resolve spontaneously within 1–2 years.** However, because they are unsightly and can be spread, many patients want immediate treatment. Treatment depends on the type and location of the warts, the age of the patient, the extent of the lesions, the patient's motivation for wanting the warts removed, and the patient's immunologic status. **Genital warts** should be treated because certain types of papillomavirus have oncogenic potential. HPV-16, 18, 31, and 33 have been found in cervical cancers.

   (1) **Salicylic acid in collodion** or **salicylic acid plasters**

   (2) **Cryosurgery** or **electrodesiccation** (in combination with **podophyllin),** for the treatment of genital warts

(3) Other treatments

(a) Topical tretinoin

(b) **Oral cimetidine** (25–40 mg/kg/day for 2 months). Cimetidine has been shown to inhibit suppressor T-cell formation and to increase delayed hypersensitivity responses. Studies have reported more than 80% of widespread, recalcitrant warts in children cleared after the administration of cimetidine.

(c) **Surgical excision** and **laser therapy** are not curative, and are associated with the risk of scarring.

B. Malignant neoplasms

1. **Melanoma.** Although only approximately 3% of skin cancers are melanomas, **melanomas cause 66% of deaths from all skin cancers.** Melanomas frequently metastasize widely to regional lymph nodes, skin, liver, lungs, or the brain.

a. Clinical features

(1) Melanomas are **usually black or dark brown** but can be flesh-colored. They sometimes have blue, pink, or red components.

(2) The lesions are **irregular in outline** with an **outward spreading of pigment.** If the lesion changes in size over a relatively short period of time, malignant degeneration needs to be considered.

(3) Although most commonly seen on the **skin,** a melanoma can occur anywhere on the body, including the **eye** and mucous membranes of the **genitalia, anus,** or **oral cavity.**

b. **Prognosis** can be estimated by the thickness of the lesion. A melanoma entirely within the epidermis carries a very good prognosis. As the thickness progresses beyond the epidermis, the prognosis diminishes. The likelihood of survival is further diminished if the melanoma is on the upper back, upper arm, neck, or scalp.

c. **Treatment. Early detection is the key to successful treatment of melanoma.** Over the past 30 years, the 5-year survival rate has increased from 25%–40% to 80%. Melanoma patients **need to be referred to a dermatologist or surgeon** for complete excision and follow-up.

2. **Squamous cell** and **basal cell carcinomas** are the most common neoplasms of the skin. Metastasis is rare.

a. Clinical features

(1) The lesions are **asymptomatic, but may itch or bleed.** The patient seeks treatment because the lesions do not heal.

(2) The lesions present on areas that are usually exposed to the sun (e.g., the face, head, neck, and, in men, the trunk).

b. **Treatment** involves complete eradication of the cancer. Options include:

(1) **Excision with clear margins**

(2) **Electrodesiccation with curettage**

(3) **5-Fluorouracil**

(4) **Cryosurgery**

(5) **Radiation therapy**

(6) **Mohs micrographic surgery**

(7) **Laser vaporization**

3. **Kaposi's sarcoma** is **the most common HIV-related malignancy.**

a. **Clinical features.** The lesions are **purplish** and **nonblanching** in fair-skinned people, and **brown** in dark-skinned people. They may be located on the skin and mucous membranes; in the mouth, lesions are usually on the hard palate.

b. **Treatment** is usually handled by infectious disease specialists or oncologists. Various medications, such as **vincristine** and **vinblastine,** are used, but may be palliative only.

IV. SYSTEMIC DISEASES THAT AFFECT THE SKIN

A. **Exanthems** are **skin eruptions that occur as a result of an acute viral or coccal infection.**

   1. Viral exanthems include measles, fifth disease, and varicella.

   a. Clinical features

   (1) Measles

   (a) Following an incubation period of 9–21 days, the patient develops a **prodrome (cough, coryza, conjunctivitis, fever)** lasting 2–5 days.

   (b) **Koplik's spots** on the buccal mucosa may precede the characteristic rash by a couple of days.

   (c) **Rash.** The lesions start out **erythematous and macular** and **become papular.** They usually begin in the hairline and progress downward toward the feet, becoming increasingly confluent. They fade in the same sequence as they appear.

   (2) **Fifth disease (erythema infectiosum)** is caused by **human parvovirus B19** and mainly affects **children between the ages of 3 and 12 years.**

   (a) Prodrome. Following an **incubation period of 9–21 days**, a prodromal stage of 2–5 days occurs. Fifth disease has **few prodromal symptoms;** the **sudden onset of macular erythema of the cheeks** (a "slapped cheek" appearance) may be noted.

   (b) **Rash.** As the facial rash begins to diminish, an erythematous maculopapular eruption spreads over the extensor aspects of the extremities. This eruption later fades with a central clearing, creating a distinctive **marbled appearance.**

   (3) Varicella (chicken pox)

   (a) Prodrome. Following an incubation period of 9–21 days, a prodromal stage (characterized by cough, coryza, conjunctivitis, or fever) develops and persists for 2–5 days.

   (b) **Rash.** The lesions begin as faint macules, which progress to vesicles on an erythematous base within 24 hours. The vesicles rapidly become pustular, umbilicated, and then crusted.

   (c) **Laboratory findings.** Many health care providers feel that **seeing a patient with lesions in all three stages at the same time is diagnostic.** The diagnosis can be confirmed if necessary by a **direct fluorescent antibody test;** a **Tzanck preparation** may also be helpful.

   b. **Treatment.** Because most viral exanthems are self-limiting, treatment is mainly supportive.

   (1) Supportive therapy

   (a) **Antipyretics** and **hydration** form the mainstay of supportive therapy. **Aspirin or products with aspirin as an ingredient should never be used in children because they increase the risk of Reye syndrome.**

   (b) **Antipruritics** may be prescribed if the patient appears to be itching. Topical agents (e.g., **calamine, phenols, lotions**) may be soothing but do not appear to promote healing. **Oatmeal baths** also may make the patient more comfortable.

   (2) **Specific treatment for varicella.** The patient might benefit from **acyclovir** therapy if started very early (i.e., within the first 24 hours). The dosage is 20 mg/kg (maximum, 800 mg/dose), four times daily for 5 days. The newer agents valacyclovir and famciclovir are also effective and less expensive.

   2. Bacterial exanthems include **scarlet fever.**

   a. Clinical features

   (1) **Rash.** A rash consisting of **tiny erythematous papules** that **blanch under pressure** appears on the second day on the **upper torso** and **spreads to the remainder of the trunk**, sparing the face, palms, and soles.

   (2) **Strawberry tongue.** The patient's face is flushed. A whitish-yellow layer develops over the red papillae of the tongue ("white strawberries"); the tongue then turns a beefy red color and is described as "strawberry tongue."

    b. Treatment entails **aggressive antibiotic therapy,** because the causative organism can cause rheumatic fever, glomerulonephritis, and other serious complications. Penicillin or erythromycin may be used in doses appropriate to the child's age and weight.

B. Psoriasis is a chronic, inflammatory, scaling condition of the skin that may also involve the mucous membranes. It is **thought to be a genetic disorder,** although only approximately one third of patients have family members with the condition. It appears that the earlier the onset of the disease, the more severe it will be; early onset also seems to increase the risk of developing **psoriatic arthritis.**

    1. Clinical features. The symptoms are mild, consisting of **mild itching,** but the **lesions are unsightly.**

        a. Psoriasis patches are usually **raised, reddened areas with distinct margins and loosely adherent silvery scales.** Peeling away a scale produces specks of bleeding from the capillaries **(Auspitz's sign).**

        b. Patches are most often found on the **elbows, knees,** and **scalp,** but can be anywhere on the body. Patients with extensive disease also have **nail involvement,** varying from tiny pits to separation from the nail beds. **Psoriatic arthritis,** if it develops, usually **begins in the distal joints of the hands and feet.**

    2. Treatment

        a. Steroids

            (1) Topical corticosteroids and **topical vitamin D preparations** are useful for mild cases**.**

            (2) Intralesional instillation of steroids sometimes helps.

            (3) Systemic steroids help, but sometimes the disease flares up after withdrawal.

        b. Coal tar or **salicylic acid preparations** are effective in controlling or removing scales.

        c. Ultraviolet B phototherapy, psoralens plus ultraviolet A radiation, and **methotrexate** have been **effective but carry some risk** for the patient. Hepatic enzyme levels and white blood cell (WBC) counts should be monitored in patients undergoing this type of therapy.

C. Ulcers. Diabetic ulcers, stasis (venous) ulcers, or arterial leg ulcers may develop on the lower limb.

    1. Clinical features

        a. Diabetic ulcers tend to be **deep, punched-out lesions** over the **malleoli,** the **plantar surfaces of the feet,** or the **toes.** They are usually painless because of associated neuropathies.

        b. Stasis (venous) ulcers follow chronic venous stasis. Initially, the skin has a **brown, mottled appearance,** and the area is itchy and dry. Eventually, the tissue breaks down and forms an ulcer, usually over the **inner side of the ankle** or the **distal third of the shin.**

            (1) These ulcers tend to be **wide but not deep,** with **irregular, undulating edges** and a **clean base.**

            (2) There is usually not much pain, but if there is, **elevating the affected limb eases the pain.** (This is in contrast to arterial ulcers, which become more painful on elevation.)

            (3) Because the problem is with the veins, **pedal pulses** are present.

        c. Arterial leg ulcers do not usually become as large as venous ulcers and are not preceded by the brown, mottled appearance of stasis.

            (1) Arterial ulcers are often **very painful.**

            (2) Pulses may be absent, and the **foot will be cold.**

            (3) A **Doppler flow ultrasonogram** should be obtained to confirm the blockage.

    2. Treatment. All lower limb ulcers are somewhat difficult to treat. Treatment depends on which type of ulcer is being treated.

        a. Diabetic and **arterial ulcers** are treated similarly, and **neither heals well.**

            (1) Lifestyle changes include smoking cessation and moderate exercise to enhance blood flow.

            (2) Débridement is necessary if the wound is necrotic, and then dressings are applied. **Wet-to-dry dressings** or the **hydrogels** are standard because wounds heal better in a moist environment. The newer hydrogels (also called hydrocolloids) maintain moisture, enhance granulation, promote débridement, and improve rates of epithelialization.

(3) **Antibiotic therapy** (e.g., topical mupirocin) is indicated if there is evidence of infection.

b. **Stasis (venous) ulcers** are treated with **elevation** and **compression** to enhance venous return.

(1) The affected limb should be **whirlpooled, the lesion painted with gentian violet,** and then **an Unna boot should be applied weekly.**

(2) **Wraps or support hose** may also be used for compression. One hint for using wraps or support hose is to apply them while the leg is elevated and before the veins fill again.

(3) **Antibiotic therapy.** If there are signs of infection, the wound needs to be treated with antibiotic therapy.

D. **Tickborne illnesses.** The two most common tickborne illnesses are Lyme disease and Rocky Mountain spotted fever (RMSF).

1. **Lyme disease** is caused by *Borrelia burgdorferi*. This spirochete is carried by the *Ixodes* tick and is transmitted to the host when the tick has been embedded in the skin for 24 hours or more.

a. **Clinical features**

(1) **Stage 1.** A "bull's-eye" rash forms at the site of the tick inoculation within days to weeks of the initial bite.

(2) **Stage 2. Neurologic symptoms** (e.g., meningitis, encephalitis, chorea, cranial neuritis) or **cardiologic symptoms** (e.g., atrioventricular block, cardiomegaly) develop weeks to months later.

(3) **Stage 3. Arthritis** may occur even later.

b. **Treatment**

(1) In any tickborne illness, **the tick must be removed.** It is best to use a forceps to remove the tick because the infectious fluid or feces from the tick may infect the person removing it.

(2) **Pharmacotherapy**

(a) **Stage 1. Doxycycline** (100 mg twice daily) or **amoxicillin** (500 mg 3 times daily for 10 days to 2 weeks) is appropriate.

(b) **Stage 2 or 3.** If the patient presents with stage 2 or 3 disease, **doxycycline** or **amoxicillin** can be administered for **4–6 weeks,** or the **dosages can be increased** (doxycycline, 100 mg twice daily or amoxicillin, 1000 mg 3 times daily).

c. **Prevention.** Patients who live in endemic areas should be taught to **perform tick checks** on themselves and companions.

2. **RMSF** is caused by the coccobacillus ***Rickettsia rickettsii*** and is transmitted by a bite from either a **dog tick** (*Dermacentor variabalis*) or a **wood tick** (Dermacentor andersoni), depending on the part of the country.

a. **Clinical features.** Symptoms appear within 2 days to 2 weeks from the time of the tick bite.

(1) **Prodrome.** The prodrome includes **flu-like symptoms** (e.g., malaise, loss of appetite, chills, fever). Some patients also experience **myalgias, conjunctival erythema, nausea,** and **photophobia.**

(2) **Rash.** A rash composed of **erythematous macules and papules** develops, beginning on the wrists and ankles and spreading inward to involve the trunk. The rash becomes **hemorrhagic and purpuric** and often involves the palms and soles.

(3) **Other organ system involvement** can occur. Rickettsia infection may become disseminated and lead to vasculitis of the arterioles, capillaries, and venules in the skin, brain, heart, and kidneys. Rickettsia damages the endothelial cells, resulting in medial necrosis, endothelial hypertrophy, and proliferation, which, along with platelet and fibrin thrombosis, causes vascular occlusion.

b. **Treatment.** If not treated, RMSF can be fatal; mortality rates range from 15%–80%. **Aggressive treatment as early as possible is recommended;** treatment should be started before laboratory results are available.

(1) **The tick must be removed.**

(2) **Pharmacotherapy**

(a) **Tetracycline** (500 mg 4 times daily) should be started. **Tetracycline should not be used** in children 8 years or younger or in pregnant women. Doxycycline or chloramphenicol should be used instead.

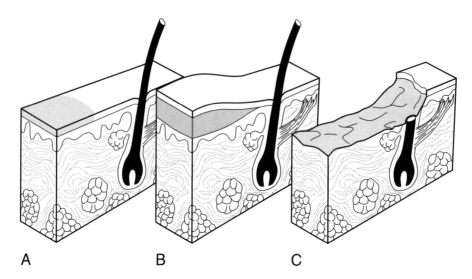

Figure 13-1. Types of burns. (A) First degree. (B) Partial thickness. (C) Full thickness.

        (b) In patients with more severe illness, **hospital admission** and **intravenous chloramphenicol** may be necessary, and should be continued for at least 5–7 days.

    (3) Fluid replacement is indicated.

   c. Prevention is the same as for Lyme disease.

V. BURNS AND OPEN WOUNDS need to be evaluated according to the **extent of injury, the age of the patient,** and **any associated illnesses or injury**.

  A. Burns. Figure 13-1 illustrates the 3 types of burns.

    1. Any blisters should not be broken, but left intact if at all possible. If the blisters have been broken, the wound should be carefully débrided. If the burn is severe enough that there is an eschar formation, the **eschar should be débrided** to allow proper healing.

    2. Silver sulfadiazine is applied topically.

  B. Open wounds

    1. Tetanus immunization should be given any time the skin has been broken, unless the patient has been inoculated in the past 10 years. [Some emergency department physicians believe the tetanus immunization is needed even more often if the offending agent (e.g., rusty nail, barbed wire) has caused what is sometimes termed a "barnyard" injury.]

    2. Inspection and cleansing. Open wounds should be cleansed well and closed if the patient presents within 6–8 hours of sustaining the injury, and if there is no sign of infection. Wounds should be **irrigated well.** Wounds should not be closed after 8 hours or if there are signs of infection.

    3. Antibiotic therapy

      a. Most **"clean" injuries** do not require antibiotics.

      b. **"Dirty" wounds** (e.g., gunshot wounds, human bites) are usually treated with **cephalosporins. Penicillin, tetracycline,** or **amoxicillin-clavulanic acid** is recommended for the treatment of animal bites.

  C. Hematomas may be treated with ice packs.

  D. Contusions and **abrasions** need to be cleansed and a topical antibiotic ointment applied.

Comprehensive Examination

Directions: *Each of the numbered items or incomplete statements in this section is followed by answers or by completions of the statement. Select the ONE lettered answer or completion that is BEST in each case. Some of the numbered items or incomplete statements are negatively phrased, as indicated by a capitalized word such as NOT, LEAST, or EXCEPT. For these items, select the ONE lettered answer or completion that is BEST in each case.*

1. A 78-year-old man is found to have iron deficiency anemia. Of the following conditions, which is the most likely cause?
   A. Poor nutritional intake of iron
   B. Carcinoma of the colon
   C. Consumption of starch or clay
   D. Lack of intrinsic factor

2. A patient with anemia is found to have a mean corpuscular hemoglobin (MCH) of 28 picograms (pg) and a mean corpuscular volume (MCV) of 88 pg. Of the following types of anemia, which is most consistent with these findings?
   A. Iron deficiency
   B. Folic acid deficiency
   C. Anemia of chronic disease
   D. Thalassemia

3. Treatment of folic acid deficiency includes which of the following?
   A. Administration of erythropoietin
   B. Supplementation with intrinsic factor
   C. Correction of chronic bleeding
   D. Avoidance of alcohol

4. A patient presents with a complaint of headaches and dizziness. Further questioning reveals that he also has a sensation of fullness in his head and face and he experiences severe itching after bathing. Physical examination reveals blood pressure of 180/84, plethoric facies, and splenomegaly. What finding would you expect in his laboratory evaluation?
   A. Thrombocytosis
   B. Leukocytopenia
   C. Decreased serum B_{12}
   D. Macrocytic erythrocytes

5. A 5-year-old child is brought in for evaluation of fatigue, abrupt onset of fever, headache, and bone pain. His mother states that he has been uncharacteristically quiet for the past several weeks. In considering a diagnosis of leukemia for this child, what is the most likely type?
   A. Acute myelogenous leukemia (AML)
   B. Acute lymphocytic leukemia (ALL)
   C. Chronic myelogenous leukemia (CML)
   D. Chronic lymphocytic leukemia (CLL)

6. A patient diagnosed with Hodgkin's lymphoma is found to have positive nodes in the supraclavicular and hilar areas without splenic involvement. He has no fever, night sweats, or weight loss. According to the Ann Arbor Criteria, his disease can be correctly staged as
   A. IA
   B. IB
   C. IIA
   D. IIIB

7. Of the following therapeutic agents, which is used in the prevention of *Pneumocystis carinii* infection in the patient with AIDS?
   A. Zidovudine
   B. Rifabutin
   C. Ganciclovir
   D. Pentamidine

8. A 6-year-old child treated recently for an upper respiratory infection is brought in by his parents for evaluation of sudden skin changes on the lower extremities. Physical examination reveals both petechiae and purpura. How should the patient be managed?
   A. The parents should be reassured and the child monitored
   B. Corticosteroid therapy should be initiated
   C. The patient should be referred for an emergency splenectomy
   D. The parents should be advised to use children's aspirin for pain and fever

9. Hemophilia A (classic hemophilia) is associated with which coagulation factor?
   A. II
   B. VIII
   C. IX
   D. X

10. A 3-year-old child is brought in for evaluation of red and swollen eyelids. In addition to these findings, examination reveals ptosis, proptosis, conjunctivitis, and decreased range of motion in the eye muscles. His mother states that she has been treating him with acetaminophen and an over-the-counter decongestant for a severe upper respiratory infection. Of the following, what is the organism most likely to be responsible for the child's eye findings?
A. *Staphylococcus aureus*
B. *Moraxella catarrhalis*
C. *Streptococcus pyogenes*
D. *Haemophilus influenzae*

11. It is September and school has recently reopened. You have seen 4 children this morning with bilateral red eyes. The conjunctivae are injected and there is limbic sparing. All the children have copious watery discharge and three of the four exhibit preauricular lymphadenopathy. What is the most likely cause of this condition?
A. Viral conjunctivitis
B. Bacterial conjunctivitis
C. Allergic conjunctivitis
D. Iritis

12. Which of the following is a sensorineural cause of hearing loss?
A. Cerumen impaction
B. Noise exposure
C. Otosclerosis
D. Otitis media

13. Which of the following tests is used to establish a diagnosis of vertigo?
A. The Weber test
B. The Rinne test
C. The Hallpike maneuver
D. Caloric testing

14. A 24-year-old male patient presents with a painful, erythematous inflammation along the left lower palpebral margin that began about 24 hours ago. What is the first line of treatment?
A. Incision and drainage
B. Initiation of systemic antibiotics
C. Referral for elective excision
D. Warm compresses

15. Chest radiograph in a patient with chronic obstructive pulmonary disease (COPD) is likely to show
A. hyperinflation of the lungs and flattened diaphragms
B. small opacities in the upper lung fields
C. mediastinal shift and presence of pleural air
D. blunting of the costophrenic angles

16. Which of the following treatments for reflux esophagitis increases gastric emptying?
A. Ranitidine
B. Bethanechol
C. Omeprazole
D. Nifedipine

17. In differentiating ulcerative colitis from Crohn's disease, which finding would make a diagnosis of ulcerative colitis more likely?
A. Gradual onset of symptoms
B. Primarily right-sided distribution
C. Tenesmus
D. Development of toxic megacolon

18. The most common cause of chronic or recurrent abdominal pain in the United States is
A. ulcerative colitis
B. Crohn's disease
C. gastritis
D. irritable bowel syndrome (IBS)

19. A 65-year-old woman presents with a complaint of constipation for the past 3–4 months. Prior to that time, she normally had one stool per day. What is the next step in the management of this patient?
A. Evaluate her for colon cancer
B. Advise her to increase her fiber and fluid intake
C. Recommend that she increase her exercise
D. Discuss intermittent use of over-the-counter laxatives

20. A patient who has severe pain and bright red blood per rectum on defecation in the absence of other symptoms most likely has
A. hemorrhoids
B. an anal fissure
C. ulcerative colitis
D. Crohn's disease

21. What is the most common cause of chronic pancreatitis in the United States?
A. Cholelithiasis
B. Hyperlipidemia
C. Peptic ulcer disease
D. Alcohol abuse

22. A 45-year-old woman presents to the emergency department with severe right upper quadrant pain. This began as colicky pain, but is now steady and more intense. The pain radiates to the right shoulder. She is feverish and has vomited 3 times. The most likely diagnosis is
A. acute cholecystitis
B. acute pancreatitis
C. perforated duodenal ulcer
D. gastroenteritis

23. What is the most common cause of acute hepatitis in the United States?
A. Alcohol use
B. Viral infection
C. Autoimmune disease
D. Hereditary disorders

24. A positive antigen against hepatitis B serum antigen (anti-HBs) indicates
A. acute infection
B. ongoing infection
C. immunity
D. highly contagious state

25. Which of the following causes of infectious diarrhea is associated with bloody and purulent stools?
A. Norwalk virus
B. *Staphylococcus aureus* toxin
C. *Giardia lamblia*
D. *Shigella* species

26. Which of the following is a cause of respiratory alkalosis?
A. Hyperventilation
B. Myasthenia gravis
C. Chronic obstructive pulmonary disease
D. Brain stem injury

27. A laboratory report specifies the following values: blood urea nitrogen (BUN) 12 mg/dl; creatinine 1 mg/dl; sodium 144 mEq/L; potassium 3.0 mEq/L; chloride 100 mEq/L; bicarbonate 12 mEq/L. What is the anion gap for this patient?
A. 29
B. 32
C. 35
D. 53

28. A 23-year-old man presents with a complaint of severe dysuria and a profuse yellowish urethral discharge. Gram stain reveals gram-negative intracellular diplococci. The recommended treatment for this patient includes
A. amoxicillin and probenecid
B. benzathine penicillin
C. ceftriaxone and azithromycin
D. doxycycline

29. In a man older than 35 years of age, what is the most common organism implicated in epididymitis?
A. *Chlamydia trachomatis*
B. *Neisseria gonorrhoeae*
C. *Mycobacterium tuberculosis*
D. *Escherichia coli*

30. What is the most common presenting symptom of bladder cancer?
A. Hematuria
B. Bladder irritability
C. Bladder infection
D. Urethral discharge

31. Electrocardiographic changes indicating ischemic heart disease include which of the following?
A. Q waves
B. Down-sloping ST-segment depression
C. U waves
D. Wide and bizarre QRS complexes

32. Development of Q waves in leads II, III, and aVF suggest a myocardial infarction in what location?
A. Posterior
B. Anterolateral
C. Inferior
D. Anteroseptal

33. "Holiday heart" is precipitated by excessive alcohol use and withdrawal. What is the associated arrhythmia?
A. Paroxysmal supraventricular tachycardia
B. Atrial flutter
C. Ventricular flutter
D. Atrial fibrillation

34. What is the recommended treatment for asymptomatic premature ventricular contractions?
A. None at all
B. β-blockers
C. Calcium channel blockers
D. Sodium channel blockers

35. What is the preferred treatment for patients who are symptomatic with sick sinus syndrome?
A. Digitalis
B. Permanent pacing
C. Surgical or radiofrequency ablation
D. β-blockers

36. A patient presents for evaluation of an ulcer over the medial malleolus. The surrounding skin is edematous, shiny, atrophic, and darkly pigmented and the ulcer has ragged edges with undermining. Her feet are warm and the pedal pulses are full. Sensation is intact. What is the most likely cause of this ulcer?
A. Arterial insufficiency
B. Underlying diabetes mellitus
C. Chronic venous insufficiency
D. Persistent application of pressure ulcers

37. A teenaged boy presents to the clinic for evaluation of a rash. The rash is primarily on the trunk and consists of small oval, salmon-colored, slightly raised lesions in a skinfold distribution. When scratched, the lesions show a fine scale. He has no other symptoms, but says he had a single larger lesion about a week prior to this eruption. What is the most likely diagnosis?
A. Tinea versicolor
B. Rubella
C. Pityriasis rosea
D. Secondary syphilis

38. A patient is suspected to have a disorder of the aortic valve. In order to best hear a murmur in this area, the patient should be instructed to
A. sit upright and lean forward
B. lie in the left lateral position
C. execute a Valsalva maneuver
D. breathe in fully

39. The drug of choice for treating an infected human bite wound is
A. a cephalosporin
B. penicillin
C. tetracycline
D. amoxicillin-clavulanic acid

40. Which cardiac marker is the LEAST sensitive in detecting myocardial infarction?
A. Troponin T
B. Isoenzyme of creatine kinase containing M and B subunits (CK-MB)
C. Lactate dehydrogenase (LDH)
D. Total creatine kinase

41. All of the following are characteristics of malignant melanoma EXCEPT
A. irregular borders
B. asymmetry
C. size greater than 6 mm
D. uniform color

42. Tetralogy of Fallot consists of all of the following anomalies EXCEPT
A. subaortic septal defect
B. left ventricular outflow obstruction
C. overriding aorta
D. right ventricular hypertrophy

43. Initial laboratory testing in a patient who is found to have a low hemoglobin or hematocrit should include all of the following EXCEPT
A. hemoglobin electrophoresis
B. red cell indices
C. red cell distribution width
D. corrected reticulocyte count

44. All of the following eye disorders are associated with insidious loss of vision EXCEPT
A. cataracts
B. macular degeneration
C. retinal detachment
D. open-angle glaucoma

45. Common findings of acute appendicitis in a previously healthy young person include all of the following EXCEPT
A. localization of pain to the right lower quadrant
B. low-grade fever
C. vomiting and diarrhea
D. positive psoas sign

46. A male patient presents with erythema and scale formation that is more evident at the margin of the eyelid and involves the skin immediately adjacent to the eyelashes. He complains of mild pruritus and conjunctival erythema. This scenario is descriptive of which of the following conditions?
A. Acute dacryocystitis
B. Blepharitis
C. Conjunctivitis
D. Keratitis

47. A 65-year-old man who smokes cigarettes has a history of chronic cough productive of phlegm occurring on most days for 6 months. What is the most likely diagnosis?
A. Pneumonia
B. Asthma
C. Pulmonary embolism
D. Chronic bronchitis

48. Which of the following persons is most at risk for hypertension?
A. A sedentary black woman
B. An overweight white man
C. A black male smoker
D. A white woman with elevated serum cholesterol

49. Dysphagia with intermittent chest pain is most commonly associated with which of the following conditions?
A. Esophageal stenosis
B. Scleroderma
C. Esophageal spasm
D. Zenker's diverticulum

50. The patient is a 28-year-old man who has had multiple anonymous unprotected sexual encounters with both men and women. He has no history of intravenous drug use and has no medical complaints. Which of the following is an appropriate first step in evaluating this patient?
    A. A CD4+ count
    B. A skin test for tuberculosis
    C. Screening for cytomegalovirus (CMV)
    D. HIV enzyme-linked immunosorbent assay (ELISA) and Western blot test

51. What is the primary reason folic acid supplementation is recommended prior to conception?
    A. It decreases the incidence of neural tube defects
    B. It improves folic acid anemia
    C. It corrects an underlying acid–base imbalance
    D. It enhances the nutritional status of the mother

52. Which of the following is an uncommon cause of hematuria?
    A. Glomerulonephritis
    B. Renal failure
    C. Kidney stones
    D. Bladder cancer

53. A 49-year-old male truck driver presents with severe, diffuse neck pain, and pain in his right shoulder and arm. He has paresthesias and numbness in the fingers. He has no history of trauma. On physical examination, pain is found to be increased by extension of the neck and relieved by flexion. Radiographs show osteophytes and disk space narrowing, and changes in the joints of Luschka and the facet joints. What is the most likely diagnosis?
    A. Muscle spasm in the extensor muscles of the neck with radiculopathy
    B. Herniated nucleus pulposus (HNP)
    C. Ankylosing spondylitis
    D. Cervical spondylosis

54. A 67-year-old man presents to the emergency department with acute paralysis and decreased sensation of the right lower extremity. These are most consistent with an occlusion of the
    A. anterior circulation of the brain
    B. internal carotid artery
    C. middle cerebral artery
    D. posterior circulation of the brain

55. A 13-year-old girl has been menstruating for about 1 year without any difficulties. For the past 2 months, however, she has experienced cramping and diarrhea for the first 2 days of her periods severe enough to keep her out of school. She states she has never had sexual intercourse. Her physical examination is normal. What should be the next step in managing this patient?
    A. Perform a work-up for possible pelvic pathology
    B. Tell her that menstrual discomfort is a normal part of life
    C. Prescribe oral contraceptives
    D. Advise her to start a nonsteroidal anti-inflammatory drug (NSAID) just before menses

56. Patients with schizophrenia, schizophreniform disorder, or brief psychotic disorder present with common symptoms. The differential diagnosis is based on
    A. the age of the patient at the time of initial symptom onset
    B. the severity and duration of the symptoms
    C. the presence of organicity
    D. the extent of dissociation

57. Which of the following is a feature of Graves' disease?
    A. Far more common in men than in women
    B. Usually a disease of old age
    C. Rarely found in people with a positive family history
    D. Occurs in people with other autoimmune disorders

58. A 3-year-old boy in good general health develops an erythematous vesicle that ruptures and forms a thick, yellowish crust around his lips. The most likely diagnosis is
    A. acne vulgaris
    B. dermatophytosis
    C. oral candidiasis
    D. impetigo

59. How much protein is excreted into the urine with nephrotic syndrome?
    A. Less than 1 gram per day
    B. 1–2 grams per day
    C. 2–3 grams per day
    D. More than 3 grams per day

60. A female patient presents to the clinic with a chief complaint she describes as "a curtain being pulled down" over her eyes, and loss of vision in the right eye. She denies pain or redness but states that recently she noticed "floaters." The most likely diagnosis would be

    A. central retinal vein occlusion

    B. central retinal artery occlusion

    C. retinal detachment

    D. temporal arteritis

61. Patients with chronic congestive heart failure (CHF) would be expected to exhibit

    A. an elevated liver enzyme profile and left-sided cardiomegaly

    B. a deficient liver enzyme profile and left-sided cardiomegaly

    C. an elevated liver enzyme profile and right-sided cardiomegaly

    D. a deficient liver enzyme profile and right-sided cardiomegaly

62. If a patient and her husband seek medical attention because they have been unable to conceive after one year, what should the first step be?

    A. They should be counseled to relax, and eventually pregnancy will probably occur.

    B. Measures should be instituted for an infertility work-up.

    C. Basal body temperature graphs should be taken and folic acid supplementation begun.

    D. They should be told to seek counseling for an underlying sexual dysfunction.

63. The patient is a 32-year-old married female elementary school teacher and mother of 2 children who comes in concerned about increasing nervousness, exhaustion, diarrhea, and menstrual problems. Further questioning reveals heat intolerance, sweating, and weight loss of about 10 pounds despite increased appetite. She was well at her annual physical examination 11 months ago. On physical examination, she is found to be tachycardic with a fine resting tremor, hyperreflexia, and warm, moist hands. What is the most likely diagnosis?

    A. Pheochromocytoma

    B. Panic attacks

    C. Thyrotoxicosis

    D. Amphetamine abuse

64. Which set of presenting symptoms would you expect to see in a patient with schizophrenia?

    A. Delusions, hallucinations, and disorganized speech

    B. Irritability, hypervigilance, and sleep disturbances

    C. Grandiosity, psychomotor agitation, and flight of ideas

    D. Suicidal ideation, terminal insomnia, and significantly depressed mood

65. Dark-field examination is used to test for which disease?

    A. Gonorrhea

    B. Herpes

    C. Syphilis

    D. Chlamydia

66. What is the major reversible risk factor for chronic obstructive pulmonary disease (COPD)?

    A. Smoking

    B. Infection

    C. Pollutants

    D. Allergies

67. Of the following, the most definitive diagnostic finding in ischemic heart disease would be

    A. angina during a cardiac stress test

    B. narrowed coronary arteries demonstrated by angiography

    C. chest radiograph showing a left shift in the cardiac silhouette

    D. electrocardiogram (ECG) showing down sloping ST–segment depression

68. The patient is a 26-year-old man with known HIV disease and a helper cell (CD4) count of 190 cells/mm^3. He complains of pain on swallowing for 2 days. Physical examination is unremarkable except for nontender lymphadenopathy of cervical and occipital nodes and a few white plaques on the tonsillar pillars. What regimen should be administered initially?

    A. Fluconazole, 200 mg every day

    B. Acyclovir, 400 mg twice a day

    C. Dexamethasone elixir, 1 mg (10 ml) twice a day

    D. Foscarnet, 60 mg/kg every 8 hours

69. A 36-year-old woman presents looking for assistance with "worsening premenstrual syndrome (PMS)." Her symptoms include premenstrual inability to cope with her job, irritability, and depression. Her menses are regular with mild cramping and she has no other symptoms. Her physical examination is normal. The first step in her treatment should be
  A. referral to a psychologist or psychiatrist
  B. prescription of an antidepressant medication
  C. charting symptoms on a calendar and returning for a follow-up visit
  D. referral to a gynecologist for hysterectomy

70. At 20 weeks' gestation
  A. the uterus will be at the umbilicus; quickening is probable
  B. the uterus will be midway between the symphysis and the umbilicus; no quickening will have occurred
  C. the uterus will be at the umbilicus; no quickening will have occurred
  D. the uterus will be at the symphysis with positive fetal heart tones

71. A patient who is typically in excellent health is brought to the emergency department reporting sudden onset of acute, severe, generalized headache pain, described as "the worst headache I've ever had." Initial examination reveals elevated blood pressure and a temperature of more than 101° F. The most likely diagnosis is
  A. classic migraine headache
  B. subarachnoid hemorrhage
  C. aseptic meningitis
  D. subdural hemorrhage

72. The treatment of choice for acute exertion-induced angina in ischemic heart disease is
  A. sublingual propranolol
  B. sublingual nitroglycerin
  C. daily aspirin anticoagulant therapy
  D. slow-release transdermal nifedipine

73. A 78-year-old woman presents with mild dyspnea and fatigue. Other than moderate osteoarthritis for which she takes over-the-counter ibuprofen, she is well. Initial blood work shows a hypochromic-microcytic anemia. Her serum ferritin is low and the total iron binding capacity is elevated. What is the next appropriate step in caring for this patient?
  A. Initiate treatment with ferrous sulfate
  B. Perform a stool guaiac test
  C. Advise her to increase iron in her diet
  D. Perform a work-up for anemia of chronic disease

74. A 65-year-old man presents with dysphagia for solid food that was first noticed 2 months ago and has progressed rapidly since that time. What would be the most crucial question in the history?
  A. Does the patient require pillows to avoid substernal pain at night?
  B. Has the patient ever had ulcer disease?
  C. Does the patient smoke cigarettes?
  D. Has the patient had a change in bowel habits?

75. A 52-year-old man with arthritis has a routine urinalysis that shows 3+ proteinuria. What is the most likely cause?
  A. Minimal change disease
  B. Acute interstitial nephritis
  C. Multiple myeloma
  D. Orthostatic proteinuria

76. A 22-year-old woman presents to your office with vague complaints of lower abdominal pain and vaginal spotting. Her past history includes chlamydial infection, and she is using condoms for contraception. Her last regular menstrual period was 6 weeks ago. The most important test to order in this circumstance would be
  A. a test for chlamydia
  B. hemoglobin
  C. a serum human chorionic gonadotropin (hCG)
  D. urinalysis

77. A 10-year-old girl is referred by her school nurse for evaluation of truncal rotation with forward bending and a 20° curve measured by scoliometer. The patient has a family history of idiopathic scoliosis, and physical examination confirms a 20° right thoracic curve with an immature Risser stage. Which of the following is the correct recommendation?
  A. No follow-up is required as curves of 0°–20° are normal at this age
  B. Follow-up is required every 6 months with forward bending test and scoliometer test to check for progression
  C. Serial observation with repeat radiographs on a 36″ anteroposterior film is required every 3–4 months
  D. Referral to a specialist is required for consideration of bracing and close follow-up

78. A 68-year-old retired male engineer is brought in by his wife who is concerned about his increasing apathy and depression. She tells you his normally excellent appetite has disappeared, yet he seems to have put on weight. He is unable to add much in the way of history, but does admit to "wishing it all would end." Physical examination reveals, bradycardia, dry skin, hyporeflexia, and pallor. Which one of the following tests should be ordered first?

A. Administer a depression inventory

B. Draw blood for a serum thyroid-stimulating hormone (TSH) level

C. Perform a fingerstick glucose test immediately

D. Order an adrenocorticotropic hormone (ACTH) stimulation test

79. A 20-year-old man reports to have had several seconds of twitching of his right thumb, followed by similar twitching of the right hand, then the right arm, and finally the right side of his face. The most likely cause of this activity would be

A. complex partial seizure

B. benign tremor

C. simple partial seizure

D. febrile seizure

80. Social and occupational functioning are negatively impacted in all schizophrenic conditions. In reviewing charts of schizophrenic patients, you run across an anomaly that calls the diagnosis of schizophrenia into question. Which of the following patient profiles would you label as anomalous?

A. A patient who has been unable to hold any job for an extended period

B. A patient who could never maintain a marital relationship

C. A patient unable to withdraw from schooling even after completing several degrees

D. A patient unable to sustain friendships

81. A 20-year-old woman develops flu-like symptoms, including malaise, anorexia, chills, and fever. Soon thereafter, a hemorrhagic and purpuric rash develops, beginning on the patient's wrists and ankles and spreading inward to involve the trunk. During the course of the interview, the patient reveals that she, her husband, and their two young children had returned from a camping trip earlier in the week. The four had shared a tent. What is the most likely diagnosis?

A. Lyme disease

B. Varicella

C. Rocky Mountain spotted fever (RSMF)

D. Measles

82. On a routine physical examination, the patient asks you to evaluate a "bump" on his left eyelid. On examination, there is a painless, non-tender, 2-mm firm nodule without any signs of inflammation. There is no visible "point" or "head." You determine that the abnormality is

A. hordeolum

B. chalazion

C. entropion

D. xanthelasma

83. A 32-year-old woman arrives at the emergency room in an ambulance in respiratory distress. Family members say that the patient has been sick for several days with an upper respiratory infection. This morning, while asleep, the patient vomited. The patient continues to deteriorate in the emergency room, and develops hypoxemia that is refractory to oxygen therapy. What is the most likely diagnosis?

A. Pneumonia

B. Adult respiratory distress syndrome (ARDS)

C. Pulmonary embolus

D. Asthma

84. Which of the following would be a typical set of presenting symptoms in a patient with aortic stenosis?

A. Cough, distended neck veins

B. Nocturia, paroxysmal dyspnea

C. Congestion, nocturia, headache

D. Fatigue, systolic ejection murmur

85. Which of the following diseases is associated with *Helicobacter pylori* (HP)?

A. Gastric lymphoma

B. Esophageal adenocarcinoma

C. Type A gastritis

D. Cholangitis

86. A 47-year-old man is admitted with nephrotic syndrome. He reports pedal edema in the mornings, progressing to midcalf edema the remainder of the day. On physical examination there are no signs of congestive heart failure, but mild ascites and 4+ lower extremity edema. Laboratory studies show blood urea nitrogen (BUN) 10 mg/dL, creatinine 1.0 mg/dL, urinalysis 4+ protein. The 24-hour urine sample contains 9.6 grams of protein. The most likely diagnosis is

A. membranous nephropathy

B. post-streptococcal glomerulonephritis

C. amyloidosis

D. diabetes mellitus

87. An absolute contraindication to postmenopausal estrogen replacement therapy (ERT) is

A. undiagnosed abnormal vaginal bleeding

B. estrogen receptor-negative breast cancer

C. fibrocystic breast changes

D. family history of stroke or deep venous thrombosis

88. A patient is diagnosed with chronic generalized seizures requiring anticonvulsant therapy. Initial therapy might include
A. ethosuximide
B. carbamazepine combined with valproic acid
C. carbamazepine alone
D. valproic acid combined with phenytoin

89. A man brings his 28-year-old wife to your office 4 weeks after a stillbirth. She is oriented to person, place, and time and appears to be a pleasant, well-kept individual who is alert and with appropriate affect. The husband indicated that for approximately two weeks after the unsuccessful pregnancy his wife engaged in promiscuous behavior, and had informed her husband that God had appeared to her and told her that she had been punished for past transgressions. The husband indicated that when he recommended that his wife see a health care provider, she disappeared for three days. On returning home, the patient recognized that she had been confused after losing her child but recalls nothing of the events that followed. The patient has been free of any symptoms for the past week. An appropriate diagnosis would be
A. psychotic disorder not otherwise specified
B. schizophreniform disorder
C. schizophrenia—paranoid type
D. brief psychotic disorder

90. A mother brings her 4-week-old infant in for a routine well-child examination. She states that the baby's eye has been red and watery and seems to be bothering the child. On examination you notice increased tearing, slight crusting on the lid, and slight erythema to the conjunctiva. The most likely diagnosis is
A. foreign body
B. conjunctivitis
C. nasal lacrimal duct obstruction
D. blepharitis

91. Which one of the following would you expect to find in a patient with adult respiratory distress syndrome (ARDS)?
A. Purulent, foul-smelling sputum and hemoptysis
B. Myalgia, fatigue, and a nonproductive cough
C. Tachypnea, frothy pink or red sputum, and rales
D. Fever, night sweats, and weight loss

92. The typical murmur observed in mitral stenosis is
A. a loud first heart sound and an opening snap following S_2
B. a whistling during systolic ejection accompanied by a split second heart sound
C. a soft, high-pitched blowing crescendo heard during expiration
D. a soft, high-pitched blowing that extends throughout systole and is heard best near the apex

93. A 37-year-old woman is delighted when she comes into your office because her home pregnancy test was positive. Her last menstrual period (LMP) was 7 weeks ago, and she and her husband had been attempting pregnancy for the past 3 years. She does report a small amount of spotting in the past week. On examination, her uterus is not enlarged. Her urine pregnancy test in your office was also positive. Your next laboratory tests would include
A. a quantitative serum human chorionic gonadotropin (hCG) and a transvaginal ultrasound
B. a qualitative serum hCG and a transvaginal ultrasound
C. a quantitative serum hCG and an abdominal ultrasound
D. a qualitative serum hCG and an abdominal ultrasound

94. A 25-year-old man was playing football. As he was ready to throw the ball, with the humerus extended and externally rotated, he sustained a hard blow to his arm. He came to the sidelines cradling the arm with the opposite hand. After he lay down, his shoulder spontaneously reduced. What is the recommended treatment?
A. The shoulder should be immobilized with a figure-of-eight splint for 4 weeks, followed by range of motion and strengthening exercises
B. Passive range of motion exercises should be begun to avoid a frozen shoulder
C. The shoulder should be immobilized for 2–4 weeks, followed by range of motion exercises and a return to normal activity
D. A Lachman's test should be performed to check for stability; if the shoulder is stable, treat conservatively; if the shoulder is unstable, the patient should be referred to a specialist

95. A patient makes an appointment because of a bright red-orange rash that has developed underneath her breasts. Examination reveals that the rash is surrounded by papules and pustules. A 10% potassium hydroxide (KOH) preparation reveals hyphae and spores. What is the most likely diagnosis?
A. Cutaneous candidiasis
B. Tinea corporis
C. Tinea cruris
D. Malassia furfur

96. The most common cause of noncongenital aortic stenosis is
   A. rheumatic heart disease
   B. prolonged hypertension
   C. atherosclerosis
   D. senile degeneration of valve tissue

97. Hashimoto's thyroiditis
   A. is more common in women than in men
   B. results from exposure to radiation
   C. is caused by pituitary disease
   D. is a consequence of untreated neonatal hypothyroidism

98. A 24-year-old woman presents with a complaint of blurred vision and weakness in her legs. You note that several months ago she had other vague complaints of altered vision and transient balance problems that resolved without treatment or formal evaluation. You are suspicious that she might have multiple sclerosis. Which of the following would be most helpful in establishing this diagnosis?
   A. Computed tomography scan of the head
   B. Magnetic resonance imaging with gadolinium
   C. Serum electrophoresis
   D. Auditory evoked potentials

99. A 54-year-old man presents with nausea and burning abdominal pain which improves with eating. Which of the following will best diagnose the problem?
   A. Barium swallow
   B. Esophageal manometry
   C. Hepato-iminodiacetic acid (HIDA) scan
   D. Endoscopy

100. A 32-year-old woman with a history of previous preterm delivery calls the office. She is now at 28 weeks' gestation and complains of low back pain. She should be advised to
   A. rest and use heat for her back
   B. go to the hospital laboratory for a urinalysis and culture
   C. report to the office for an examination
   D. take an analgesic for her pain and call if it continues

101. When interpreting the results of thyroid function tests, the clinician must keep in mind that
   A. phenytoin may increase the thyroxine (T_4) level
   B. high estrogen states decrease both triiodothyronine (T_3) and T_4
   C. cirrhosis of the liver increases T_4
   D. acute psychiatric problems may increase T_4

102. A patient with long-standing, relapsing–remitting multiple sclerosis presents with an acute exacerbation consisting of pronounced unsteadiness of gait and optic neuritis. The patient is on no medication routinely. The most effective therapy to address these acute symptoms would be
   A. interferon-β
   B. oral prednisone
   C. copolymer
   D. intravenous corticosteroids

103. An acute, spreading inflammation of the dermis and subcutaneous tissue that is often caused by a bacteria is most likely
   A. candidiasis
   B. varicella
   C. cellulitis
   D. measles

104. A sudden onset of painless unilateral loss of vision and a cherry-red fovea with a pale retina is a classic presentation of which of the following?
   A. Macular degeneration
   B. Angle-closure glaucoma
   C. Central retinal artery occlusion
   D. Open-angle glaucoma

105. A 78-year-old man has decreased urination. Some days he passes large amounts of urine; other days he passes none at all. On physical examination, his blood pressure is 180/90 but otherwise normal. His laboratory studies show a blood urea nitrogen (BUN) of 12 mg/dL, creatinine of 4.2 mg/dL, and urinalysis shows occasional white blood cells. The most likely cause of his renal insufficiency is
   A. obstructive uropathy
   B. acute glomerulonephritis
   C. acute interstitial nephritis
   D. chronic renal failure of unknown etiology

106. A 3-year-old child grabs a tree limb with her right outstretched hand to stop herself from falling out of a tree. The child later complains of pain in the elbow and wants to hold the right hand with the palm facing down. Radiographs show no evidence of fracture. What injury is most likely?
   A. The radial head has slipped out of the annular ligament
   B. The muscles comprising the extensor wad have been strained or torn
   C. The radioulnar joint bursa has ruptured, limiting supination
   D. A tear in the long head of the biceps tendon has occurred

107. An elderly male patient with a history of hypertension is experiencing progressive memory loss, has become disoriented on occasion, and is no longer able to do carpentry work as a hobby. A complete laboratory profile, including complete blood cell count, serum electrolytes, blood glucose levels, and thyroid studies, is normal, and a computed tomography of the head reveals no abnormalities. The most likely cause of this patient's signs and symptoms is
  A. Alzheimer's disease
  B. senile dementia
  C. vascular dementia
  D. multi-infarct dementia

108. Major depressive disorders, manic disorders, and bipolar disorders fall under which of the following clinical entities?
  A. Mood disorders
  B. Anxiety disorders
  C. Schizophrenic disorders
  D. Manic-depressive disorders

109. Which one of the following is characterized by pale macules that will not tan and is caused by *Malassezia furfur*?
  A. Tinea capitis
  B. Tinea corporis
  C. Tinea cruris
  D. Tinea versicolor

110. A 62-year-old man who is a retired ironworker complains of tinnitus and a gradual loss of hearing. He states that he is missing parts of words or sentences. He most likely has
  A. cerumen impaction
  B. otitis media
  C. otitis externa
  D. presbycusis

111. A 50-year-old patient with a childhood history of rheumatic fever presents with dyspnea and pulmonary congestion. Physical examination reveals thready carotid pulses and a whistling systolic ejection murmur. Which of the following tests would you order?
  A. Echocardiogram to confirm aortic stenosis
  B. Cardiac catheterization to confirm mitral stenosis
  C. Chest radiograph to confirm tricuspid valve disease
  D. Electrocardiogram (ECG) to confirm congestive heart failure

112. The patient is a 26-year-old woman who has developed sudden-onset, profuse vomiting associated with abdominal cramps. She has been eating her normal diet, and prepares most of her food at home, but did eat a commercially prepared eclair 3 hours before her illness began. What is the most likely etiology?
  A. *Staphylococcus aureus*
  B. *Clostridium perfringens*
  C. Enterotoxic *Escherichia coli*
  D. *Shigella*

113. The patient is a 60-year-old woman who stopped menstruating about 8 years ago. She elected not to take hormone replacement therapy (HRT). She comes in for evaluation after the occurrence of bloody staining in her underwear. Should the bleeding be from the vagina, the test most commonly used to determine its cause is
  A. Pap smear
  B. endometrial biopsy
  C. pelvic ultrasound
  D. computed tomography (CT) scan of the pelvis

114. In the emergency room, a 38-year-old gravida 6, para 4, Ab 1 presents at 37 weeks' gestation with decreased fetal movement and vaginal bleeding. No ultrasound has been performed during the pregnancy. On examination, fetal heart tones are present at 90 beats per minute (BPM); maternal blood pressure is 150/100; maternal pulse is 120 BPM, and a moderate amount of blood is visible on the external genitalia. After calling the obstetrical service, the next step should be to
  A. establish intravenous access, send blood for type and crossmatch, and order coagulation studies
  B. perform a careful digital examination
  C. order an ultrasound to check the location of the placenta
  D. prepare the patient for an immediate cesarean section

115. When ordering and interpreting thyroid function tests, the clinician should know that
  A. thyroid-stimulating hormone (TSH) is secreted by the hypothalamus
  B. the most active thyroid hormone is thyroxine (T_4)
  C. triiodothyronine (T_3) is derived from peripheral deiodination of T_4
  D. the active thyroid hormones are bound to thyroid-binding globulin (TBG)

116. What disease presents with the triad of tinnitus, vertigo, and hearing loss?
  A. Tic douloureux
  B. Amaurosis fugax
  C. Bell's palsy
  D. Meniere's disease

117. A 26-year-old man comes to the emergency room complaining of the acute onset of ipsilateral chest pain and dyspnea. Physical examination reveals unilateral chest expansion, decreased tactile fremitus, hyperresonance, and diminished breath sounds. The most likely diagnosis is
  A. pleural effusion
  B. asthma
  C. pneumothorax
  D. emphysema

118. A 62-year-old man has been hospitalized and treated for sepsis for 1 week. He has a sudden onset of oliguria, nausea, vomiting, shortness of breath, weakness, and orthostatic hypotension. His laboratory studies show a blood urea nitrogen (BUN) of 40, creatinine of 4.2, increased urine sodium, and increased fractional excretion of sodium and dilute urine. What is the most likely diagnosis?
  A. Acute tubular necrosis
  B. Hypovolemia
  C. Urinary tract infection
  D. Nephrotoxicity

119. How effective is Rh immunoglobulin in prevention of sensitization?
  A. 69%
  B. 79%
  C. 89%
  D. 99%

120. A 73-year-old woman was watering her lawn when she tripped over the hose and landed on the ground with most of the impact on her right hyperflexed hand. Radiographs show a break in the distal radius with the distal fragment minimally displaced toward the volar aspect. Which statement applies to this fracture?
  A. The complications of such a fracture will be associated with median nerve and radial artery damage
  B. Common names for this fracture are Colles' fracture or silver fork deformity
  C. The fracture can be treated best by wrapping with a bulky dressing until the swelling subsides and then casting in a long-arm cast for 6 weeks
  D. If the fracture is stable, it can be casted without trying to reduce the minimally displaced fracture

121. A 40-year-old man presents with a 2-week history of severe headaches in the area of his right eye, occurring several times during the day. He has no pain now, but reports that his last episode was earlier in the day and he noted redness and tearing from the right eye. He experienced similar headaches several months ago, but they seemingly resolved until now. He has taken no medication. He most likely has
  A. common migraine headaches
  B. an acute sinusitis
  C. cluster headaches
  D. classic migraine headaches

122. A mood episode is
  A. the result of hallucinations
  B. the result of delusions
  C. a psychotic episode in the presence of a neurologic disorder
  D. a description of the symptoms that make up a patient's mood state

123. When examining a patient's nasal mucosa, you note a clear, watery discharge and pale, boggy mucosa. The mucosa also appears cyanotic. These findings are consistent with
  A. allergic rhinitis
  B. vasomotor rhinitis
  C. rhinitis medicamentosa
  D. atrophic rhinitis

124. A 62-year-old man who smokes is found to have a lung mass that originated in the central bronchi and has metastasized to the regional lymph nodes with cavitation. The most likely diagnosis is
  A. squamous cell carcinoma
  B. small (oat) cell carcinoma
  C. adenocarcinoma
  D. bronchogenic carcinoma

125. The patient complains of gradual onset of dysphagia for solid foods. Smooth, conical tapering of the esophagus is seen on barium radiograph. These findings are consistent with what diagnosis?
  A. Cancer of the lower esophageal sphincter
  B. Achalasia
  C. Hiatal hernia
  D. Esophageal spasm

126. A 36-year-old man presents with a 2-day history of right flank pain and hematuria. Physical examination shows that he is unable to sit still and has costovertebral angle tenderness. Plain film of the abdomen reveals a 6-mm lucency over the right psoas. What is the best management plan?
  A. Send the patient home, instruct him to drink fluids, strain urine, and take oral analgesics
  B. Manage the patient in the emergency room with intravenous fluids and parenteral analgesia
  C. Admit the patient to the hospital and give him intravenous antibiotics and analgesia
  D. Refer the patient for lithotripsy

127. A 16-year-old girl reports to your office complaining of irregular bleeding and cramps. She may have passed some gray-colored substance. She is unsure of her last menstrual period and is not using contraception although she is sexually active. On examination, her uterus is tender and 4 weeks in size. No adnexal masses are appreciated. The cervix appears closed. A moderate amount of blood is noted in the vagina. Her urine pregnancy test is positive. To exclude an incomplete abortion in this situation, you would
  A. rely on history and physical examination for diagnosis
  B. order a serum human chorionic gonadotropin (hCG)
  C. order a transvaginal ultrasound
  D. order both a serum hCG and an ultrasound

128. A 31-year-old woman who is 7 months' pregnant has intense night pain in the thumb, index, and middle fingers. What is the best recommendation for this patient?
  A. Endoscopic carpal tunnel release
  B. Nonsteroidal anti-inflammatory medications should be given until delivery and surgical release can be performed
  C. Volar wrist splinting should be done at night and with activity, and vitamin B$_6$ should be given daily
  D. No treatment will be helpful in pregnancy-related carpal tunnel syndrome

129. Which of the following is most likely to represent a malignancy?
  A. A hot nodule on radioactive iodine (RAI) uptake
  B. A nodule in a patient with a history of neck irradiation
  C. Multiple nodular lesions
  D. A slowly growing nodule

130. A young woman with well-documented migraine headaches has had fair success at aborting headache episodes once or twice a month with oral sumatriptan and experiences no adverse effects. She is now having more frequent migraine attacks and is occasionally exceeding the recommended number of doses of her sumatriptan. Her examination is normal. What would be the most appropriate change in her medication?
  A. Continue with the sumatriptan tablets but supplement with oral codeine as needed
  B. Substitute subcutaneous sumatriptan for the oral tablets
  C. Authorize injectable meperidine hydrochloride (Demerol) in the emergency department when needed
  D. Prescribe a β-blocker in an attempt to reduce the frequency of her headaches while she continues to use sumatriptan as directed

131. Patients who present with inflated self-esteem, decreased need for sleep, and a need to keep on talking are likely to be diagnosed as
  A. schizophrenic
  B. suicidally depressed
  C. manic
  D. delusional

132. Which one of the following outcomes occurs in a patient diagnosed with kyphoscoliosis?
  A. Increased lung compliance because of progressive ateletasis
  B. Decreased work of breathing and decreased stiffness of the chest wall
  C. Increased lung volume secondary to hyperinflation
  D. Acute respiratory failure

133. Electrocardiogram (ECG) findings in sinus tachycardia show
  A. normal PQRS at a rate of 300+ beats per minute (BPM)
  B. prolonged PR interval at 100–160 BPM
  C. normal PQRS at a rate of 100–160 BPM
  D. no organized atrial activity with an irregular ventricular rate of 100–180 BPM

134. A 22-year-old white woman presents with supraclavicular lymphadenopathy and intermittent fevers for 6 months. Physical examination reveals a 1.5-cm left supraclavicular node and a mediastinal mass, but no other demonstrable lymphadenopathy. Laboratory evaluation demonstrates Reed-Sternberg cells. What is the appropriate diagnosis?
  A. Hodgkin's disease
  B. Non-Hodgkin's lymphoma
  C. Chronic myelogenous leukemia (CML)
  D. Acute lymphocytic leukemia (ALL)

135. The patient is a 66-year-old man who visited the clinic last week for dyspepsia of about 5 months' duration associated with a 10-pound weight loss. His symptoms have not improved with treatment. What is the next step in diagnosing this patient's condition?
  A. Complete blood cell count (CBC) and Hemoccult
  B. Amylase, lipase
  C. Electrocardiogram (EKG), Holter monitor
  D. Barium swallow

136. How long should acute prostatitis be treated with antibiotics?
  A. 7–10 days
  B. 14 days
  C. 1 month
  D. Longer than 2 months

137. Headache, nausea, rapid weight gain, and swelling in the upper extremities in late pregnancy are probably the result of
  A. late third-trimester benign symptomatology
  B. preeclampsia
  C. nephrotic syndrome
  D. congenital adrenal insufficiency

138. While playing basketball, a 16-year-old boy sustained an injury to the little finger. He is unable to fully extend the distal joint. Radiographs the day of the injury show no intra-articular fracture or subluxation. What is the best course of action?
  A. Radiographs should be repeated in 10–14 days to rule out fracture
  B. The distal joint should be actively exercised daily to prevent loss of motion
  C. Flexor tendon injury should be suspected and referred to a specialist
  D. Extension splinting of the distal joint should be done for at least 6 weeks

139. A patient complains of frequent, generalized headaches described as dull and aching. They appear to have started after a minor automobile accident when the patient's car was involved in a rear-end collision. There appears to be no history of acute emotional stress. Examination reveals no neurologic deficit and mild localized tenderness in the occipital region with full range of motion of the neck. These are presumed to be tension headaches and are best initially treated with
  A. tricyclic antidepressants
  B. aspirin, acetaminophen, or a nonsteroidal anti-inflammatory drug (NSAID)
  C. a soft collar
  D. acetaminophen with codeine

140. According to the DSM-IV criteria, what is the difference between manic and hypomanic episodes?
  A. Social and occupational functioning are not markedly impaired in the hypomanic
  B. Unrestrained sexual sprees occur with manic episodes
  C. Hospitalization is generally required with hypomanics
  D. Patient is easily distractable in the manic episode

141. What is the most common presentation of psoriasis?
  A. An inflammatory follicular, papular, and pustular eruption
  B. Raised, reddened areas with distinct margins and loosely adherent silvery scales
  C. Superficial flaccid vesicles that erupt, forming a thick, yellowish crust
  D. Erythematous, hard, tender lesions in hair-bearing areas of the head, neck, or body

142. Which of the following imaging studies is most helpful and practical for differentiating sinusitis from rhinitis without sinus involvement?
  A. Magnetic resonance imaging
  B. Plain sinus radiographs
  C. Sinus ultrasound
  D. Positron emission tomography

143. An 82-year-old man presents with pleuritic chest pain, dyspnea, cough, and hemoptysis following an injury to his left thigh 1 week ago. In the diagnostic evaluation of this patient
  A. a normal lung perfusion scan virtually rules out clinically significant thromboembolism
  B. arterial blood gas measurements will show a mildly acute respiratory acidosis
  C. the most common abnormality found on chest radiograph is an air bronchogram
  D. Doppler ultrasonography is associated with false-negative results

144. The characteristic electrocardiogram (ECG) pattern in second degree atrioventricular block shows
  A. uniform QRS complexes of ventricular origin occurring at more than 100 beats per minute (BPM)
  B. prolonged PR interval with a ventricular rate of 100–160 BPM
  C. increased ratio of P waves to QRS complexes
  D. widened QRS complexes with an irregular ventricular rate of 100–180 BPM

145. The patient is a 35-year-old woman who just completed a 7-day course of antibiotic therapy with ciprofloxacin for a urinary tract infection. She now complains of watery diarrhea occurring for the past day or so. What is the most likely diagnosis?
  A. *Cryptosporidium*
  B. *Clostridium difficile*
  C. *Vibrio cholera*
  D. *Giardia*

146. Which of the following medications is the most common and safest for use in the seizures associated with eclampsia?
- **A.** Hydralazine
- **B.** Magnesium sulfate
- **C.** Diazepam
- **D.** Carbamazepine

147. A 45-year-old insulin-dependent diabetic man has experienced progressive pain and catching sensation in the distal joint of the thumb, sometimes requiring use of the other hand to extend or flex the painful joint. The condition is most likely
- **A.** gamekeeper's thumb
- **B.** trigger thumb
- **C.** diabetic neuropathy
- **D.** hypoplastic thumb

148. Which of the following statements is TRUE regarding thyroid cancer?
- **A.** Thyroid function tests are most often normal in thyroid cancer
- **B.** The most common thyroid malignancy is medullary thyroid carcinoma
- **C.** Patients with thyroid cancer usually present with painful neck swelling and hoarseness
- **D.** Papillary carcinoma is associated with distant metastasis

149. While working a fast track clinic, you are asked to see a patient brought in by the police. Clothing and personal hygiene suggest that this individual is a transient. The patient is actively hallucinating; is not oriented to day, date, or time; has flat affect; and is actively engaging in inappropriate sexual behavior making it impossible to obtain an accurate personal or medical history. The appropriate diagnosis is
- **A.** schizophreniform disorder
- **B.** psychotic disorder not otherwise specified (NOS)
- **C.** delusional disorder
- **D.** schizoaffective disorder

150. What is the best treatment for a pyogenic granuloma?
- **A.** Electrodesiccation and curettage or excision
- **B.** Topical antibiotics
- **C.** Oral cephalosporins
- **D.** Both topical and oral antibiotics

151. Which organisms are most likely to cause acute sinusitis?
- **A.** *Haemophilus influenzae, Moraxella catarrhalis, Staphylococcus aureus*
- **B.** *Streptococcus pneumoniae, H. influenzae, M. catarrhalis*
- **C.** *H. influenzae, M. catarrhalis,* anaerobes
- **D.** Anaerobes, *S. aureus, H. influenzae*

152. The most common cause of atypical community-acquired pneumonia is
- **A.** *Mycoplasma pneumoniae*
- **B.** *Pseudomonas aeruginosa*
- **C.** *Streptococcus pneumoniae*
- **D.** *Haemophilus influenzae*

153. Monomorphic ventricular tachycardia consists of
- **A.** waves of ventricular depolarization and the presence of prominent neck vein pulsations up to 300 beats per minute (BPM)
- **B.** widened QRS complexes with an irregular ventricular rate of 100–180 BPM
- **C.** prolonged PR interval with a ventricular rate of 100–160 BPM
- **D.** 3 or more consecutive uniform QRS complexes of ventricular origin occurring at more than 100 BPM

154. Which of the following is true about the treatment of diverticular disease?
- **A.** Increased dietary fiber is a part of the treatment
- **B.** Barium enema is the best procedure for both diagnosis and treatment of an acute episode of diverticulitis
- **C.** Patients with a history of diverticulitis must be monitored more closely for colon cancer
- **D.** Acute diverticulitis episodes often require hospitalization for intravenous antibiotic therapy, bowel rest, and analgesics

155. Which urinary symptoms are irritative symptoms due to bladder mucosa inflammation?
- **A.** Increased frequency, urgency, and nocturia
- **B.** Hesitancy and straining
- **C.** Double voiding
- **D.** split stream urination

156. The patient is a 30-year-old woman with a history of fairly regular menstrual cycles. She presents to you with a history of a 2-week delay of menses and left-sided abdominal pain. She is not sexually active at present and takes no medications. Her examination is normal except for a left adnexal mass. Ultrasound confirms the presence of a 6-cm ovarian cyst. The most appropriate next step in managing this patient is
- **A.** following her for 1–2 months
- **B.** referring her for urgent laparoscopy
- **C.** starting her immediately on high-dose oral contraceptives
- **D.** obtaining a serum level of CA-125

157. The most common complication of multiple pregnancy is
- **A.** gestational diabetes
- **B.** pregnancy-induced hypertension (PIH)
- **C.** preterm birth
- **D.** cord accidents

158. A 25-year-old man has played 5 basketball games this weekend. He stopped participating in the last game because of pain in his left knee. The pain was exacerbated by running and jumping. Palpation of the knee reveals tenderness near the anterior inferior border of the knee. The pain is increased in extension, not in flexion. The most likely diagnosis is
A. prepatellar bursitis
B. iliotibial band friction syndrome
C. patellar tendon rupture
D. patellar tendinitis

159. The patient is a 55-year-old woman of Mexican descent. She is 4'10" tall and weighs 165 pounds. She comes to the free clinic today for treatment of her fourth "yeast infection" in a year. A wet prep and potassium hydroxide (KOH) preparation demonstrate the presence of spores and hyphae only. In addition to treating the infection, the most important task you should accomplish at this visit is
A. obtain a random plasma glucose
B. screen her for gonorrhea and syphilis
C. teach her about vaginal hygiene
D. culture vaginal scrapings on Saboraud's medium

160. A 50-year-old male business executive presents with several months' history of tremor involving his hands. He notes that the tremor is more noticeable when he is under stress at work, but that if he has a glass of wine at lunch or with dinner, the tremor resolves nearly entirely. He is concerned about the tremor and desires treatment. Appropriate initial therapy would be
A. amantadine
B. levodopa/carbidopa
C. benztropine
D. low-dose propranolol

161. Mary, a 41-year-old patient with a long history of treatment for a bipolar disorder, complains that she has been having reoccurring episodes of depression and mania. While she does not express concern over the depth of the mood states she is experiencing, she is concerned with the rapidity with which the mood swings occur. A review of her record indicates a recent change in her treatment regimen. The most likely explanation for Mary's presenting complaint is a change in her treatment regimen to
A. antidepressants
B. lithium
C. electroconvulsive therapy
D. anticonvulsants

162. Each of the following statements about acne vulgaris is true EXCEPT
A. lesions can be open comedones or closed noninflammatory comedones
B. erythematous, fluid-filled, and tender cysts may form
C. acne is most commonly found on the buttocks, feet, and hands
D. tetracyclines, benzoyl peroxides, and retinoids are the drugs of choice

163. Which of the following organisms most commonly causes epiglottitis?
A. Group A β-hemolytic streptococcus
B. *Haemophilus influenzae* type B
C. *Mycoplasma pneumoniae*
D. *Chlamydia trachomatis*

164. A radiographic finding for atypical community-acquired pneumonia is
A. lobar infiltrate
B. segmental unilateral lower lung zone infiltrate
C. patchy or streaky opacities
D. cavitary infiltrate in the lung apex

165. Class I antiarrhythmia drugs include
A. Na$^+$ channel blockers like procainamide
B. β-adrenergic antagonists like propranolol
C. slow K$^+$ channel blockers like bretylium
D. calcium channel blockers like nifedipine

166. Macrosomia is associated with
A. gestational diabetes
B. pregnancy-induced hypertension (PIH)
C. multiple pregnancies
D. smoking

167. The most likely diagnosis for the anteroposterior radiograph (see Fig., p. 221) is
A. Anterior dislocation of the hip
B. Posterior dislocation of the hip
C. Anterior dislocation and fraction of the hip
D. Posterior dislocation and fracture of the hip

168. The patient is a 14-year-old girl of Scandinavian descent whose mother brings her in for evaluation. She is worried that the girl seems to be in the bathroom constantly and is drinking more than usual. Despite a markedly increased appetite, she has lost weight over the past few weeks. The girl herself seems a bit withdrawn and apathetic, but admits to "needing to pee a lot." You suspect a diagnosis of
A. bulimia nervosa
B. non–insulin-dependent diabetes mellitus (NIDDM)
C. Addison's disease
D. insulin-dependent diabetes mellitus (IDDM)

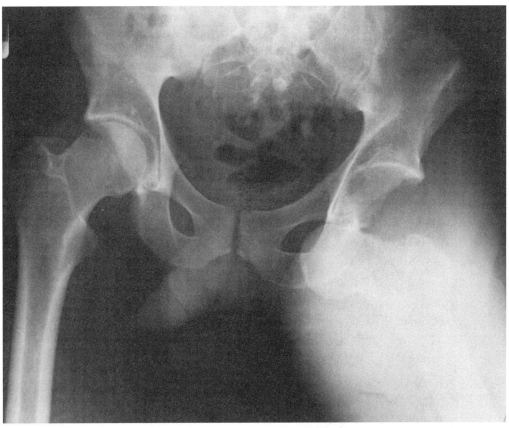

Question 167

169. All are true of squamous cell and basal cell carcinomas EXCEPT
   A. the lesions usually present on areas that are usually exposed (e.g., the face, head, neck, and trunk)
   B. the lesions are generally asymptomatic and do not itch or bleed
   C. the lesions generally do not heal
   D. metastasis in both basal cell and squamous cell is rare

170. Which of the following is the most appropriate therapy for a tension pneumothorax?
   A. Observation
   B. Insertion of chest tube
   C. Insertion of large-bore needle
   D. Thoracotomy

171. Which of the following conditions would be inappropriate for permanent cardiac pacing?
   A. Premature ventricular contractions
   B. Atrial fibrillation
   C. Atrioventricular block
   D. Sick sinus syndrome

172. Which of the following is a classic physical finding associated with peptic ulcer disease?
   A. Burning epigastric pain associated with eating, or with an empty stomach
   B. Burning epigastric pain occurring when lying flat
   C. Sharp, stabbing pain without radiation occurring immediately after meals
   D. Sharp, stabbing pain with radiation to the back occurring

173. Transurethral resection of the prostate (TURP) is the treatment of choice for which disease?
   A. Benign prostatic hyperplasia (BPH)
   B. Prostate cancer
   C. Bladder cancer
   D. Chronic prostatitis

174. The most important complication of untreated Rh incompatibility is
   A. maternal anaphylaxis
   B. fetal hemolytic anemia or death
   C. development of antibodies to the Rh factor
   D. fetal–maternal hemorrhage

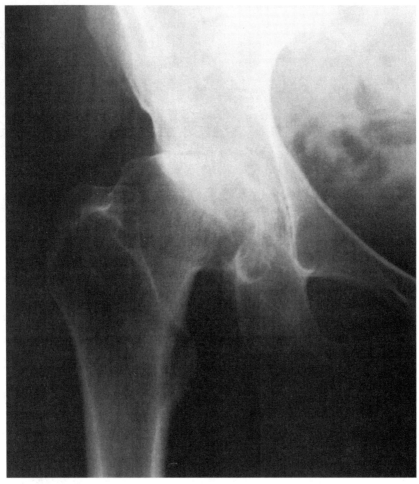

Question 175

175. A 73-year-old woman walks into your clinic complaining of chronic lower back pain and inability to fully extend the left knee when walking. Examination reveals decreased flexion, no internal rotation or external rotation of the hip, and the knee has 5°–90° of motion with crepitation. The radiograph of the pelvis (see Fig.) shows what prominent finding?
   A. Rheumatoid arthritis with steroid-induced osteonecrosis
   B. Osteoarthritis with joint space narrowing
   C. Lytic changes in both the acetabulum and femoral head
   D. Normal findings for a patient of this age

176. A 65-year-old African-American woman has just been diagnosed with non–insulin-dependent diabetes mellitus (NIDDM). She had few complaints other than vague vision difficulties and feeling thirsty all the time. She weighs 265 pounds. The appropriate next step in getting her diabetes under control is

   A. immediate referral to an ophthalmologist
   B. initiating sulfonylurea treatment of her hyperglycemia
   C. starting her on a weight loss diet and exercise program
   D. starting her on regular and neutral protein Hagedorn (NPH) insulin in low doses

177. Compulsions are defined as
   A. mental acts that the patient feels compelled to perform
   B. mental acts that are performed either to prevent distress or control anxiety
   C. repetitive behaviors that the patient feels forced to perform to avoid an undesirable consequence
   D. thought intrusions based on real problems experienced by the patient

Items 178 through 182

Directions: Each set of matching questions in this section consists of a list of lettered options followed by several numbered items. For each numbered item, select the ONE lettered option that is most closely associated with it. Each option may be selected once, more than once, or not at all.

- **A.** Varicella
- **B.** Measles
- **C.** Scarlet fever
- **D.** Pityriasis rosea
- **E.** Fifth disease

For each patient, select the most appropriate diagnosis.

178. A 4-year-old girl develops a tiny, erythematous rash that appears on the upper torso and spreads to the remainder of the trunk, sparing her face, palms, and soles. Examination of the oral cavity reveals a "strawberry tongue."

179. A 3-year-old boy develops a solitary, round, pink lesion with a raised border and fine, adherent scales in the margin. Approximately 1 week later, oval, salmon-colored, slightly raised maculopapular lesions in a "Christmas tree" distribution appear on the boy's trunk.

180. A 6-year-old girl is brought to the clinic because her mother noticed an erythematous, macular rash that began in the hairline and progressed downward. A tiny, punctate, whitish rash with an erythematous base is noted on the buccal mucosa, over the lower molars.

181. An 8-year-old girl develops a vesicular rash. The lesions become pustular, umbilicated, and then crusted. At the time of presentation, lesions in all three stages are visible.

182. A 5-year-old girl suddenly develops a macular, erythematous rash on her cheeks that looks like sunburn.

Directions: Each of the numbered items or incomplete statements in this section is followed by answers or by completions of the statement. Select the ONE lettered answer or completion that is BEST in each case. Some of the numbered items or incomplete statements are negatively phrased, as indicated by a capitalized word such as NOT, LEAST, or EXCEPT. For these items, select the ONE lettered answer or completion that is BEST in each case.

183. The majority of cases of epistaxis originate in which area of the nose?
- **A.** Lateral turbinates
- **B.** Medial turbinates
- **C.** Nasal wall
- **D.** Kiesselbach's plexus

184. A 69-year-old patient presents with exertional dyspnea, a dry cough of insidious onset, digital clubbing, and fatigue. You diagnose the patient as having interstitial lung disease and expect the chest radiograph to show
- **A.** diffuse ground-glass appearance
- **B.** patchy diffuse infiltrates
- **C.** unilateral high diaphragm
- **D.** blurring of posterior diaphragm

185. One of the most common predisposing factors for dilated cardiomyopathy is
- **A.** genetically transmitted defects
- **B.** fibrotic collagen-defect diseases
- **C.** infective endocarditis
- **D.** excessive alcohol consumption

186. Which of the following is associated with small-bowel obstruction?
- **A.** Flatulence
- **B.** Frequent, low-pitched bowel sounds
- **C.** Abdominal distention
- **D.** Vomiting of undigested food

187. Hyperkalemia is a life-threatening disorder. The severity of the disorder can be monitored by changes in the electrocardiogram (ECG). Which ECG finding indicates the most serious condition?
- **A.** Peaked T waves
- **B.** Flattened P waves and prolonged PR interval
- **C.** Widened QRS complex
- **D.** Sine wave pattern

188. A 24-year-old woman presents to your office 6 months postpartum. She delivered by cesarean section elsewhere and is nursing full time. She has been living in a homeless shelter and has not had an examination since her delivery. She denies sexual intercourse since the delivery but is concerned because she has not started to menstruate. On examination, galactorrhea is present bilaterally. Her abdominal incision appears well-healed. On pelvic examination, the vaginal walls and external genitalia appear slightly atrophic. The uterus and adnexa are unremarkable. Her pregnancy test is negative. The most likely explanation for her amenorrhea is
- **A.** anovulation secondary to breast feeding
- **B.** a false negative pregnancy test
- **C.** anovulation secondary to stress (suppression hypothalamic-pituitary axis)
- **D.** scarring of the uterus (Asherman's syndrome)

189. A 43-year-old woman with vasculitis fell while getting out of her vehicle and was unable to bear weight on the right leg. She has exquisite tenderness over the lateral ankle with palpation. Radiographs will most likely show what condition?
  A. Fracture of the lateral malleolus
  B. Fracture of the dome of the calcaneus and medial malleolus
  C. Fracture of the dome of the talus and lateral malleolus
  D. Fracture of the medial malleolus

190. The patient is a thin, apathetic-appearing 36-year-old white man. He has come in for evaluation of "constant nausea." His skin seems darker than you remember and he appears to have lost about 15 pounds since you last saw him 18 months ago. The only reason he came in is because his wife forced him to. She tells you she had to make the appointment and drive him in because he was "too tired" to lift up the phone. He has been missing work, something he formerly loved. He seems to have some darkly pigmented areas on the buccal mucosa. Following a thorough physical examination, what is the next step in this patient's work-up?
  A. Biopsy the oral lesions
  B. Order an adrenocorticotropic hormone (ACTH) stimulation test
  C. Get a serum thyroid-stimulating hormone (TSH) level
  D. Administer a depression inventory

191. A patient had been diagnosed with mild Parkinson's disease several years earlier, and has never taken any medication for the symptoms. He presents now for follow-up with much more disabling symptoms, having fallen numerous times while walking or bending over. He has a very slow shuffling gait and coarse tremors of both upper extremities as well as in his lips. A trial of what medication regimen should be considered?
  A. Amantadine
  B. Benztropine
  C. Propranolol
  D. Levodopa/carbidopa

192. Alprazolam (Xanax) has historically been the only FDA-approved medication for which of the following anxiety disorders?
  A. Obsessive-compulsive disorders
  B. Panic disorder
  C. Generalized anxiety disorder
  D. Post-traumatic stress disorder

193. A 32-year-old woman presents to your office with dyspnea of insidious onset and chest discomfort as well as fatigue and exertional dyspnea. Pulmonary function testing shows some impairment of gas exchange and evidence of lung restriction. You suspect sarcoidosis; the diagnosis is confirmed by
  A. chest radiograph
  B. transbronchial lung biopsy
  C. mediastinotomy
  D. bronchoalveolar lavage

194. Hypertrophic obstructive cardiomyopathy
  A. is associated with increased risk of sudden cardiac death even in young adults
  B. is rarely lethal
  C. is associated with increased risk of morbidity only in patients older than 55 years of age
  D. is almost always asymptomatic

195. The best diagnostic method for cholecystitis is
  A. Sonogram
  B. Abdominal flat plane radiograph
  C. Hepato-iminodiacetic acid (HIDA) scan
  D. Endoscopic retrograde cholangiopancreatography (ERCP)

196. A 19-year-old woman presents to your office 5 days postpartum complaining of heavy bleeding. She is febrile at 101.4°F, her blood pressure is 124/80 and her pulse is 100. Her abdomen is tender in the suprapubic region, and blood is present on the external genitalia. Bimanual examination reveals a soft, boggy, enlarged uterus. Her hemoglobin is 10.7 g/dL and hematocrit is 32%. The most likely diagnosis would be
  A. endometritis and possible retained placental fragments
  B. laceration of the cervix
  C. thrombophlebitis
  D. pelvic inflammatory disease

197. An 18-year-old woman recently was an un-seatbelted passenger involved in a motor vehicle accident. She sustained a right posterior hip dislocation. She now presents with lateral foot pain 1 week after initiating full weight bearing on the right leg. Radiographs (see Figs., p. 225) are obtained and confirm which of the following injuries?
  A. old fracture of the third metatarsal
  B. old fracture, but substantial soft-tissue swelling; treatment will be indicated for reflex sympathetic dystrophy secondary to trauma
  C. new fracture of the third metatarsal
  D. stress fracture of the third metatarsal

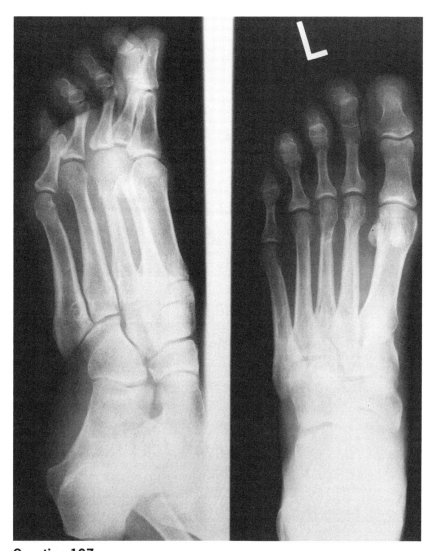

Question 197

198. A common laboratory finding in acute adrenal insufficiency includes
  A. hyponatremia
  B. hypokalemia
  C. hypocalcemia
  D. hyperglycemia

199. Throughout the past year a 12-year-old boy has been noted to have a variety of motor tics involving his facial features and shoulders. His teachers have reported frequent disruptive verbal utterances in the classroom as well, but he remains an excellent student. The most likely diagnosis is
  A. simple partial seizures
  B. Tourette's syndrome
  C. benign familial tremor
  D. acting out behavior

200. The patient you are asked to see was brought to the emergency room after having ingested a substance at a fraternity party. His friends called emergency medical services after he complained of having trouble breathing, and alleged that he saw Babe Ruth making passes at his girlfriend. The history and physical examination findings indicate that the patient has no prior history of a mental disorder and there is no organic cause for the symptoms. The patient is currently in good spirits, is oriented, and has stable vital signs. This patient was probably experiencing effects of
  A. substance abuse
  B. substance dependence
  C. substance intoxication
  D. substance withdrawal

201. The corneal light reflex test and the cover test are used to determine the presence of which of the following abnormalities?
A. Strabismus
B. Amblyopia
C. Central retinal artery occlusion
D. Central retinal vein occlusion

202. The outstanding respiratory symptom in kyphoscoliosis is
A. Exertional dyspnea
B. Hypoventilation
C. Chest pain
D. Productive cough

203. Both folic acid deficiency and vitamin B_{12} deficiency can cause anemia. Which of the following is a distinguishing characteristic of B_{12} deficiency in contrast to folate deficiency?
A. Has a mean corpuscular volume (MCV) more than 100
B. Commonly associated with peripheral neuropathies
C. May cause glossitis
D. Causes a megaloblastic anemia

204. Which type of hepatitis can be transmitted by the fecal-oral route?
A. Hepatitis B
B. Hepatitis C
C. Hepatitis D
D. Hepatitis E

205. The patient is a 14-year-old girl whose Pap smear indicates a low-grade squamous intraepithelial lesion (LSIL). You should
A. refer her for cervical conization
B. follow her with Pap smears every 4 months
C. refer her promptly for colposcopy
D. treat any infection and repeat the Pap

206. The most accurate method of diagnosing multiple pregnancy is
A. increased serum alpha-fetoprotein
B. auscultating two fetal heart tones
C. ultrasound examination
D. large for gestation age on examination

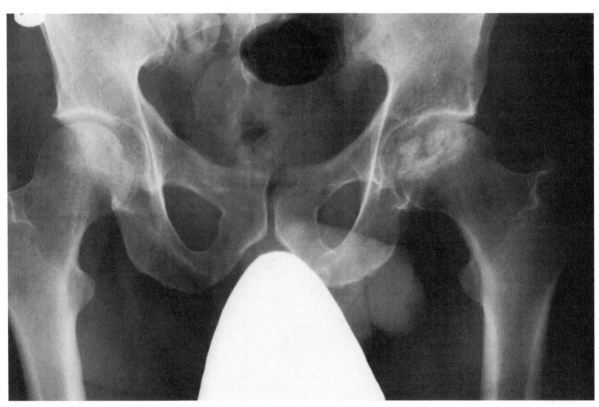

Question 207

207. A 21-year-old man develops left groin pain and left knee pain while playing basketball. He was diagnosed as having a groin pull and started on nonsteroidal anti-inflammatory drugs (NSAIDs) with protective weight bearing 2 weeks ago. He has no history of predisposing factors for systemic disease. He has returned because of increased pain in the groin and pain with weight bearing. The radiograph (see Fig., p. 226) shows evidence of what condition?
  A. Osteonecrosis of the femoral head
  B. Osteoarthritis of the femoral head and acetabulum
  C. Acute osteomyelitis
  D. Chronic osteomyelitis

208. What is the most common cause of Cushing's syndrome (hypercortisolism)?
  A. An adrenocorticotropic hormone (ACTH)-secreting pituitary tumor
  B. Ectopic ACTH production by a malignancy such as a pheochromocytoma
  C. An adrenocortical tumor
  D. Exogenous administration of corticosteroid drugs

209. A child is brought to you with a tentative diagnosis of attention-deficit/hyperactivity disorder (ADHD). In relating the child's behavioral profile to you, the parents indicate that they are at their wits' end and would dearly love to have their child medicated with Ritalin. The parents indicate that approximately 10 months ago their 11-year-old son started exhibiting maladaptive behaviors that included constant chattering, fidgeting, difficulty in interacting with others at school, and trouble remaining seated in the classroom. The private school he attends has indicated that the child is on the verge of being expelled. What factor would contraindicate a diagnosis of ADHD?
  A. The child is too old for a diagnosis of ADHD to be made
  B. The child is male
  C. The child failed to exhibit symptoms of the condition until after age 7 years
  D. The child's behavior is consistent with a diagnosis of ADHD and Ritalin should be prescribed

210. A 55-year-old woman presents with a chief complaint of abrupt onset of excruciating pain in the right eye, associated with visual blurring and halos around lights. Her examination revealed a narrowed anterior chamber and the cornea was steamy. Her likely diagnosis would be
  A. temporal arteritis
  B. acute iritis
  C. acute angle-closure glaucoma
  D. acute keratitis

211. A 23-year-old man presents with a 1-day history of rhinorrhea, coryza, a slight fever, and a nonproductive cough. The most likely etiology of this illness is
  A. anaerobic streptococcus
  B. aerobic streptococcus
  C. *Bacteroides* species
  D. virus

212. For which of the following conditions would the use of positive inotropic drugs be appropriate?
  A. Hypertrophic cardiomyopathy
  B. Restrictive cardiomyopathy
  C. Dilated cardiomyopathy
  D. Infectious pericarditis

213. A double contrast barium enema shows cobblestone filling defects with segmental areas of involvement. This finding is consistent with what diagnosis?
  A. Diverticulosis
  B. Crohn's disease
  C. Colon cancer
  D. Ulcerative colitis

214. A 30-year-old woman presents with asymptomatic hypertension of 3 months' duration. Her past medical history and family history are unremarkable. Blood pressure is 180/110 mmHg and pulse rate is 72 BPM. Physical examination reveals a high-pitched bruit on the left side of the abdomen and no diaphoresis. Laboratory studies reveal a blood urea nitrogen (BUN) of 11 mg/dL, creatinine 0.9 mg/dL, cholesterol 180 mg/dL, glucose 98 mg/dL, and a normal urinalysis. The most likely cause of her hypertension is
  A. essential hypertension
  B. renal failure
  C. adrenal medullary tumor
  D. renal artery stenosis

215. The patient is a married, nulliparous 28-year-old woman who stopped her oral contraceptives 8 months ago in order to become pregnant. Her husband is 30 years old. Her previous examinations have all been normal and she has no history of sexually transmitted disease. She comes in for her annual physical examination worried about infertility. Finding nothing on physical examination, the next step should be
  A. reassuring her and asking her to return if she does not become pregnant in the next 4 months
  B. sending her husband for a complete examination by a urologist
  C. ordering a hysterosalpingogram
  D. referring her to a gynecologist for laparoscopy

216-218.

A 32-year-old woman, gravida 2, para 1, with previous vaginal delivery presents at 38 weeks' gestation. On examination, her cervix is 5 centimeters dilated and 40% effaced.

216. This patient is in the
    A. first stage of labor
    B. second stage of labor
    C. third stage of labor
    D. fourth stage of labor

217. Cervical dilation slowed remarkably over the next 6 hours and the fetus did not descend into the pelvis. Augmentation of labor with oxytocin failed to dilate the cervix further. This probably represents
    A. Dystocia
    B. Abnormal presentation
    C. Inadequate pelvis
    D. Maternal fatigue

218. The fetus experienced persistent bradycardia on fetal monitoring. The next best step would probably be to
    A. perform a cesarean section
    B. deliver by forceps
    C. increase administration of oxytocin
    D. continue watchful waiting

219. A new female patient, who appears quite obese, presents with a chief complaint of "feeling lousy." In the course of her initial examination, it is noted that she has a blood glucose level of 325, her blood pressure with a wide cuff is 160/110, and she has wide, purplish striae on her breasts, upper arms, abdomen, buttocks, and thighs. What should your tentative diagnosis be?
    A. Hypertension
    B. Diabetes mellitus, type II
    C. Cushing's syndrome
    D. Hypothyroidism

220. The patient you are asked to see is in for a prescription refill. A review of his records indicates that his current medication is to control a diagnosed case of major depression. The record indicates that the patient was plagued by guilt feelings, suffered from terminal insomnia, and reported that he had been preoccupied with thoughts of death. During the interview the patient presents as a contented self-starting dynamo who has a bubbly personality and a propensity to talk. Before the patient leaves, you ask him to return for a diagnostic reevaluation because of the
    A. inappropriate feelings of guilt
    B. pervasive feeling of unbounded energy
    C. terminal insomnia
    D. thoughts of death

221. Which of the following should be done to manage a chemical burn to the eye?
    A. Immediate patching and referral to an ophthalmologist
    B. Irrigation with copious amounts of sterile water for 30 minutes
    C. Fluorescein staining
    D. Tonometry

222. Which of the following cardiac abnormalities is one of the more common complications associated with obstructive sleep apnea?
    A. Pulmonary hypertension
    B. Sinus arrhythmia
    C. Cor pulmonale
    D. Systemic hypertension

223. The patient brought to the emergency department complains of chest pain that has gradually increased over the last 36 hours. The pain is severe when taking a large breath but is relieved by sitting up and leaning forward. Physical examination reveals fever (100.1°F), no pulmonary wheezing or rales, and a left thoracic friction rub. Complete blood cell count results show elevated monocytes. You suspect
    A. pulmonary embolus
    B. bacterial pneumonia
    C. pericarditis
    D. restrictive cardiomyopathy

224. What is the most common cause of acute pancreatitis?
    A. Alcohol abuse
    B. Diabetes mellitus
    C. Perforated ulcer
    D. Cholelithiasis

225. An important clinical finding that is indicative of pyelonephritis is
    A. urethral discharge
    B. hematuria
    C. white cell casts
    D. pyuria

226. A 22-year-old woman comes in with a "yeast infection that won't go away." She has treated it several times with an over-the-counter antifungal agent. On examination, you find that she has a frothy, yellow-green, malodorous discharge, with petechial lesions on the cervix. If laboratory evaluation confirms your clinical suspicion, the appropriate treatment is
    A. a vaginal preparation of 2% ketoconazole
    B. 2 grams of metronidazole by mouth in a single dose
    C. clindamycin 2% cream intravaginally
    D. doxycycline 100 mg twice a day by mouth for 7 days

227. Prior to allowing a patient to attempt a vaginal birth after cesarean section, it is vital to obtain records regarding
- **A.** previous prenatal record
- **B.** nature of previous surgical incision
- **C.** medical history
- **D.** results of prenatal diagnostic tests

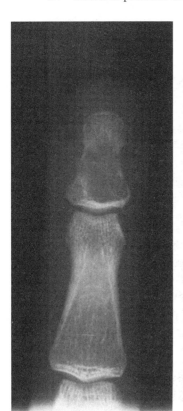
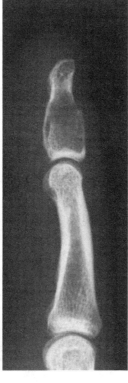

Question 228

228. A 24-year-old man has an acute onset of pain in the finger. Radiographs (see Fig.) shows
- **A.** pathologic fracture
- **B.** old fracture with new fracture through exostosis
- **C.** new fracture with callus formation
- **D.** chronic osteomyelitis

229. Which of the following drugs is associated with calcium deficiency?
- **A.** Sulfasalazine
- **B.** Phenytoin
- **C.** oral contraceptives
- **D.** Isoniazid

230. Compression of the lateral femoral cutaneous nerve (meralgia paresthetica) secondary to obesity or advanced pregnancy produces pain, paresthesias, or numbness of the
- **A.** bottom of the foot
- **B.** anterolateral aspect of the calf
- **C.** lateral aspect of the thigh
- **D.** anteromedial aspect of the thigh

231. Systemic complaints associated with tuberculosis include
- **A.** cough, dyspnea, expiratory wheezing, and chest tightness
- **B.** dyspnea, orthopnea, anorexia, and edema
- **C.** cough, weight loss, hemoptysis, and fatigue
- **D.** cough, chills, fever, and rust-colored sputum

232. The most common cause of infective endocarditis is
- **A.** *Streptococcus viridans*
- **B.** *Staphylococcus aureus*
- **C.** *Enterococcus faecalis*
- **D.** *Mycoplasma pneumoniae*

233. Which of the following is true of the treatment of cirrhosis?
- **A.** Hydration with normal saline is key to reestablishing electrolyte balance
- **B.** Beta-interferon may be used to stimulate nodular regeneration
- **C.** Damage to the liver is generally reversible with proper treatment
- **D.** Removal of toxins and treatment of complications are all that is generally indicated

234. Breast milk differs from formula or cow's milk because it contains
- **A.** sugar
- **B.** fat
- **C.** antibodies
- **D.** iron

235. Osteoporosis is best prevented by
- **A.** physical activity and calcium supplement intake of 1500 mg per day and alendronate 10 mg a day
- **B.** physical activity; conjugated estrogen 0.62 mg a day or its equivalent and continued indefinitely
- **C.** calcium supplementation and etidronate 400 mg a day
- **D.** physical activity; calcitonin intranasal spray 200 IU per day

236. A patient presents to the emergency department with acute headache, stiff neck, and fever. A lumbar puncture reveals turbid cerebrospinal fluid with 2400 white blood cells (mostly neutrophils), protein of 200 mg/dl, and cerebrospinal fluid glucose of 40 mg/dl. This patient must be treated for
- **A.** Guillain-Barré syndrome
- **B.** bacterial meningitis
- **C.** aseptic meningitis
- **D.** cryptococcal meningitis

237. Which of the following is the most important aspect of managing epistaxis?
- **A.** Immediate insertion of anterior packing
- **B.** Compression of the mobile portion of the nose
- **C.** Localizing the site of bleeding
- **D.** Immediate insertion of posterior packing

238. A 63-year-old man presents with chronic production of sputum, which is often foul-smelling, and hemoptysis. Which of the following are the most likely physical findings with this condition?
A. Decreased breath sounds and early inspiratory crackles
B. Chest tightness and wheezing
C. Chest crackles and digital clubbing
D. Pleural pain and friction rub

239. Which of the following individuals is most at risk for pulmonary embolus?
A. A sedentary woman with recent total hip replacement
B. An athletic woman immobilized following anterior cruciate ligament injury
C. A male smoker receiving radiation therapy for lymphatic tumor
D. A 75-year-old man with chronic angina

240. What enzyme is most useful in the diagnosis of early acute pancreatitis?
A. Lactic dehydrogenase
B. Alkaline phosphatase
C. Amylase
D. Alanine aminotransferase

241. Which statement is true about the treatment of prostate cancer?
A. Chemotherapy is an effective treatment modality
B. Tumor grading is more important than staging for treatment
C. All stages of disease may benefit from prostatectomy
D. Stage D disease is treated with hormonal manipulation

242. The patient is a 17-year-old girl who presents with right lower abdominal pain and a fever of 102°F. Her last menstrual period began 7 days ago and was associated with unusually severe dysmenorrhea. She has recently had unprotected intercourse with a new boyfriend. On physical examination you note leukorrhea, tenderness in the right adnexa, a right adnexal mass, and cervical motion tenderness. She vomits as you examine her. You should
A. treat her with oral ceftriaxone 250 mg intramuscularly and have her return in 2–3 days
B. get an emergency consult for surgical treatment of ectopic pregnancy
C. hospitalize her; start cefoxitin 2 g and doxycycline 100 mg intravenously
D. await the results of gonorrhea culture and a monoclonal antibody test for chlamydia

243. A patient who is one week postpartum calls complaining of persistent leg pain and swelling. Her pregnancy was complicated with pregnancy-induced hypertension (PIH). She has been careful to rest since the delivery because her husband brought her to her mother's house, a 6-hour drive away. She doesn't recall any trauma to the leg. The most important differential would be
A. deep venous thrombosis
B. superficial thrombophlebitis
C. dependent edema
D. persistent hypertension

244. A 28-year-old woman fell on an outstretched hand while playing tennis. She demonstrates exquisite pain with palpation of the anatomical snuff-box. Radiographs show no evidence of fracture. Which statement below is NOT true?
A. Radiographs should be taken again 10–12 days post injury
B. Non-union and osteonecrosis are common complications of scaphoid fractures
C. If anatomical snuff-box tenderness is present, treat as scaphoid fracture until proved otherwise
D. Bone scans show decreased uptake in the area of fracture

245. The most common neurologic complication in patients with Paget's disease of bone is
A. conductive and sensorineural hearing loss
B. symmetrical peripheral neuropathy in a stocking–glove distribution
C. ataxia
D. paraplegia

246. A 14-year-old patient presents with a 3-day history of headache, stiff neck, fever, sore throat, and mild nausea. The patient's oral temperature is 100.1°F and examination reveals a fine, erythematous rash on the trunk. Cerebrospinal fluid is essentially normal, with a few lymphocytes noted. With a presumptive diagnosis of viral (aseptic) meningitis, what therapy is appropriate for this patient?
A. Acetaminophen, 650 mg every 3–4 hours for the fever
B. Codeine, 65 mg every 4–6 hours as required for headache
C. Phenobarbital, administered orally, to suppress seizures
D. A third-generation cephalosporin, administered intravenously

247. A 65-year-old man is diagnosed with a large pleural effusion. What is the most likely radiographic finding in this patient?
- **A.** Presence of pleural air
- **B.** Mediastinum shifts away from the effusion
- **C.** Flattened diaphragms
- **D.** Air bronchograms

248. During a routine yearly physical, you detect a pulsating abdominal mass in the central upper abdomen. You suspect an abdominal aortic aneurysm. To confirm your suspicion, your first diagnostic test would be
- **A.** abdominal ultrasound
- **B.** angiography
- **C.** electrocardiogram (ECG)
- **D.** magnetic resonance imaging

249. Physical findings in irritable bowel syndrome (IBS) might include which of the following?
- **A.** Tender, palpable sigmoid colon
- **B.** Decreased resonance on percussion over the abdomen
- **C.** Occult blood in the stool
- **D.** Pain referred to the flanks

250. A patient with a known solitary lesion of the lung presents with hyponatremia and increased urine osmolality without edema or hypotension. The most likely diagnosis is
- **A.** syndrome of inappropriate antidiuretic hormone (SIADH)
- **B.** nephrotic syndrome
- **C.** congestive heart failure
- **D.** hypothyroidism

251. Which of the following occurs in 8%–10% of pregnancies and is the leading cause of neonatal death not due to congenital anomalies?
- **A.** Gestational diabetes
- **B.** Preterm delivery
- **C.** Pregancy-induced hypertension
- **D.** Abruptio placentae

252. Which of the following statements is NOT true?
- **A.** Greenstick fractures are subtle, nondisplaced, bending fractures (ulna and fibula most commonly involved)
- **B.** The most common locations of fractures in children are the humerus, tibia, and femur
- **C.** Injuries to the ligamentous attachments of the bone are most likely to cause ligamentous tears
- **D.** Children's fractures heal much quicker and less immobilization is required

253. Brain abscesses most typically result from
- **A.** postoperative sepsis
- **B.** hematogenous spread from soft tissue infections
- **C.** direct spread from local infection
- **D.** head trauma

254. Which of the following drugs can cause a rash in a patient who has Epstein-Barr virus (mononucleosis)?
- **A.** Tetracycline
- **B.** Ampicillin
- **C.** Amoxicillin
- **D.** Sulfa

255. Which of the following disorders is NOT one of the diseases that comprise chronic obstructive pulmonary disease (COPD)?
- **A.** Bronchiectasis
- **B.** Emphysema
- **C.** Chronic bronchitis
- **D.** Asthma

256. Hoarseness due to compression of the laryngeal nerve is likely to occur in
- **A.** aortic stenosis or abdominal aortic aneurysm
- **B.** aortic stenosis or pulmonary edema
- **C.** pericarditis or pulmonary edema
- **D.** mitral stenosis or thoracic aortic aneurysm

257. The patient is a 14-year-old boy who was playing softball when he began to experience intermittent abdominal pain. The pain has now intensified and become constant, localizing to the right lower quadrant. Which of the following should be included in the physical examination?
- **A.** The physician should place his hand on the patient's right knee and ask him to flex the knee
- **B.** The abdomen should be examined with deep palpation beginning in the right lower quadrant
- **C.** The patient should be carefully evaluated for Murphy's sign
- **D.** The patient should be given a full musculoskeletal examination

258. The most common cause of chronic renal failure is
- **A.** diabetes
- **B.** glomerulonephritis
- **C.** polycystic kidney disease
- **D.** benign prostatic hyperplasia

259. Which of the following signs or symptoms necessitates delivery in term pregnancy?
- **A.** Braxton Hicks contractions
- **B.** Bloody show
- **C.** Rupture of membranes
- **D.** Cervical dilatation 2–3 centimeters

260. A 37-year-old woman presents to the emergency room complaining of chest tightness, breathlessness, and wheezing. Which of the following should NOT be used in this patient?

A. Cromolyn sodium

B. β-blockers

C. Inhaled corticosteroids

D. Theophylline

261. Which of the following is a correct pairing of type of shock and its cause?

A. Cardiogenic—hypertension

B. Hypovolemic—anaphylactic reaction

C. Obstructive—myocardiopathies

D. Neurogenic—loss of electrolytes

262. Which of the following meets the Centers for Disease Control and Prevention criteria for "presumptive AIDS diagnosis"?

A. *Pneumocystis carinii* pneumonia with evidence of HIV infection

B. Kaposi's sarcoma at any age with evidence of HIV infection

C. Cytomegalovirus retinitis with evidence of HIV infection

D. Invasive cervical cancer with evidence of HIV infection

263. What is the single most helpful test in evaluation for malabsorption?

A. Albumin test

B. 72-hour fecal fat test

C. Stool test for white blood cells (WBCs)

D. Endoscopy

264. A patient is admitted to the hospital with hypernatremia. Her blood pressure is 120/80 mm Hg, and her pulse is 80 BPM and regular, without orthostasis or edema. She is diagnosed with diabetes insipidus. Which laboratory results are the most consistent with this diagnosis?

A. Decreased urine sodium and decreased urine osmolality

B. Increased serum glucose and increased urine osmolality

C. Decreased urine sodium and increased urine osmolality

D. Increased urine sodium and increased urine osmolality

265. A 20-year-old woman comes into the office with a possibility of ruptured membranes at 36 weeks' gestation. Her fetus is in the breech position. There is obvious evidence of amniotic fluid because a large amount of watery, clear, nitrazine-positive liquid is evident on the external genitalia. On bimanual examination, a ropelike, elongated, soft mass is palpated in the vagina. This probably represents

A. compound presentation

B. prolapsed umbilical cord

C. placenta previa

D. cephalohematoma

266. Patients with rheumatoid arthritis share the following common features EXCEPT

A. destructive synovitis

B. osteopenia

C. permanent articular damage

D. heel pain and Achilles tendinitis

267. Which of the following lipid-lowering agents has been shown to be associated with reduction in total mortality?

A. Probucol

B. Gemfibrozil

C. Cholestyramine

D. Niacin (nicotinic acid)

268. A normally healthy, athletic adult patient presents with a complaint of acute low back pain that occasionally radiates down to his right foot. There is no history of trauma. On examination he appears to be uncomfortable, but not in acute distress. You note a weakness of dorsiflexion of his right foot and toes. Appropriate initial management of this patient would include

A. bed rest with nonsteroidal anti-inflammatory drug (NSAID) analgesics

B. magnetic resonance imaging to rule out intervertebral disc prolapse

C. referral immediately to a neurosurgeon

D. admission to a hospital and initiation of physical therapy

269. A 21-year-old college sophomore is brought into the emergency room by her friends. The patient appears incoherent and does not want to be bothered. After spending additional time with the patient, you note that she is emotionally labile, is not oriented to person or place, and expresses paranoid fantasies. Physical examination reveals a well-nourished female with needle marks on the inside of her left thigh. The appropriate working diagnosis should be

A. paranoid schizophrenia

B. bipolar mood disorder

C. delusional disorder

D. drug-induced psychosis

270. A 72-year-old man who has worked in coal mines for 30 years presents with dyspnea, inspiratory crackles, and digital clubbing. After pulmonary function tests and chest radiograph are completed, your diagnosis is pneumoconioses. All of the following are pneumoconioses caused by injurious inhalants EXCEPT
  A. byssinosis
  B. silicosis
  C. asbestosis
  D. sarcoidosis

271. Which of the following is a recognized risk factor for atherosclerotic cardiovascular disease?
  A. Female sex
  B. Cigarette smoking
  C. Total cholesterol less than 200 mg/dl
  D. Under 45 years of age

272. What is the treatment for celiac disease?
  A. Gluten-free diet
  B. Tetracycline
  C. Corticosteroids
  D. Pancrease

273. Which of the following is used to differentiate between organic and psychogenic impotence?
  A. Medical and sexual history
  B. Pelvic arteriography
  C. Nocturnal penile tumescence testing
  D. Trial of penile-injected vasoactive substance

274. Factors associated with increased likelihood of breast cancer include
  A. multiple births
  B. delayed menarche
  C. early menopause
  D. delayed childbearing

275. A 15-year-old expectant mother at 36 weeks' gestation has an increase in her baseline blood pressure from 100/70 to 140/85 and is complaining of difficulty removing her rings. A random urinalysis showed pH 5.0; microscopic examination of white blood cell count (WBCs) 0–1/high-powered field (hpf) and red blood cell count (RBCs) 0–1/hpf; negative nitrates and $3^+/4^+$ protein urine dipstick. All of the following laboratory studies would be important in managing this patient EXCEPT
  A. complete blood cell count (CBC) with a differential and platelets
  B. 24-hour urinalysis for protein
  C. liver function tests
  D. urine culture

Directions: Each group of items in this section consists of lettered options followed by a set of numbered items. For each item, select the ONE lettered option that is most closely associated with it. Each option may be selected once, more than once, or not at all.

Items 276 through 279
  A. A soft, nontender, transilluminant tumor
  B. A tumor located on the dorsal, distal interphalangeal joint
  C. A soft, nontender, mobile tumor
  D. A tumor that frequently causes pathological fractures

Choose the best description for these benign conditions.

276. Enchondroma

277. Mucous cyst

278. Ganglion

279. Lipoma

Directions: Each of the numbered items or incomplete statements in this section is followed by answers or by completions of the statement. Select the ONE lettered answer or completion that is BEST in each case. Some of the numbered items or incomplete statements are negatively phrased, as indicated by a capitalized word such as NOT, LEAST, or EXCEPT. For these items, select the ONE lettered answer or completion that is BEST in each case.

280. After initially complaining of 2 days of a burning pain in the right upper back, a patient presents with a vesicular, erythematous rash in the painful area, extending from the paraspinal area to the axilla. Herpes zoster is diagnosed. What is the role of acyclovir in the management of this case?
  A. Reduce the likelihood of postherpetic neuralgia
  B. Control the chronic pain syndrome
  C. Reduce the duration and severity of the eruption
  D. Prevent spread of the eruption

281. In talking to your patient, you realize that he is agitated and appears preoccupied with something other than his appointment with you. On questioning, the man indicates that his girlfriend, who also happens to be your patient, has threatened to leave him. Your patient indicates that his plans for the future have been ruined and that his only option is to teach his girlfriend a lesson by shooting her with the handgun in his car. When you try to assess the lethality of your patient, he abruptly leaves. Your legal responsibility, as reaffirmed under the *Tarasoff v. Regents of University of California*, is to
   A. record the encounter in the patient's record
   B. limit your notes in the patient's record to the presenting problem
   C. immediately inform the patient's girlfriend and the appropriate authorities about the impending threat
   D. protect patient–practitioner confidentiality at all costs

282. Which of the following is a rare cause of otitis externa?
   A. Fungi
   B. *Pseudomonas*
   C. Enterobacteriaceae
   D. *Proteus*

283. All of the following are appropriate for the treatment and management of pneumoconioses EXCEPT
   A. avoidance of exposure
   B. corticosteroids
   C. smoking cessation
   D. antibiotics

284. A patient presents to the emergency department with sudden-onset pain of one hour's duration (which he describes as "aching under my breast bone") along with restlessness, dyspnea, and nausea. The diagnosis most consistent with this presentation is
   A. costochondritis
   B. reflux esophagitis
   C. pulmonary embolism
   D. myocardial infarction

285. The patient is a 62-year-old woman who presents with sudden-onset left lower quadrant abdominal pain. Which of the following will be first on your differential diagnosis?
   A. Colon cancer
   B. Appendicitis
   C. Crohn's
   D. Diverticulitis

286. A 43-year-old diabetic man presents with a 5-year history of impotence. Which treatment will likely be most effective?
   A. Sex therapy
   B. Testosterone injections
   C. Finasteride
   D. Penile prosthesis

Directions: *Each group of items in this section consists of lettered options followed by a set of numbered items. For each item, select the ONE lettered option that is most closely associated with it. Each option may be selected once, more than once, or not at all.*

Questions 287 through 290
   A. Alpha-fetoprotein 3 (AFP 3)
   B. Amniocentesis
   C. Chorionic villus sampling (CVS)
   D. All of the above

Choose the prenatal screening test most appropriate for each description.

287. Offered routinely to all pregnant women

288. Useful in screening for Down syndrome

289. Cannot be used to detect neural tube defects

290. Associated with the greatest risk of fetal limb defects

Directions: *Each of the numbered items or incomplete statements in this section is followed by answers or by completions of the statement. Select the ONE lettered answer or completion that is BEST in each case. Some of the numbered items or incomplete statements are negatively phrased, as indicated by a capitalized word such as NOT, LEAST, or EXCEPT. For these items, select the ONE lettered answer or completion that is BEST in each case.*

291. Which of the following statements is TRUE regarding secondary causes of lipid abnormalities?
   A. Hypothyroidism is associated with decreased total cholesterol
   B. Cirrhosis of the liver is associated with increased total cholesterol
   C. A sedentary lifestyle is associated with decreased high-density lipoprotein (HDL) cholesterol
   D. Alcohol use is associated with decreased HDL cholesterol

292. A young female patient presents with a vague history of transient double vision, difficulty chewing, and weakness in her legs noted while climbing stairs. The symptoms seem to wax and wane throughout the day and may not recur for weeks. Examination reveals only a slight ptosis. What is the likely diagnosis?
   A. Cerebral neoplasm
   B. Cerebrovascular disease
   C. Amyotrophic lateral sclerosis
   D. Myasthenia gravis

293. Isaac Jones is a 75-year-old wheelchair-bound disabled veteran who lost the use of his legs during the Korean conflict. Since the death of his wife 5 years ago, two of Mr. Jones's adult daughters have cared for him. Within the last year you have noted that Mr. Jones has become more withdrawn during his checkups, with his daughters taking over more of the conversation. A finding that proves particularly vexing is the minor bruises suffered by Mr. Jones. While his daughters disagree on how the bruising occurred, they do agree that there has been an overall physical and cognitive deterioration in his condition. They believe he may be showing the early manifestations of Alzheimer's. Your course of action should be to
  A. offer the case to family social services as a suspected case of abuse
  B. refer the case to a specialist in geriatrics for his or her opinion
  C. evaluate Mr. Jones for Alzheimer's
  D. schedule Mr. Jones for a 90-day follow-up to assess any changes in his condition

294. Which of the following is a rare causative organism for otitis media?
  A. *Moraxella catarrhalis*
  B. *Pseudomonas aeruginosa*
  C. *Haemophilus influenzae*
  D. *Streptococcus pneumoniae*

295. A 49-year-old man is diagnosed with sleep apnea. Treatment consists of all of the following EXCEPT
  A. hypnotic medications
  B. weight reduction
  C. alcohol avoidance
  D. continuous positive airway pressure (CPAP)

296. "Classic" electrocardiogram changes in myocardial infarction include peaked T waves, Q waves, T-wave inversions, and
  A. ST-segment elevations
  B. a shortened QT interval
  C. U waves
  D. a widened QRS complex

297. A 12-year-old African-American boy is brought in by his mother. He complains of pain in his left upper quadrant and in the bones of his right leg. A complete blood count reveals a moderate anemia and a slight leukocytosis and thrombocytosis. What test should be ordered next?
  A. Hemoglobin electrophoresis
  B. A reticulocyte count
  C. Total iron binding capacity
  D. Serum ferritin

298. Which of the following is true about the diagnosis of colorectal cancer?
  A. Carcinoembryonic antigen (CEA) is specifically associated with this type of cancer
  B. Occult blood is a specific marker for the disease
  C. Flexible sigmoidoscopy may be used in screening for the disease
  D. Barium swallow is the test of choice to detect obstruction

299. A 35-year-old man complains of a painless scrotal mass. Physical examination reveals a nontender mass in the left hemiscrotum that reduces in size with the patient in the supine position. You believe it to be a varicocele. Which characteristic of the mass would best confirm your suspicions?
  A. Transilluminable
  B. "Bag of worms" texture
  C. Reappearance with Valsalva maneuver
  D. Accompanying abdominal tenderness

300. All of the following are risk factors for cervical neoplasia EXCEPT
  A. human papillomavirus infection
  B. early age at first intercourse
  C. cigarette smoking
  D. upper socioeconomic status

301. Glossitis, cheilosis, and sore mouth are common symptoms of
  A. vitamin E deficiency
  B. vitamin B deficiencies
  C. vitamin K deficiency
  D. vitamin C deficiency

302. The mainstay of treatment for myasthenia gravis is
  A. edrophonium
  B. pyridostigmine
  C. corticosteroids
  D. immunosuppressive agents

303. Martha was referred to you by her minister for severe depression. Your workup indicated that she was probably suffering from a major depressive disorder serious enough that hospitalization might be required for electroconvulsive therapy if the selective serotonin reuptake inhibitor (SSRI) you prescribed did not result in improvement. After 8 weeks on the SSRI, Martha is starting to show improvement. Your next course of action with Martha is to
  A. refer her for psychotherapy
  B. monitor her progress even closer because she is now at a greater risk for suicide
  C. congratulate her on the improvement and, as a visible sign of her progress, allow her to schedule follow-ups as needed
  D. maintain her current treatment regimen

304. Which of the following procedures, examinations, or treatments would be CONTRAINDICATED in a patient with a suspected penetrating injury of the eye?
   A. Schiøtz tonometer
   B. Orbital radiograph
   C. Tetanus toxoid
   D. Broad-spectrum antibiotics

Items 305 through 309

Directions: Each group of items in this section consists of lettered options followed by a set of numbered items. For each numbered item, select the one lettered option that is the recommended tuberculosis treatment. Each option may be selected once, more than once, or not at all.
   A. Isoniazid 300 mg/d; rifampin 600 mg/d; pyrazinamide 20–30 mg/kg/d (not to exceed 2 g); ethambutol 15–25 mg/kg/d (until drug susceptibilities are available)
   B. Isoniazid 300 mg/d; rifampin 600 mg/d
   C. Isoniazid 300 mg daily for 6–12 months
   D. Isoniazid 300 mg daily for 12 months
   E. Isoniazid 10 mg/kg/d (not to exceed 300 mg/d for 12 months); rifampin 15 mg/kg/d (not to exceed 600 mg for 12 months); streptomycin 20 mg/kg/d

305. Extrapulmonary infection in children

306. Latent infection in non–HIV-infected adults

307. Active infection—initial phase in adults

308. Active infection—continuation phase in adults

309. Latent infection in HIV-infected adults

Directions: Each of the numbered items or incomplete statements in this section is followed by answers or by completions of the statement. Select the ONE lettered answer or completion that is BEST in each case. Some of the numbered items or incomplete statements are negatively phrased, as indicated by a capitalized word such as NOT, LEAST, or EXCEPT. For these items, select the ONE lettered answer or completion that is BEST in each case.

310. A patient in the coronary care unit for treatment of an acute myocardial infarction develops fever, leukocytosis, and a pericardial friction rub. He is likely suffering from
   A. Wolff-Parkinson-White syndrome
   B. Dressler's syndrome
   C. Adams-Stokes syndrome
   D. Bradbury-Eggleston syndrome

311. The patient is a 4-week-old infant whose mother brings him in with projectile vomiting of ingested material. On physical examination, a 2.5-cm mobile mass is detected in the epigastrium. The child is immediately referred to surgery, with what working diagnosis?
   A. Hirschsprung's disease
   B. Hypertrophic pyloric stenosis
   C. Esophageal atresia
   D. Diaphragmatic hernia

312. The most important laboratory test used to evaluate the cause of male infertility is
   A. serum testosterone
   B. serum glucose
   C. semen analysis
   D. scrotal ultrasound

313. Which of the following women should NOT be screened for cervical cancer according to the American Cancer Society consensus guidelines?
   A. A 14-year-old who is sexually active
   B. A 17-year-old who is not yet sexually active
   C. An 18-year-old regardless of sexual activity
   D. A 70-year-old who is sexually monogamous

Questions 314 through 317

Directions: Each group of items in this section consists of lettered options followed by a set of numbered items. For each numbered item, select the one lettered option that is the most appropriate. Each option may be selected once, more than once, or not at all.
   A. Placenta previa
   B. Abruptio placentae
   C. Neither
   D. Both

314. Associated with advanced age, smoking, and high parity

315. Cesarean section is often the preferred route of delivery

316. Painless bleeding

317. Ultrasound is very accurate in making diagnosis

Items 318 through 321

Directions: Each group of items in this section consists of lettered options (set in a figure) followed by a set of numbered items. For each numbered item, select the one lettered option that is most closely associated with it.

Match the radiographic findings with a diagnosis.

    318. Osteoporosis
    319. Osteoarthritis
    320. Metastatic bone disease
    321. Osteosarcoma

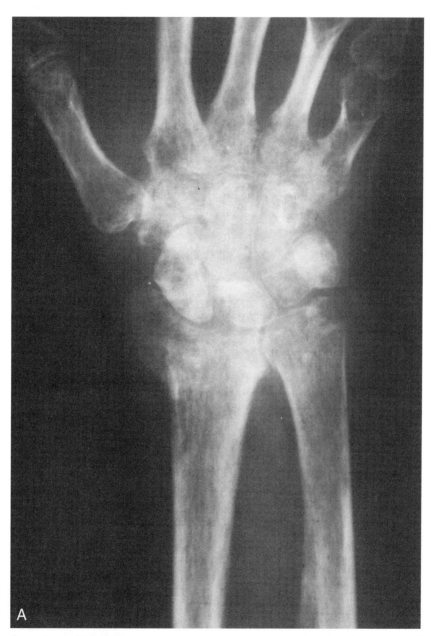

Questions 318–321

(continued on next page)

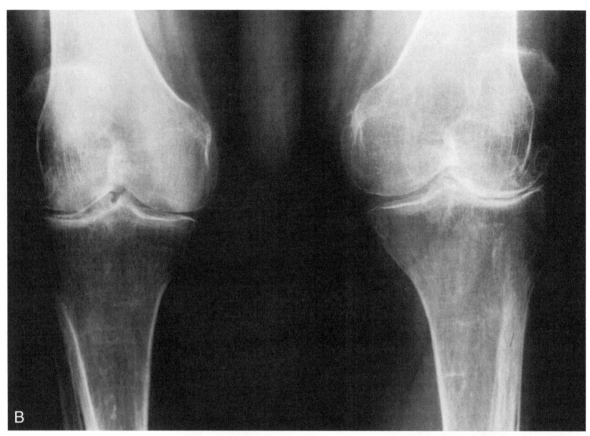

Questions 318–321

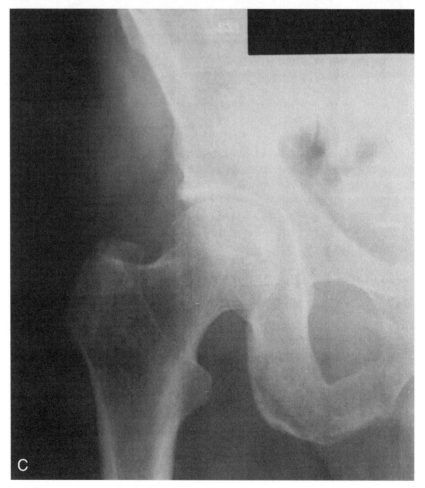

Questions 318–321

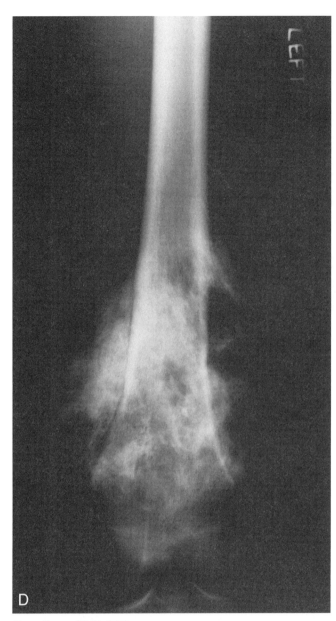

Questions 318–321

Directions: Each of the numbered items or incomplete statements in this section is followed by answers or by completions of the statement. Select the ONE lettered answer or completion that is BEST in each case. Some of the numbered items or incomplete statements are negatively phrased, as indicated by a capitalized word such as NOT, LEAST, or EXCEPT. For these items, select the ONE lettered answer or completion that is BEST in each case.

322. Which of the following is a common cause of thiamine deficiency?
- **A.** Alcoholism
- **B.** Lack of intrinsic factor
- **C.** Biliary atresia
- **D.** Fat malabsorption syndromes

323. In a patient with Brown-Séquard's syndrome, what is the neurologic examination most likely to reveal?
- **A.** Ipsilateral motor disturbance with accompanying impairment of proprioception and contralateral loss of pain and temperature below the lesion
- **B.** Flaccid paralysis and loss of sensation below the level of the lesion
- **C.** Lower motor neuron deficit and loss of pain and temperature, but a sparing of posterior column functions
- **D.** Contralateral motor disturbance and impaired proprioception, and ipsilateral loss of pain and temperature below the lesion

324. Antidepressants are effective for each of the following conditions EXCEPT
- **A.** cyclothymic disorder
- **B.** bulimia
- **C.** anorexia
- **D.** uncomplicated grief

325. Which of the following is classified as a "cyanotic" congenital heart anomaly?
- **A.** Atrial septal defect
- **B.** Patent ductus arteriosus
- **C.** Ventricular septal defect
- **D.** Hypoplastic left heart syndrome

326. Complications of ulcerative colitis include which of the following?
- **A.** Toxic megacolon
- **B.** Fistulas
- **C.** Malabsorption
- **D.** Hemorrhoids

327. A 32-year-old man presents with a painless testicular mass. Ultrasound reveals a suspicious intratesticular echogenic focus. Biopsy shows a seminomatous tumor. The most effective therapy is
- **A.** orchiectomy only
- **B.** radiation
- **C.** chemotherapy with cisplatin
- **D.** nerve-sparing retroperitoneal lymph node dissection

Questions 328 through 331.

Directions: Each group of items in this section consists of lettered options followed by a set of numbered items. For each numbered item, select the lettered option that is the most appropriate. Each lettered item may be selected once, more than once, or not at all.
- **A.** Dizygotic twin
- **B.** Monozygotic twin

Match A or B to the correct diagnosis.

328. Most common twin gestation

329. Occurs randomly

330. Increased with family history, fertility drugs, and above average health and weight of mother

331. Formed from one egg

Directions: Each of the numbered items or incomplete statements in this section is followed by answers or by completions of the statement. Select the ONE lettered answer or completion that is BEST in each case. Some of the numbered items or incomplete statements are negatively phrased, as indicated by a capitalized word such as NOT, LEAST, or EXCEPT. For these items, select the ONE lettered answer or completion that is BEST in each case.

332. A work-up for screening for allergic rhinitis may commonly use all of the following EXCEPT
  A. nasal smear
  B. skin testing
  C. radioallergosorbent testing (RAST)
  D. complete blood cell count (CBC)

333. A constellation of findings including subaortic septal defect, right ventricular outflow obstruction, an overriding aorta, and right ventricular hypertrophy is known as
  A. tetralogy of Fallot
  B. patent ductus arteriosus
  C. transposition of the great vessels
  D. coarctation of the great vessels

334. In a patient in whom you suspect Zollinger-Ellison syndrome, the test you will need to obtain to confirm the diagnosis is
  A. angiography
  B. gastrin level
  C. secretin level
  D. endoscopy

335. An 18-year-old man complains of a painless lesion on his penis and dysuria for two days. He spent the last two weeks on spring break in Florida. During that time he had multiple sex partners, including a prostitute, and did not use condoms. He is flying home tomorrow and wants some medicine before he leaves. Your pharmacologic therapy should include all EXCEPT
  A. benzathine penicillin
  B. ceftriaxone
  C. azithromycin
  D. acyclovir

Items 336 through 339

  A. Nonerosive arthritis involving 2 or more peripheral joints
  B. First metatarsal phalangeal joint involvement
  C. Arthritis, urethritis, and conjunctivitis
  D. Irregularity and pitting of the nail

Match the condition to its associated finding.

336. Psoriatic arthritis

337. Reiter's syndrome

338. Systemic lupus erythematosus (SLE)

339. Gout

340. Papilledema may be caused by all of the following EXCEPT
  A. malignant hypertension
  B. chronic subdural hematoma
  C. hemorrhagic stroke
  D. acute subdural hematoma

341. A 26-year-old man presents with fever, cough, dyspnea, and arthralgias. On physical examination, he has splinter hemorrhages and palatal petechiae. He admits to using intravenous drugs. Echocardiography is likely to demonstrate endocarditis of which valve?
  A. Aortic
  B. Mitral
  C. Pulmonic
  D. Tricuspid

342. Factors that may predispose to Barrett's esophagitis include
  A. Zenker's diverticulum
  B. reflux esophagitis
  C. achalasia
  D. esophageal atresia

343. Which of the following are the most common primary central nervous system tumors?
  A. Gliomas
  B. Meningiomas
  C. Pituitary adenomas
  D. Neurofibromas

344. A man who is a 60-pack-year smoker presents with the chief complaint of calf pain, which now prevents him from walking the quarter of a mile to his mailbox. The pain is relieved by stopping and resting. The likely diagnosis is
  A. arterial insufficiency
  B. venous insufficiency
  C. varicose veins
  D. deep venous thrombosis

345. A secretory diarrhea will be seen in which of the following disease processes?
  A. *Clostridium difficile*
  B. Ulcerative colitis
  C. Pancreatic insufficiency
  D. *Salmonella*

346. Tumors involving the temporal lobe of the brain typically manifest themselves by
  A. ataxia, incoordination, and pyramidal and sensory deficits of the limbs
  B. crossed homonymous hemianopia or a partial visual field defect
  C. contralateral disturbances of sensation and may cause sensory seizures or impaired stereognosis
  D. seizures, olfactory or gustatory hallucinations, depersonalization, emotional and behavioral changes

347. All of the following are associated with hypocalcemia EXCEPT
  A. tetany
  B. Chvostek's sign
  C. Trousseau's sign
  D. depressed deep tendon reflexes

348. A 78-year-old female patient whose hypertension has been poorly controlled comes in with a complaint of awakening at night gasping for air. She has also noted some swelling of her ankles and a cough. The most likely diagnosis is
  A. asthma
  B. pulmonary embolus
  C. congestive heart failure
  D. atherosclerosis

349. Sleep apnea causes disordered and inefficient sleep that results in excessive daytime sleepiness. Sleep apnea is managed most effectively by
  A. taking stimulants during the day
  B. maintaining an open airway utilizing continuous positive pressure through the nasopharynx
  C. taking short-acting hypnotics at bedtime
  D. taking clonazepam at bedtime

350. All of the following are diagnostic criteria for diabetes mellitus in nonpregnant women EXCEPT
  A. random plasma glucose more than 200 mg/dl with classic symptoms
  B. hemoglobin A_{1C} of 2.6 mmol/L
  C. two fasting plasma glucose levels more than 140 mg/dl
  D. after 75 mg oral glucose, plasma glucose more than 200 mg/dl at 2 hours and at least once between 0 and 2 hours

351. Prazosin falls into which class of antihypertensives?
  A. Central sympatholytics
  B. β-Blockers
  C. Calcium channel blockers
  D. α-Adrenergic antagonists

352. A patient with a long history of type II diabetes complains of many months of marked pain in both feet, noting decreased sensation to touch and temperature up to his ankles. Which of the following would NOT be appropriate management for this condition?
  A. Aggressive management of serum glucose
  B. Careful foot care to avoid pressure or thermal injury
  C. Pain control with a tricyclic antidepressant
  D. High-dose corticosteroids

353. Which of the following statements regarding brain injury is NOT true?
  A. The degree of retrograde and posttraumatic amnesia is directly related to the severity of brain injury
  B. Loss of consciousness for over 2 minutes implies a worse prognosis
  C. Prognosis is directly related to the site and severity of brain damage
  D. There is no relationship between the degree of amnesia in head injury and the severity of brain injury

354. Appropriate treatment for inflammatory pericarditis is
  A. pericardiocentesis
  B. an antibiotic that is effective against *Staphylococcus*
  C. nonsteroidal anti-inflammatory agents
  D. diuretics

355. Insomnia describes a number of problems related to sleep, including difficulty falling asleep, staying asleep, and awakening too early in the morning. Which of the following is NOT commonly implicated in chronic insomnia?
  A. Psychiatric disorders, including depression
  B. Heavy smoking
  C. Diabetes
  D. Alcohol abuse

356. Of the following, the most appropriate recommended regimen for a patient with deep venous thrombosis is
  A. heparin for 3–6 months
  B. heparin for 7–10 days, followed by coumadin for approximately 11 weeks
  C. heparin for 7–10 days, followed by aspirin indefinitely
  D. coumadin for 3–6 months

357. Which of the following is NOT part of the classic tetrad of signs in Parkinson's disease?
- **A.** Intention tremor
- **B.** Bradykinesia
- **C.** Rigidity
- **D.** Resting tremor

358. A 65-year-old male patient began experiencing chest pain approximately 20 hours before arriving at the emergency room. Should the cause of his chest pain prove to be myocardial infarction, which of the following treatments would NOT be appropriate to initiate?
- **A.** Aspirin
- **B.** Nitroglycerin
- **C.** Streptokinase
- **D.** Morphine

Items 359 through 363

359. Sore throat, generalized lymphadenopathy, fatigue
- **A.** Viral pharyngitis
- **B.** Streptococcal pharyngitis
- **C.** Acute epiglottitis
- **D.** Tracheobronchitis
- **E.** Mononucleosis

360. Sore throat, chills, painful dysphagia, and excessive secretions with drooling; can be life-threatening

361. Pharyngeal exudates, enlarged and tender anterior cervical nodes, fever, leukocytosis

362. Sore throat, coryza, nasal congestion, mild fever, and minimal cervical lymphadenopathy

363. Persistent cough, fever, headache, sore throat, and coryza

364. Initial treatment of reflux esophagitis includes all of the following EXCEPT
- **A.** nitroglycerin
- **B.** cisapride
- **C.** cimetidine
- **D.** omeprazole

ANSWERS AND EXPLANATIONS

1. **The answer is B** [Chapter 4 I D 1 a (2)].
In an adult, the most common cause of iron deficiency anemia is chronic blood loss, particularly from the gastrointestinal tract. Anemia may, therefore, be the first sign of a colon cancer. In the United States, poor nutritional intake is rarely the cause of iron deficiency in adults, although it may occur in children, particularly those bottle-fed with a formula not supplemented with iron. The consumption of materials such as laundry starch or clay is called pica and is a symptom of anemia rather than a cause. Lack of intrinsic factor is a cause of vitamin B_{12} deficiency anemia rather than iron deficiency anemia.

2. **The answer is C** [Chapter 4 I E 1 a (1); Table 4-2].
Both a mean corpuscular hemoglobin (MCH) of 28 picograms (pg) and a mean corpuscular volume (MCV) of 88 pg fall within the normal range, making this a normochromic, normocytic anemia. Anemias of chronic disease are most often normochromic and normocytic. Iron deficiency anemia is usually microcytic and hypochromic, whereas folic acid deficiency is macrocytic. Thalassemia presents most often as a microcytic, hypochromic anemia.

3. **The answer is D** [Chapter 4 I F 2 d (2)].
Avoidance of alcohol and folic acid metabolism antagonists is important in the treatment of folic acid deficiency. In addition, patients should increase dietary intake of food rich in folic acid (fresh, leafy vegetables) or receive folic acid supplements. Erythropoietin is given to patients with anemia associated with kidney failure, because they can no longer manufacture sufficient supplies of this substance, which is ordinarily produced by the kidney. Lack of intrinsic factor is a part of vitamin B_{12} deficiency, rather than folic acid deficiency anemia. Patients who lack intrinsic factor are treated with intramuscular B_{12}. The lack of intrinsic factor makes it impossible for them to absorb oral B_{12}. Chronic bleeding is a factor in iron deficiency anemia and must be corrected in its treatment.

4. **The answer is A** [Chapter 4 II B 2, 3, 4, C 1].
The patient's history and physical examination are consistent with a diagnosis of polycythemia. Typical laboratory findings include thrombocytosis, leukocytosis, elevated leukocyte alkaline phosphatase, elevated serum B_{12}, and normal red cell morphology.

5. **The answer is B** [Chapter 4 III A 2 a (2), b (1)].
Leukemias can present in persons of any age, but generally increase in incidence with age. Acute lymphocytic leukemia (ALL) is more common in children than acute myelogenous leukemia (AML). Chronic myelogenous leukemia (CML) may occur in people of any age, but occurs most often in young to middle-aged adults, whereas chronic lymphocytic leukemia (CLL) rarely occurs before age 30. Its incidence increases with age.

6. **The answer is C** [Chapter 4 Table 4-3].
Stage II includes 2 or more involved nodes on the same side of the diaphragm, whereas stage I includes a single node and stage III includes nodes on both sides of the diaphragm with splenic involvement. B symptoms include fever, night sweats, and loss of 10% or

more of body weight. Disease in patients without these symptoms is classified as A.

7. The answer is D [Chapter 4 IV D 2 b].
Aerosolized pentamidine, trimethoprim-sulfamethoxazole, and dapsone may each be used for the prevention of *Pneumocystis carinii* pneumonia. Zidovudine is used in the prevention of transmission of HIV from an infected mother to her unborn child. Rifabutin, clarithromycin, or azithromycin are used in *Mycobacterium avium* prophylaxis, whereas ganciclovir is used prophylactically following exposure to cytomegalovirus.

8. The answer is A [Chapter 4 V D 2 a, 4 a].
The child most likely has acute idiopathic thrombocytopenic purpura (ITP). This is found most commonly in children of both sexes and is associated with a preceding viral upper respiratory infection. Most cases resolve spontaneously. Some patients may require corticosteroids or splenectomy. Platelet antagonists such as aspirin should be avoided.

9. The answer is B [Chapter 4 V G 1].
Classic hemophilia is also known as factor VIII disease or hemophilia A. Hemophilia B (Christmas disease) involves a deficiency of factor IX. Vitamin K-dependent factor deficiency disorders involve factors II, VII, IX, and X.

10. The answer is D [Chapter 1 I A 5 a (3)].
The child's presentation is consistent with orbital cellulitis, a condition that may be caused by sinusitis, dental infections, facial infections, or infections of the globe, eyelids, or lacrimal system. In children under the age of 4, the most common causative agents include *Haemophilus influenzae* and *Streptococcus pneumoniae*. *Streptococcus pyogenes* may cause cellulitis and necrotizing fasciitis. *Staphylococcus aureus* causes a variety of skin conditions, including abscesses, cellulitis, and toxic shock syndrome. *Moraxella catarrhalis* is more often associated with respiratory infections than with skin infections.

11. The answer is A [Chapter 1 I C 1 a, b].
Viral conjunctivitis is most common in midsummer to early fall. It is highly contagious and is more common in children than in adults. It is characterized by conjunctival injection with limbic sparing, copious watery discharge, and preauricular lymphadenopathy. Bacterial conjunctivitis usually presents with copious, purulent discharge and eyes that are "glued" shut in the morning. Allergic conjunctivitis is characterized by itching of the eyes, scanty discharge, and mild conjunctival injection, whereas iritis presents as a red eye with limbic involvement and is not contagious.

12. The answer is B [Chapter 1 II A 2].
Sensorineural losses are due to disruption in the nerves of mechanics of hearing. Noise exposure is a possible

cause, along with neural degeneration, decreased cilia, and problems with the ossicles. Conductive losses are those that involve impaired transmission of sound. Causes include impacted cerumen, otitis media or externa, and otosclerosis.

13. The answer is C [Chapter 1 II D 3].
The Hallpike maneuver (quickly turning the patient's head by 90° while he or she is in the supine position) reproduces vertigo and may elicit fast nystagmus. It also can localize the anatomic lesion causing the vertigo. The Weber and Rinne tests differentiate between sensorineural and conductive hearing loss. Caloric testing helps in the understanding of normal and abnormal physiology of the vestibular system.

14. The answer is D [Chapter 1 I B 2 b (3)].
Acute-onset painful inflammation of the lid margin is typical of a hordeolum or sty, for which the mainstay of treatment is warm compresses. Topical antibiotics may be used. Incision and drainage is reserved for hordeola not responding to conservative treatment. Excision by an ophthalmologist is reserved for chalazion, a painless, indurated lesion deep from the margin.

15. The answer is A [Chapter 2 I C 1].
The chest radiograph in chronic obstructive pulmonary disease (COPD) usually shows hyperinflation of the lungs and flattened diaphragms, although this finding is neither specific nor sensitive enough for chest radiograph to be used as a screening tool. Small opacities in the upper lung fields are found in coal workers' pneumoconiosis. Mediastinal shift and pleural air may be found with pneumothorax, whereas costophrenic angle blunting may be found in pleural disease.

16. The answer is B [Chapter 5 I A 4 b (3)].
Bethanechol is a prokinetic drug that increases gastric emptying. Others include metoclopramide and cisapride. These agents may be combined with H_2 blockers. Ranitidine is a histamine blocker. Omeprazole is a proton pump inhibitor, which suppresses acid. Calcium channel blockers such as nifedipine decrease lower esophageal sphincter pressure and should be avoided in the patient with reflux.

17. The answer is C [Chapter 5 Table 5-2].
Bloody, pus-filled diarrhea with tenesmus is a characteristic finding of ulcerative colitis. Both ulcerative colitis and Crohn's disease may present with gradual onset and patients with either disease may develop toxic megacolon. Crohn's disease is primarily right sided and has a characteristic "skip" pattern, whereas ulcerative colitis has continuous involvement.

18. The answer is D [Chapter 5 III E 1 b].
Irritable bowel syndrome (IBS), which is defined as hypersensitivity to intestinal distention, is the most

common cause of chronic or recurrent abdominal pain in the United States. IBS is more commonly found in women than men and is usually an intermittent, lifelong problem. Gastritis is common in alcohol users, persons who take nonsteroidal anti-inflammatory drugs, and those infected with *Helicobacter pylori*. Crohn's disease and ulcerative colitis are relatively uncommon.

19.   The answer is A [Chapter 5 IV A 1 b].
Any patient over 50 years of age with new-onset constipation should be evaluated for colon cancer prior to initiating treatment for constipation. Furthermore, constipation lasting more than 2 weeks or not responding to lifestyle modification should have an evaluation to determine the underlying cause. Most cases of constipation will respond to increased fiber and fluid intake and to increased exercise. Over-the-counter laxatives are usually not necessary with appropriate lifestyle modifications.

20.   The answer is B [Chapter 5 IV D 1].
Anal fissures are linear lesions in the rectal wall, leading to severe pain on defecation accompanied by bright red bleeding. Hemorrhoids may also present with bright red bleeding, with rectal discomfort and itching, and possibly a mucoid discharge. Ulcerative colitis may begin with rectal involvement, but usually presents with bloody diarrhea and tenesmus. Crohn's disease usually involves the terminal ileum and the right colon. Blood may be present in the stool.

21.   The answer is D [Chapter 5 V C 1 a].
Ninety percent of cases of chronic pancreatitis in the United States are caused by alcohol abuse. Some cases will resolve if alcohol consumption is decreased. Other causes include cholelithiasis, peptic ulcer disease, hyperparathyroidism, and hyperlipidemia.

22.   The answer is A [Chapter 5 VI A 2].
The typical presentation of acute cholecystitis is colicky right upper quadrant or epigastric pain that becomes steady and more intense. The pain may radiate to the right shoulder or subscapular area. Nausea, vomiting, and low-grade fever are common. Constipation and a mild paralytic ileus may occur. Acute pancreatitis may present in a variety of ways, including deep epigastric pain with nausea and vomiting; however, it more typically radiates through to the back. Perforated duodenal ulcer presents with an abrupt change of vague, gnawing, epigastric pain to severe pain of peritonitis. The pain of gastroenteritis is crampy and usually confined to the abdomen.

23.   The answer is B [Chapter 5 A 1 b].
The most common cause of acute hepatitis in the United States is viral infection, followed by toxins (in-

cluding alcohol) as the second most common cause. Chronic hepatitis may be caused by viral infections, inherited disorders, autoimmune disease of the liver, or hepatic effects of systemic disease.

24.   The answer is C [Chapter 5 VII A 2 c (4)].
The presence of antigen against hepatitis B serum antigen (anti-HBs) indicates immunity by past infection or immunization. Hepatitis B core antibody (anti-HBc) indicates acute hepatitis, whereas hepatitis B serum antigen (HBsAg) indicates ongoing infection of any duration. A high level of hepatitis B envelope antigen (HBeAg) indicates active infection that is highly contagious, whereas anti-Hbe indicates a lower titer.

25.   The answer is D [Chapter 5 Table 5-1].
Invasive *Shigella*, *Campylobacter*, and enterohemorrhagic *Escherichia coli* are all associated with purulent, bloody diarrhea accompanied by cramping. The viral diarrheas generally present with watery diarrhea, whereas *Staphylococcus aureus* toxin is associated with cramping and some non-bloody diarrhea. *Giardia* may or may not cause diarrhea. It typically causes bloating and flatulence.

26.   The answer is A [Chapter 6 V B 1 d].
Alkalosis is defined as decreased partial pressure of carbon dioxide (P_{CO_2}) in the blood and increased blood pH (alkalemia). Respiratory alkalosis is associated with excessive elimination of CO_2 from the lungs. Causes include anxiety and other causes of hyperventilation, salicylate intoxication, hypoxia, gram-negative septicemia, primary central nervous system dysfunction, and hepatic insufficiency. Myasthenia gravis, chronic obstructive pulmonary disease (COPD), and brain stem injury all reduce pulmonary function and CO_2 clearance, leading to acidosis.

27.   The answer is B [Chapter 6 V C 3 b].
The anion gap is calculated to determine levels of unmeasured ions. The anion gap is calculated by subtracting the sum of the serum bicarbonate and the serum chloride from the serum sodium.

28.   The answer is C [Chapter 6 VII B 4 b, c].
Intracellular gram-negative diplococci indicate gonococcal urethritis. The treatment of choice for gonorrhea is ceftriaxone (125 mg administered intramuscularly); however, concurrent treatment for chlamydia should be initiated, as coinfection is common. This may be accomplished with erythromycin (500 mg, 4 times daily) or doxycycline (100 mg, 2 times daily for 7 days). An anti-chlamydia regimen that is recommended when compliance may be an issue is azithromycin (1 g administered orally). Due to widespread bacterial resistance, the penicillins should

no longer be used as first-line therapy for gonorrhea; however, benzathine penicillin G is the treatment of choice for primary, secondary, and early latent syphilis.

29. The answer is D [Chapter 6 VII F 1 b].
Escherichia coli is the most common organism causing epididymitis in men older than 35 years of age, whereas *Chlamydia trachomatis* and *Neisseria gonorrhoeae* are more common in younger men. *Mycobacterium tuberculosis* was once a common cause of epididymitis, but is rarely a cause in the United States at this time.

30. The answer is A [Chapter 6 X B 2 a].
Blood in the urine is the most common presenting symptom in bladder cancer. Bladder irritability and infection are other presenting symptoms. Urethral discharge is a presenting symptom of urethritis.

31. The answer is B [Chapter 3 VI C 2].
Development of horizontal or down-sloping ST-segment depression is one of the most sensitive clinical signs of ischemic heart disease. Q waves develop in the course of a myocardial infarction. U waves are associated with hypokalemia and wide, bizarre QRS complexes with aberrant ventricular contractions.

32. The answer is C [Chapter 3 Table 3-2].
Changes in leads II, III, and aVF suggest an inferior myocardial infarction. Posterior and anteroseptal infarctions are suggested by changes in V1 and V2, whereas anterolateral infarctions show changes in V4, V5, and V6.

33. The answer is D [Chapter 3 X A 1 d].
So-called "holiday heart" is atrial fibrillation precipitated by excessive alcohol use and withdrawal. Atrial fibrillation is the most common chronic arrhythmia. None of the other arrhythmias are associated with excessive alcohol use.

34. The answer is A [Chapter 3 X B 4 a; Table 3-7].
Asymptomatic premature ventricular contractions (PVCs) are usually not treated. Symptomatic PVCs may be treated with β-blockers or sodium channel blockers. Calcium channel blockers are used in treatment of supraventricular tachycardias.

35. The answer is B [Chapter 3 XI D 1].
Most patients with sick sinus syndrome who have syncope, dizziness, confusion, heart failure, palpitations, or angina require permanent pacing. Digitalis and β-blockers may cause sick sinus syndrome. Surgical and radiofrequency ablation is used for arrhythmias caused by ectopic foci.

36. The answer is C [Chapter 3 XV D 2; Chapter 13 IV C 1 b, c].
This is the classic presentation of the patient with chronic venous insufficiency leading to ulceration. Neuropathic ulcers found in diabetic patients are accompanied by decreased sensation in the feet and paresthesias. While they may occur around the ankles, they are more typically on the plantar surfaces and toes. In arterial insufficiency, the foot is cold and pale or mottled, with absent pulses. Ulcers associated with arterial insufficiency have a punched-out appearance. Pressure ulcers occur on the sacrum, elbows, heels, and similar areas.

37. The answer is C [Chapter 13 II A 1 b (2) (a)].
The first lesion is the so-called "herald patch," pathognomonic for pityriasis rosea. The subsequent rash has a typical "Christmas tree" distribution along the natural skin folds. Of unknown etiology but thought to be viral, the rash resolves spontaneously in 3–8 weeks. The rash of rubella is morbilliform, starting on the face and spreading distally and is usually accompanied by systemic symptoms. Tinea versicolor appears as pale macules that will not tan. Secondary syphilis, called the "great pretender" because it mimics so many other diseases, has no herald patch.

38. The answer is A [Chapter 3 Table 3-5].
Leaning forward accentuates or brings out aortic murmurs, while the left lateral position does the same for mitral murmurs. The murmur of tricuspid regurgitation increases slightly with inspiration. Both a Valsalva maneuver and squatting accentuate findings associated with mitral prolapse and hypertrophic cardiomyopathy.

39. The answer is A [Chapter 13 V B 3 b].
"Dirty wounds" such as human bites and gunshot wounds are usually treated with cephalosporins. Animal bites may be treated with penicillin, tetracycline, or amoxicillin-clavulanic acid.

40. The answer is D [Chapter 3 Table 3-3].
The total creatine kinase is associated with many false positive results and may not even be drawn because the isoenzyme of creatine kinase containing M and B subunits (CK-MB) fraction is far more sensitive. Troponin I and T are both sensitive and should be drawn 12 hours after the onset of chest pain. Lactate dehydrogenase (LDH) is usually drawn once, at least 24 hours after the onset of pain.

41. The answer is D [Chapter 13 III B 1 a].
Features of a skin lesion that are suspicious for malignant melanoma include asymmetry, increasing size, larger than a pencil eraser (6 mm), irregular borders, and multiple colors. These lesions occur primarily on

the skin, but may occur in the eye or on the mucous membranes of the genitalia, anus, or oral cavity.

42. **The answer is B** [Chapter 3 VIII A 1 a (1)].
The 4 anomalies found in the tetralogy of Fallot include subaortic septal defect, right ventricular outflow obstruction, overriding aorta, and right ventricular hypertrophy.

43. **The answer is A** [Chapter 4 I C; Table 4-2].
Initial laboratory studies in an anemic patient include red cell indices (mean corpuscular hemoglobin, mean corpuscular volume, and mean corpuscular hemoglobin concentration) to determine the size and color of the red cells, the red cell distribution width (RDW) to determine the variability in size of red cells, and the corrected reticulocyte count to determine the bone marrow response. The hemoglobin electrophoresis is a later step in the evaluation and is used for those patients whose anemia is thought to be due to hemoglobinopathies such as those found in sickle cell anemia and the thalassemias.

44. **The answer is C** [Chapter 1 I A 2 a (2) (a)].
Retinal detachment is associated with acute onset of blurred or darkened vision that occurs over several hours. Cataracts, macular degeneration, and open-angle glaucoma are all associated with gradual loss of vision over months to years. Angle-closure glaucoma, however, is associated with acute loss of vision.

45. **The answer is C** [Chapter 5 V A 2 c].
While nausea and anorexia are common, vomiting is usually isolated and begins subsequent to the onset of pain. Diarrhea may occur, but is not common. Localization of pain to McBurney's point in the right lower quadrant usually occurs within 12 hours after onset of periumbilical or epigastric pain. Low-grade fever is common and high fever unlikely. Positive psoas and obturator signs indicate inflammation adjacent to those muscles.

46. **The answer is B** [Chapter 1, I B 2 a].
Blepharitis is an infectious or non-infectious inflammation of the palpebral edge. The infectious form usually results from *Staphylococcus aureus,* and may also cause superficial ulcerations of the skin and concurrent mild to moderate conjunctivitis. The non-infectious etiology may result from a localized form of seborrheic dermatitis. This may cause bilateral erythema of the eyelid margins with greasy scales present. Management includes lid scrubs using a cotton-tipped swab moistened with diluted baby shampoo. A topical antibiotic is applied in ointment form twice a day for 7 days. Acute dacryocystitis is an infrequent disorder that has an acute onset of unilateral pain in the medial canthal region. This is accompanied by tenderness and warmth with an occasional purulent discharge. Conjunctivitis is an inflammation of the conjunctiva that results in intense pruritus and copious discharge. There is usually ipsilateral preauricular lymphadenopathy present. Keratitis is a nonspecific inflammation of the cornea. There is usually an acute onset of unilateral pain, erythema, and decreased visual acuity. A dendritic pattern of gray-colored corneal ulcers is present.

47. **The answer is D** [Chapter 2 I A 1 b].
Chronic bronchitis is defined as a chronic productive cough occurring on most days for 3 months of the year for 2 or more consecutive years. Chronic inhalation of cigarette smoke is its major risk factor. Pneumonia is an inflammatory response of the lung parenchyma most often caused by microorganisms and presents with fever, productive cough, shortness of breath, and pleuritic chest pain. Asthma is characterized by airflow obstruction, bronchial hyperreactivity, and airway inflammation. Patients have asymptomatic periods between attacks. Pulmonary embolus has an abrupt onset with dyspnea, chest pain, hemoptysis, or syncope.

48. **The answer is C** [Chapter 3 III A 3].
The black male smoker is the only individual listed who has 3 of the known risk factors, which include age, race (elevated risk in blacks), gender (elevated risk in men), smoking, overweight, sedentary lifestyle, hyperlipidemia, and diabetes.

49. **The answer is C** [Chapter 5, I C 2 e].
Esophageal spasm is characterized by dysphagia with intermittent chest pain. Stenosis causes slowly progressive dysphagia, whereas scleroderma generally leads to reflux because of loss of tone and peristalsis. Zenker's diverticulum causes regurgitation of undigested food several hours after eating.

50. **The answer is D** [Chapter 4, IV C 1, 2].
This patient is at risk for HIV infection. The first step is to perform an enzyme-linked immunosorbent assay (ELISA), which is both sensitive and specific for HIV. Because of the potential for false positive results, a positive ELISA is usually repeated, then confirmed with the Western blot. Patients whose tests are negative must be counseled that these tests are effective only 6–12 weeks following infection; they also must be counseled about effective prevention. Whether or not he is HIV seropositive, this patient should be screened for other sexually transmitted diseases, including syphilis, gonorrhea, *Chlamydia* infection, and herpes simplex. Seropositive patients and others at risk should also be screened for tuberculosis and hepatitis B. Individual baseline testing for seropositive patients includes a complete blood count, CD4+ count, blood chemistries, toxoplasma serology, varicella zoster, and measles antibody.

51. **The answer is A.** [Chapter 8 I A 4 b].
Multiple studies have shown that folic acid supplementation ranging from 0.4 mg to 1.0 mg daily significantly reduces the risk of neural tube defects in the general population. 1.0-mg doses of folic acid are regulated to prescriptive medication because their use could mask an undiagnosed folic acid anemia. Although attention to dietary counseling is vital in preconception counseling, folic acid alone is not prescribed primarily to enhance nutritional status. The use of folic acid will not correct an underlying acid–base imbalance.

52. **The answer is B** [Chapter 6 II A 2 a; III B 4, X B 2 a].
Hematuria, red cell casts, hypertension, and edema are hallmark findings in glomerulonephritis. Bladder cancer often presents with painless hematuria. Kidney stones are often accompanied by flank pain and hematuria. In renal failure, the kidneys lose much of their functional ability, but as long as the glomerulus remains intact, hematuria is uncommon.

53. **The answer is D** [Chapter 9 IV A 1 a, b].
Cervical spondylosis usually presents in men in their 50s or 60s, typically with a history of lifting or excessive driving. Muscle spasm, herniated nucleus pulposus (HNP) or annulus bulging can be present, but the important feature identified in this case is the radiographic evidence of osteophytes (spondylitic bars) arising from the dorsal surface of the adjacent vertebral body and compressing the spinal cord. Ankylosing spondylitis is an inflammatory condition that occurs in patients in their 30s and 40s and most commonly involves the low back and hip.

54. **The answer is A** [Chapter 11 I A 2 c].
Strokes involving the anterior circulation are associated with contralateral hemispheric signs including hemiparesis and hemisensory losses. Occlusions of the middle cerebral and internal carotid arteries may cause similar signs and symptoms, but typically include a homonymous hemianopia and speech defects. Strokes in the posterior, vertebrobasilar region are commonly associated with brain stem dysfunction (i.e., coma, nausea, vomiting, and ataxia).

55. **The answer is D** [Chapter 7, I A 2 a, 4 a (1)].
Primary dysmenorrhea typically presents as a young woman's cycles become consistently ovulatory. This usually occurs within 6 months to a year or two after menarche. This dysmenorrhea is due to excess prostaglandin $F_{2\alpha}$ and E_2 release. Prostaglandins are responsible for the central abdominal or pelvic cramping (which may radiate to the back or down the thighs), diarrhea, nausea, vomiting, sweating, headache, and tachycardia some women experience with their menses. Pelvic pathology is more typically associated with secondary dysmenorrhea and is found

in older women. The first line of treatment for primary dysmenorrhea (and often for secondary) is nonsteroidal anti-inflammatory drugs (NSAIDs), begun 1–2 days before the expected onset of menses and continued at regular intervals through the first 2–3 days of the cycle. For women with mild symptoms, over-the-counter NSAIDs may be sufficient; for those with more severe symptoms, prescription-strength NSAIDs may be required. For women who also need contraception, an oral contraceptive is another appropriate first-line treatment. Heat and exercise are useful adjuncts to treatment. Young women at menarche often benefit from receiving information about their cycles and any problems that might develop. It is important to help them distinguish between what is "normal" for them and what needs further evaluation.

56. **The answer is B** [Chapter 12 II A].
The differential diagnosis of schizophrenia, schizophreniform disorder, and brief psychotic disorder is based on the severity and duration of the symptoms. To make a diagnosis of schizophrenia, the constellation of symptoms must be present for at least six months. The symptoms for schizophreniform disorder are similar to those of schizophrenia, but only three of the criteria, instead of six, need to be met. The duration of symptoms must have been present for at least a month but less than six months. For brief psychotic disorder, only one symptom needs to be present for at least a day, but less than a month.

57. **The answer is D** [Chapter 10 I A 1 b].
Patients with Graves' disease, the most common form of thyrotoxicosis, may also have other autoimmune disorders or diseases with a suspected autoimmune component, including vitiligo, myasthenia gravis, and type I diabetes. Graves' disease is found about 8 times more often in women than in men. The disease usually occurs in people between 20 and 40 years of age; evidence exists for a genetic predisposition.

58. **The answer is D** [Chapter 13 II B 2].
The most likely diagnosis is impetigo, which is caused by *Staphylococcus aureus* or group A streptococci. The lesion is characterized by a honey-colored crust. Oral candidiasis is caused by *Candida* and usually affects the buccal mucosa and resembles curdled milk. Dermatophytosis is a fungal infection that can affect the hair, nails, and skin. Acne vulgaris is an inflammatory, follicular, papular, and pustular eruption involving the sebaceous glands; this condition usually does not occur in a 3-year-old child.

59. **The answer is D** [Chapter 6 II B 1 a].
Nephrotic syndrome is defined as proteinuria greater than 3.5 grams in 24 hours per 1.73 square meter of body surface area. Proteinuria between 1 and 3 grams

per day is termed a urinary abnormality that is most commonly seen in hypertension and diabetes. The normal amount of protein in the urine is 150 mg per day.

60. **The answer is C** [Chapter 1, I A 2 a].
A retinal detachment usually has an acute onset and may result in partial or complete monocular blindness. Patients may report that for several hours prior to the onset of blindness, they sensed "floaters," flashing lights, and blurred vision. The detachment may be the result of trauma, extreme myopia as the result of an elongated eyeball length, or prior history of detachment. On examination, an area of the retina that is detached can be seen flapping in the vitreous humor. Retinal detachment is an ocular emergency and the patient should be kept supine with the head turned to the side ipsilateral to the detachment. Emergency laser therapy or cryosurgery is indicated. Central retinal vein occlusion presents as the acute onset of complete loss of vision in one eye. There are usually no associated prodromal symptoms. On examination there is a markedly edematous retina with multiple hemorrhages and dilated tortuous veins. It is usually secondary to long-standing hypertension. This is also treated as an ocular emergency with an ophthalmic consult. Central retinal artery occlusion is manifested by the acute onset of painless monocular blindness. Examination reveals a cherry-red spot in the macula, a pale optic disc, and decreased retinal artery size. This is usually the result of an arterial thromboembolic event [e.g., a prior cerebrovascular accident (CVA)]. In addition to the ocular symptoms, the patient will usually also have other sequelae of arterial thromboembolic disease. Temporal arteritis may also present with painless monocular blindness. It is almost always associated with a unilateral throbbing headache ipsilateral to the affected eye. This is also an emergency and is treated with steroids. Failure to diagnose and treat may result in permanent blindness.

61. **The answer is A** [Chapter 3 IV C].
Left-sided cardiomegaly results from myocardial hypertrophy secondary to the chronic excessive cardiac workload, while systemic congestion of the liver is associated with elevations of liver enzymes, particularly serum aspartate aminotransferase (AST).

62. **The answer is B** [Chapter 8 I A 1 c].
Infertility is defined as failure to conceive after one year of unprotected intercourse, and if a couple fits this description, measures may be instituted for an infertility workup. Frustration at a failure to conceive is very common. Although keeping basal body temperature graphs may be useful to gain more information about the status of the woman's ovulatory status, by itself it does not constitute a serious attempt at infertility eval-

uation. Folic acid supplementation should be recommended to those trying to conceive to decrease the incidence of neural tube defects. False reassurance regarding fertility or spurious assumptions regarding sexual activity are inappropriate in this situation.

63. **The answer is C** [Chapter 10 I A 2 a, b].
This patient fits the classic description of a patient with thyrotoxicosis. She might also describe restlessness, weakness, muscle cramps, palpitations, or angina pectoris. Additional physical findings might include fine hair and onycholysis. In Graves' disease, the most common cause of thyrotoxicosis, she would be expected to have a goiter, possibly with a bruit, and the classic ophthalmopathy. Pheochromocytoma is rare, occurring in less than 0.1% of patients with hypertension. Patients commonly have severe headache, palpitations, and profuse sweating. Like thyrotoxicosis, they may have nervousness, increased appetite, and weight loss. Panic attacks usually begin prior to 25 years of age and affect 3%–5% of the population. Patients typically complain of dyspnea, tachycardia, palpitations, choking sensations, nausea, and a sense of impending doom. Cocaine and amphetamines both produce an increase in central and peripheral sympathetic activity; symptoms include anxiety, tremulousness, dilated pupils, agitation, psychosis, hypertension, and diaphoresis. Given her history, amphetamine intoxication is not likely to be the source of her symptoms.

64. **The answer is A** [Chapter 12 II B].
Delusions and hallucinations provide the most restricted symptom subset to make a diagnosis of schizophrenia but the positive symptom of disorganized speech is very apparent in the more obvious cases that the practitioner will see. Irritability, hypervigilance, and sleep disturbance are symptoms of a generalized anxiety disorder. Grandiosity, psychomotor agitation, and a flight of ideas are symptoms characteristic of a manic episode. Suicidal ideation, terminal insomnia, and significantly depressed mood are part of the symptom picture characteristic of a major depressive episode.

65. **The answer is C** [Chapter 13 I C 1].
Syphilis is diagnosed by isolating and viewing spirochetes on dark-field examination. Gonorrhea is a sexually transmitted disease (STD) that is diagnosed by culture and Gram staining. Herpes, a viral skin infection, can be diagnosed using a Tzanck preparation. Chlamydia is diagnosed by specific virology testing.

66. **The answer is A** [Chapter 2 I A 2].
Smoking has been shown to be the most important risk factor associated with chronic obstructive pul-

monary disease (COPD). Cessation of smoking may prevent relentless progression of the disease and slow the decline in forced expiratory volume in 1 second (FEV_1). Although infections, pollutants, and allergies may aggravate COPD, they are not risk factors for its development.

67. **The answer is B** [Chapter 3, VI C 3].
Angina during a cardiac stress test and chest radiograph showing a left-shift in the cardiac silhouette are often seen in ischemic heart disease. Chest pain, however, may occur in conditions as varied as pericarditis, pulmonary embolus, and dilated cardiomyopathy, and left-sided cardiomegaly may occur in hypertension, congestive heart failure (CHF), aortic and mitral valve disorders, and dilated cardiomyopathy. Although electrocardiogram (ECG) showing down-sloping ST segment depression is a particularly sensitive finding, the only precise diagnostic evidence is a visual image of the narrowed vessels themselves.

68. **The answer is A** [Chapter 5, I B 1 b (1), C 4].
Fluconazole is used to treat presumptive esophageal candidiasis. The diagnosis is supported by the presence of white plaques in the mouth, although these should be swabbed and examined in a potassium hydroxide (KOH) or saline prep. Acyclovir will treat herpes simplex esophagitis, which is less common among immunosuppressed patients, although it remains part of the differential diagnosis if initial treatment is unsuccessful. Dexamethasone is contraindicated if a fungal or viral infection is present. Foscarnet will treat either cytomegalovirus or resistant herpes simplex esophagitis, but is a highly toxic medication and would never be administered without a definitive diagnosis.

69. **The answer is C** [Chapter 7, I B 3].
To be classified as premenstrual syndrome (PMS), the patient's symptoms must demonstrate a clear relationship to the luteal phase of the menstrual cycle, with a monthly symptom-free period during the follicular phase. Once the diagnosis is clearly established, treatment may include anxiolytic or antidepressant medications in some patients whose symptoms do not respond to other modalities. Simply keeping a calendar may prove useful. Patient and family education and psychosocial support are important. Fresh fruits and vegetables, minimal refined sugar, fat, and salt, avoidance of caffeine and alcohol, and daily exercise help many women with milder symptoms. Oral contraceptives, danazol, or gonadotropin-releasing hormone (GnRH) agonists to halt ovulation are more appropriate than hysterectomy and have been shown in short-term studies to be effective in some women. Psychotherapy is indicated for disorders included in the differential diagnosis of PMS such as anxiety disorder, major depression, bipolar disorder, substance abuse, and eating disorders.

70. **The answer is A** [Chapter 8 I B 2; Figure 8-1].
The primigravida often appreciates fetal activity at 20 weeks' gestation, and the multigravida at 16–18 weeks. At approximately 12 weeks, the uterus will be just above the pubic symphysis and fetal heart tones may be appreciated. At 14–16 weeks' gestation, the uterus will be midway between the pubic symphysis and the umbilicus.

71. **The answer is B** [Chapter 11 I B 2 a–d].
The patient who reports acutely "the worst headache I've ever had" should be considered to have a subarachnoid hemorrhage until proved otherwise, especially with elevated blood pressure. There is usually a history of recurrent, similar headaches with migraine, and the onset of headache and other symptoms in viral meningitis is more gradual. Subdural hemorrhage typically presents as acute back pain and there may be a history of bleeding disorder or recent lumbar puncture.

72. **The answer is B** [Chapter 3 VI D 2].
Sublingual nitroglycerin is the only medication that will provide rapid dilation of narrowed coronary vessels. Aspirin or nifedipine may be employed as long-term adjunct therapies but not for immediate acute crisis. Propranolol is not administered sublingually.

73. **The answer is B** [Chapter 4 I D 1 a (2)].
This patient's anemia is consistent with iron deficiency. In most adults in the United States, the cause of iron deficiency is chronic bleeding, especially from the gastrointestinal tract. Seeking a source of the bleeding is essential prior to initiating treatment. If her stools are heme-positive, it would be appropriate to discontinue the ibuprofen and initiate acetaminophen for the treatment of osteoarthritis; however, a postmenopausal woman (or a man) with iron deficiency anemia should be considered to have a gastrointestinal cancer until this diagnosis is definitively ruled out. It is inappropriate to initiate any kind of treatment without thorough investigation of the causes of the microcytic anemia. The laboratory findings are not consistent with a diagnosis of anemia of chronic disease.

74. **The answer is C** [Chapter 5, I D 1 c, 2].
The most important part of the history for this patient would be the smoking history. The differential diagnosis for progressive dysphagia for solid foods includes esophageal stenosis, achalasia, and esophageal cancer. Esophageal cancer will more likely present with rapid progression, and is closely related to smoking history. Bowel habits will not be significantly af-

fected by any of these unless intake is reduced. Ulcer history does not predispose to any of these conditions. The use of extra pillows is common in reflux esophagitis.

75. **The answer is B** [Chapter 6 I A 1 b, 3 b (1); Table 6-1].

All the entities listed may cause proteinuria but the most likely is acute interstitial nephritis, which can be caused by any substance that might damage the tubules, like the nonsteroidal anti-inflammatory drugs taken for arthritis pain. Minimal change disease is predominantly a disease of children. Multiple myeloma causes proteinuria by overflow of Bence Jones proteins but is usually accompanied by back pain or infection. Orthostatic proteinuria explains 90% of proteinuria in young men by changes in position.

76. **The answer is C** [Chapter 8 II A 3 a].

The most important differential diagnosis in this case is ectopic pregnancy. The patient is amenorrheic with abdominal pain and vaginal bleeding. Her past history of infection puts her at greater risk for an ectopic gestation. She is at risk for another chlamydial infection, but pelvic inflammatory disease is not likely to present an immediate threat to her health. A urinary tract infection can cause abdominal pain but is not associated with vaginal bleeding and amenorrhea. If the patient were acutely ill in appearance, a hemoglobin and hematocrit would be appropriate, along with a human chorionic gonadotropin (hCG), to exclude a ruptured ectopic pregnancy.

77. **The answer is C** [Chapter 9 V B 1 c (1), d].

Serial observation with repeat radiographs on a 36″ anteroposterior film every 3–4 months is required. Curves of 0–10° are normal and do not require follow-up. For curves 10°–15°, follow-up every 6 months with bending tests and scoliometer. For curves greater than 20°, progression is likely and referral to an orthopedist for consideration of bracing and close follow-up is necessary.

78. **The answer is B** [Chapter 10 I B 2 b, c, 3 a].

The differential diagnosis for the presenting symptoms does include depression, a complication of diabetes mellitus, and adrenal insufficiency, but the physical findings are most consistent with hypothyroidism. A serum thyroid-stimulating hormone (TSH) level is the most sensitive test for this condition. Depressed patients may also present with apathy and anorexia, but the physical findings are inconsistent with the diagnosis. A patient with diabetic ketoacidosis (associated with type I diabetes) would present with hyperpnea, nausea, vomiting, and debilitation, whereas a patient in a hyperosmolar nonketotic state (associated with

type II diabetes) would become lethargic, prostrated, and ultimately comatose. A patient with Addison's disease [diagnosed by the adrenocorticotropic hormone (ACTH) stimulation test] is likely to have darkly pigmented skin and weight loss.

79. **The answer is C** [Chapter 11 II B 2 a].

Simple partial seizures involve isolated tonic or clonic activity of a limb, and occasionally will "march" through adjacent neurons (jacksonian march), but without loss of consciousness. Complex partial seizures are followed by a short period of altered consciousness and may be preceded by an aura. Benign tremor is isolated to one area and seen more commonly in an older age-group, whereas febrile seizure is seen exclusively in childhood and associated with high fever.

80. **The answer is C** [Chapter 12 II B].

It is important to remember that social and occupational functioning are severely impacted with all types of schizophrenia. Among the problems that a clinician would expect to see with a diagnosis of schizophrenia is an inability to finish a training program. Cognitive processes are so severely impacted with schizophrenics that sustained academic achievement is not seen. A patient unable to withdraw from schooling after successful completion of a training program is exhibiting a symptom characteristic of an anxiety and not a schizophrenic disorder. Difficulty in sustaining personal and professional relationships are also symptoms of schizophrenia.

81. **The answer is C** [Chapter 13 IV D 2 a].

The patient most likely has Rocky Mountain spotted fever (RMSF), which is transmitted by a dog or wood tick bite and causes a rash and flu-like symptoms. The rash is composed of erythematous macules and papules that can involve the palms and soles. Lyme disease is also a tickborne illness, but it is associated with a "bull's-eye" rash at the site of the tick bite. Varicella is a contagious condition, characterized by umbilicated, vesicular lesions that may cover the entire body and later become crusted. Measles is an exanthem associated with a confluent rash that progresses from the hairline toward the feet.

82. **The answer is B** [Chapter 1, I B 2 c].

A chalazion presents as a painless lesion with an insidious onset. It is secondary to a chronic inflammation of an internal hordeolum of the meibomian gland. It is treated with surgical excision, usually by an ophthalmologist. A hordeolum, or common sty, has a painful presentation and exudate is usually present. It is commonly caused by *Staphylococcus aureus* and is treated with an incision and drainage (I&D) and topical antibiotics. An entropion is an inversion of the margin of the lower eyelid that is secondary to spasm or scarring. A xanthelasma is a flat or slightly raised lesion usually found on the upper or lower eyelid, which is a deposition of lipid material. It may indicate hyperlipidemia.

83. **The answer is B** [Chapter 2 IV].
Adult respiratory distress syndrome (ARDS) occurs in 3 clinical settings: sepsis, severe multiple trauma, and aspiration of gastric contents. Many patients are cyanotic with increasingly severe hypoxemia that is refractory to administered oxygen. Pneumonia in this setting may be possible, but in a young person with no comorbid illnesses, unlikely. Asthma may present acutely but more often is related to exposure to a known allergen or trigger substance. A pulmonary embolus also presents acutely, but more commonly as pleuritic chest pain, dyspnea, cough, and hemoptysis.

84. **The answer is D** [Chapter 3 IX A 1 a, 2 a; Table 3-5].
Aortic stenosis diminishes the ejection fraction. This results in decreased delivery of blood to tissues, systemic hypoxia, and, thus, symptoms of fatigue. However, there is no systemic congestion to produce cough, nocturia, paroxysmal dyspnea, or distended neck veins. Systolic ejection murmur occurs due to increased left-sided pressures against the narrowed aortic valve opening.

85. **The answer is A** [Chapter 5, II A 1 b (2), D 4 a (2)].
Gastric lymphoma is associated with *Helicobacter pylori* (HP). In addition to gastric lymphoma, HP is also associated with type B gastritis, peptic ulcer disease, and gastric adenocarcinoma. Type A gastritis is caused by autoimmune disorders. Esophageal carcinoma is associated with ingestion of toxins, including tobacco and alcohol. Cholangitis is associated with choledocholithiasis or other irritation of the biliary duct.

86. **The answer is A** [Chapter 6 II B].
Membranous nephropathy affects the basement membrane of the glomerulus and is the most common renal cause of nephrotic syndrome in adults. There is no history of prior streptococcal infection. Amyloidosis is a chronic inflammatory disease that causes plasma cell dyscrasias, which secrete amyloid fibrils into the blood. There is no sign of chronic inflammation in this patient. If the patient had diabetes, glucose would be found in the urine.

87. **The answer is A** [Chapter 7, I C 4 a (2)].
Absolute contraindications to estrogen replacement therapy (ERT) include undiagnosed vaginal bleeding, acute vascular thrombosis, undiagnosed breast mass, and a personal history of estrogen-dependent tumors. Recommendations for women with a personal history of breast cancer are controversial and should be indi-

vidualized according to tumor estrogen-receptor status, symptomatology associated with menopause, and risk for heart disease and osteoporosis.

88. **The answer is C** [Chapter 11 II D 2–3].
Monotherapy is always preferable, and a single anticonvulsant is typically administered in progressive doses until successful in preventing seizures. If a second medication is required, it may be increased to full therapeutic doses and the original medication slowly tapered in order to preserve monotherapy. The use of ethosuximide is generally limited to generalized, nonconvulsive epilepsy (absence seizures).

89. **The answer is D** [Chapter 12 II A 4].
The criteria for brief psychotic disorder include symptoms that last for less than a month with a return to premorbid functioning. This condition can occur after an extremely stressful event, but is time limited. Obviously, the patient needs to be followed on a weekly basis to ensure that symptoms do not recur. If the symptoms do recur, then the patient should be reevaluated for the possible diagnosis of schizophreniform disorder.

90. **The answer is C** [Chapter 1, I B 1].
Nasal lacrimal duct obstruction is commonly seen in the newborn from about 1–9 months of age. There is a proliferation of tears and irritation of the lid. It is treated with warm compresses and gently massaging the duct several times a day. It will usually resolve by 9 months of age. If there is no resolution with the massaging, then the duct will need to be surgically opened. Foreign body intrusion presents with pain and requires a fluorescein stain to diagnose. Conjunctivitis usually presents with purulent discharge so severe that the patient cannot open the lids; in children, it is usually viral. Conjunctivitis is highly contagious and is most common in the summer to early fall. Blepharitis is a chronic inflammation of the eyelid and is usually asymptomatic. It is treated with lid scrubs using diluted baby shampoo.

91. **The answer is C** [Chapter 2 IV B 1].
The underlying abnormality in adult respiratory distress syndrome (ARDS) is increased permeability of the alveolar capillary membranes and development of protein-rich pulmonary edema, thus producing frothy pink or red sputum. It denotes acute respiratory failure following a systemic or pulmonary insult. It is characterized by respiratory distress, bilateral infiltrates, and hypoxemia, and usually presents with tachypnea and rales. Bronchiestasis is a chronic process associated with purulent, often foul-smelling sputum and hemoptysis. Myalgia, fatigue, and nonproductive cough are consistent with atypical community-acquired pneumonia. Tuberculosis has a more chronic debilitating

course, beginning with fever and chills, accompanied by night sweats, anorexia, and weight loss.

92. **The answer is A** [Chapter 3 Table 3-5].
A loud first heart sound and an opening snap following S_2 are signs of mitral valve stenosis. A whistling during systolic ejection accompanied by a split second heart sound is associated with aortic stenosis; a soft, high-pitched blowing crescendo heard during expiration is associated with aortic regurgitation; and a soft, high-pitched blowing extending throughout systole and heard best near the apex is associated with mitral regurgitation.

93. **The answer is A** [Chapter 8 II A 3].
To exclude an ectopic gestation, often the use of both ultrasound and serial titers of human chorionic gonadotropin (hCG) are necessary. The quantitative hCG would yield a number correlating to the titer of hCG present in the maternal bloodstream. In a normally developing pregnancy, this value increases 66%–100% over 48 hours. An inappropriate increase or a plateau should increase the suspicion of an ectopic pregnancy. The transvaginal method of ultrasound is more sensitive than an abdominal approach in detecting an early ectopic gestation.

94. **The answer is C** [Chapter 9 III E 3 b].
The shoulder should be immobilized for 2–4 weeks, followed by range of motion exercises and a return to normal activity. The figure-of-eight splint is used for clavicle fractures. The Lachman's test is performed to check for knee cruciate pathology.

95. **The answer is A** [Chapter 13 II C 1 a (3)].
Candidiasis, a fungal infection, can be oral, genital, cutaneous, or systemic. Cutaneous candidiasis, which typically presents as a bright red-orange rash, is most commonly located in the axillae or under the breasts or fat folds. Tinea corporis is a superficial fungal infection involving the skin and characterized by an erythematous, annular patch with distinct borders and a central clearing. Tinea cruris is a macular erythematous fungal infection affecting the groin area in men. Tinea versicolor is characterized by a pale, macular rash that will not tan.

96. **The answer is A** [Chapter 3 IX A 1 f].
The most common cause of acquired aortic stenosis is the scarring caused by rheumatic heart disease. Prolonged hypertension and atherosclerosis do not cause aortic stenosis. Senile degeneration is responsible for a smaller fraction of cases in elderly patients.

97. **The answer is A** [Chapter 10 I B 1 b].
Hypothyroidism is usually primary to the gland itself; 99% of cases are caused either by an autoimmune thyroiditis or by prior neck irradiation. Hashimoto's thyroiditis (also known as chronic lymphocytic thyroiditis or autoimmune thyroiditis) is an autoimmune phenomenon that runs in families and is more common in women. Its incidence increases with age; patients with Hashimoto's thyroiditis are at risk for other autoimmune disorders. Pituitary and hypothalamic diseases and untreated fetal and neonatal hypothyroidism are rare causes of hypothyroidism.

98. **The answer is B** [Chapter 11 III C 1].
Magnetic resonance imaging with a contrast agent is very helpful in visualizing the characteristic plaque seen throughout the central nervous system, including the spinal cord and periventricular white matter of the brain. Unenhanced computed tomography would be helpful in ruling out other intracranial pathologies, but is less helpful in evaluating for multiple sclerosis (MS). Rather than serum, electrophoresis of the cerebrospinal fluid (CSF) would commonly demonstrate the elevated immunoglobulin G seen in MS. CSF should also be analyzed for increased myelin basic protein and evidence of oligoclonal bands. With complaints of altered vision, visual evoked responses (VER) would more likely be helpful in establishing the diagnosis.

99. **The answer is D** [Chapter 5, II C 4 a].
Endoscopy is the best method for diagnosis of peptic ulcer disease, which characteristically presents with burning pain either improved or worsened by food ingestion. Barium swallow is often used but will not detect up to 30% of ulcers. Hepato-iminodiacetic acid (HIDA) scan is for biliary disease, and esophageal manometry, for esophageal motility disorders.

100. **The answer is C** [Chapter 8 II E 1, 3].
Preterm labor has a high rate of recurrence at 17%–30%. It is vital to exclude preterm labor with any subtle signs or symptoms because early intervention may help prevent premature delivery. Both urinary tract infections and musculoskeletal pain are common problems in pregnancy.

101. **The answer is D** [Chapter 10 I A 3 d].
Numerous factors are associated with alterations in thyroid function tests. Factors decreasing thyroxine (T_4) include severe illness, cirrhosis, nephrotic syndrome, and many drugs, including phenytoin. Factors increasing thyroxine include autoimmune disease, a number of acute illnesses, high estrogen states, and many drugs. Acute psychiatric problems may be associated with either increased or decreased T_4. Morning sickness and high estrogen states such as pregnancy, estrogen replacement therapy, and oral contraceptive

use may increase both triiodothyronine (T$_3$) and T$_4$. Laboratory error should also be considered if test results seem to contrast significantly with other clinical or diagnostic information.

102. **The answer is D** [Chapter 11 III D 1].
In acute exacerbations of multiple sclerosis involving optic neuritis, high-dose intravenous corticosteroids hasten recovery and return the patient to normal function more quickly. Oral corticosteroids are not sufficient to abort acute exacerbations. Both interferon and copolymer are used as routine medications intended to reduce the frequency of relapses, but have no role in managing acute exacerbations.

103. **The answer is C** [Chapter 13 II B 1].
Cellulitis is an acute inflammation of the dermis and subcutaneous tissue most often caused by a bacterium (e.g., *Haemophilus influenzae, Streptococcus, Staphylococcus*). Cutaneous candidiasis is most commonly seen in the axillae or under the breasts or fat folds. Varicella is characterized by a contagious, umbilicated, vesicular rash that may cover the entire body and later becomes crusted. Measles is an exanthem associated with a confluent rash that progresses from the hairline toward the feet.

104. **The answer is C** [Chapter 1, I A 2 c (2)].
Central retinal artery occlusion carries a poor prognosis and is considered to be an ophthalmic emergency. A workup for valvular and atrial thrombus is warranted. Macular degeneration has an insidious onset and has the chief complaint of a gradual loss of vision. Angle-closure glaucoma is also an ophthalmic emergency and presents with painful loss of vision and a narrowed anterior chamber with a hard globe. Retinal detachment presents with the complaint of a "curtain being drawn" over the field of vision, and with a gradual loss of vision. It can happen spontaneously or secondary to trauma. Retinal detachment is also an ophthalmic emergency.

105. **The answer is A** [Chapter 6 IX B, C].
Obstructive uropathy has increasing incidence with age, especially in men. It is characterized by alternating low flow and high flow. The back pressure leads to renal insufficiency. The blood urea nitrogen (BUN) to creatinine ratio of 30:1 indicates a prerenal or postrenal cause. Acute glomerulonephritis and acute interstitial nephritis are ruled out by the normal urinalysis. In chronic renal failure, he would demonstrate signs of uremia and would likely have a higher creatinine, with a BUN to creatinine ratio of closer to 20:1.

106. **The answer is A** [Chapter 9 III E 1 b].
The radial head has slipped out of the annular ligament. At this age, the ligament is loosely attached to the neck of the radius. This allows a portion of the ligament to become trapped between the head of the radius and the capitellum of the humerus if it is pulled forcefully ("nursemaid's elbow" or "pulled elbow"). Muscles comprising the extensor wad are the extensor carpi radialis brevis, extensor carpi radialis longus, and brachioradialis. Strain of this muscle group, especially the extensor carpi radialis brevis, is called "tennis elbow." Radioulnar bursitis is caused by repeated or forcible extension of the wrist with the forearm pronated and is associated with the backhand stroke in tennis as in "tennis elbow." A torn biceps tendon is unlikely to occur in this age-group.

107. **The answer is A** [Chapter 11 IV A 2 a, 3].
In Alzheimer's disease, laboratory findings are generally normal and studies are only performed to rule out other treatable causes of dementia. Similarly, the computed tomography (CT) in Alzheimer's will be normal or may indicate cortical atrophy commonly seen in the elderly. Lacunar or multi-infarct dementia has a vascular etiology, and patients with this type of dementia have multiple lacunar or cortical infarcts on CT, with or without a history of hypertension. Alzheimer's disease accounts for 60%–80% of patients with chronic dementia; 15%–20% have a vascular etiology, and a similar number have a combination of both.

108. **The answer is A** [Chapter 12 III A].
Major depressive disorders, manic disorders, and bipolar disorders are all mood disorders. The term "manic-depressive disorder" is a generic name given to bipolar disorders (which are classified under the broader term of mood disorders). Anxiety disorders are characterized by heightened anxiety levels that, when manifested, interfere with a patient's functioning. Schizophrenic disorders are disorders of thought processes and are manifested in erroneous beliefs, perceptions, and thought processes.

109. **The answer is D** [Chapter 13 II C 3].
Tinea versicolor is a skin infection caused by a yeast, *Malassezia furfur*. The rash is best described as pale macules that will not tan. Microscopic examination of a potassium hydroxide (KOH) preparation shows hyphae and spores. Tinea corporis, tinea cruris, and tinea capitis involve the trunk, groin, and scalp, respectively. These superficial fungal infections are characterized by an erythematous, annular patch with distinct borders and a central clearing.

110. **The answer is D** [Chapter 1, II A 2 a].
Presbycusis is the most common cause of hearing loss. The incidence of presbycusis increases with age and it is more common in men than in women. It is commonly caused by exposure to loud noises. Patients may or may not benefit from hearing aids. Otitis media and

otitis externa present with pain, and, often, fever, as well as hearing loss. Cerumen impaction may present with the same complaints but would be apparent on examination. The hearing usually improves after removal of cerumen. The hearing usually improves after removal of cerumen.

111. **The answer is A** [Chapter 3 Table 3-5].
Thready pulses and systolic ejection murmur are classic signs of aortic stenosis. Although cardiac catheterization is a useful imaging technique, the systolic ejection murmer is not indicative of mitral stenosis. Chest radiograph and electrocardiogram (ECG) are inconclusive studies in valvular disorders. Echocardiogram is the least invasive method of visualizing the stenotic aortic valve.

112. **The answer is A** [Chapter 5, III A 2; Table 5-1].
Staphylococcus aureus commonly presents with rapid onset and profuse vomiting. *S. aureus* is a toxin-producing agent commonly found in food that is contaminated after cooking, and it is especially common in custards and other milk products. *Clostridium perfringens*, enterotoxic *Escherichia coli*, and *Shigella* all cause foodborne illness, but their main clinical presentation is diarrhea.

113. **The answer is B** [Chapter 7, II B 2 a].
Vaginal bleeding in a postmenopausal woman who is not on hormone replacement therapy (HRT) must be considered endometrial cancer until proved otherwise. Endometrial sampling in this woman is essential. In certain selected women, transvaginal ultrasound may be substituted. Postmenopausal women with an intact uterus should continue to have Pap smears to screen for cervical cancer; however, no consensus exists regarding the most appropriate screening interval. Computed tomography (CT) scans are generally less useful in the diagnosis of pelvic problems than they are in abdominal ones.

114. **The answer is A** [Chapter 8 II H 1 b, d, 4 b, I 1 a, 2 a, 3 b].
The differential diagnosis would include placenta previa, abruptio placentae, loss of mucous plug, trauma, and cervicitis. Because of the potentially life-threatening nature of placental problems and the unknown status of the fetus, this situation should be handled as an emergency. By establishing intravenous access and excluding blood coagulopathies, the patient would be optimally prepared in the event of acute hemorrhage. The ultrasound could then be done to find the location of the placenta and to assess the status of the fetus. The patient and fetus would probably be observed and have a firmer diagnosis before a cesarean section would be performed. A digital examination should

never be performed during the second or third trimesters of pregnancy in a bleeding patient without knowing the location of the placenta, because this could induce immediate hemorrhage from the vascular placenta.

115. **The answer is C** [Chapter 10 I A 3 a].
Thyroid-stimulating hormone (TSH) is secreted by the pituitary gland and stimulates thyroid hormone production. Triiodothyronine (T_3), the most active thyroid hormone, is derived from thyroxine (T_4). Nearly all circulating thyroid hormones are bound to thyroid-binding globulin and other serum proteins, but only the free hormones are active on a cellular level.

116. **The answer is D** [Chapter 1, II A 2 b (1)].
Meniere's disease has attacks of severe vertigo, tinnitus, and hearing loss that can last from minutes to hours and are quite debilitating. The disease is managed medically. Tic douloureux involves pressure or degeneration of the trigeminal nerve and is manifested with sharp stabbing pains along the nerve root. Bell's palsy involves paralysis of the seventh cranial nerve (CN VII). Amaurosis fugax is a temporary loss of vision due to insufficient blood flow to the retina and may be a precursor to a transient ischemic attack (TIA) or cerebrovascular accident (CVA).

117. **The answer is C** [Chapter 2 V B].
Pneumothorax is the accumulation of air in the pleural space. Causes may be spontaneous, traumatic, or iatrogenic. A small effusion may produce pleural pain and a friction rub, and a dull-to-flat percussion note over the effusion. The mediastinum is shifted away from the side of a large effusion, a development that usually occurs over time. Asthma is a bilateral process, diagnosed by pulmonary function studies and is not associated with chest radiograph findings. Emphysema is a bilateral, chronic process, with hyperinflation seen on chest radiograph. The patient is dyspneic and percussion yields increased resonance.

118. **The answer is A** [Chapter 6 I A 1 b; Table 6-1].
Acute tubular necrosis predominantly occurs in hospitalized patients and is associated with surgery or medical illness in 90% of cases. Patients present with azotemia, diuresis, then recovery. It is likely that this diagnosis is secondary to nephrotoxicity of aminoglycosides. Hypovolemia would be a prerenal cause of renal failure but laboratory studies would show decreased urine sodium, decreased fractional excretion of sodium, and concentrated urine. Urinary tract infection is an unlikely cause of oliguria.

119. The answer is D [Chapter 8 II G 1 c].
Immunoglobulin is extremely effective in preventing the future development of antibodies to the Rh factor. Approximately 15% of the population is Rh-negative. Although 98% of isoimmunizations are secondary to the Rh factor, 43 other antigens exist. Any event that may allow fetal cells to enter maternal circulation such as trauma, spontaneous abortion, therapeutic abortion, ectopic pregnancy, or amniocentesis can sensitize maternal circulation. If antibodies develop, they will attack subsequent Rh incompatible infants, which can lead to severe fetal anemia or death (fetal hydrops).

120. The answer is A [Chapter 9 III A 3].
The complications from such a fracture will result from median nerve and radial artery damage. The common name for the volarly displaced fracture is Smith's fracture. A dorsally displaced fragment is called a Colles' fracture. Treatment of a nondisplaced fracture is a long-arm cast. All displaced fractures are referred for reduction and fixation.

121. The answer is C [Chapter 11 V C 1–2].
Cluster headache can generally be differentiated from other primary headaches by their temporal pattern, occurring acutely but resolving spontaneously after 30–90 minutes even without therapy. Their periorbital location and associated eye signs also help to diagnose cluster headache. Sinus pressure or infection may produce periorbital pain, but will not resolve and recur acutely in this "cluster" pattern. Migraine headaches, while often unilateral and chronic, do not tend to occur several times in a single day and resolve without therapy.

122. The answer is D [Chapter 12 III A].
The mood episode may be characterized as the symptom picture that allows the clinician to make a diagnosis. The symptoms may be characterized as depressive, manic, or mixed depressive-manic. It is important to make the distinction between a mood state that is a function of a mood disorder and a mood state that is a function of hallucinations or delusions (i.e., characteristic of psychoses), or a medical condition (i.e., characteristic of organicity).

123. The answer is A [Chapter 1, III B 2 a].
The discharge in allergic rhinitis is thin and watery, and is usually present at certain times of the year. The mucosa is classically cyanotic and may be boggy or have polyps present. Vasomotor rhinitis is short-lived and sporadic in nature. Rhinitis medicamentosa is secondary to nasal spray abuse and appears as boggy congested mucosa. Atrophic rhinitis is a chronic inflammation with atrophy of the mucous membrane caused by severe drying.

124. The answer is A [Chapter 2 VI A 1 a (1), (2)].
Squamous cell cancer causes 30%–40% of bronchogenic carcinomas, and there is a strong association with smoking. Most of the tumors occur centrally, tend to ulcerate, and may cause bleeding. Small cell cancers commonly present as a hilar mass and mediastinal widening but cavitation is rare. Adenocarcinoma usually presents in the periphery, and may include enlarged lymph nodes, hepatomegaly, and digital clubbing. Because of the long interval between when the cancer first occurs and when it presents clinically, it is usually advanced and, thus, unresectable when it is diagnosed. Approximately 25% of cases of bronchogenic carcinoma present as a solitary pulmonary nodule, in which there is central cavitation, calcification, and satellite lesions.

125. The answer is B [Chapter 5, I C 2 d, 3 a].
Achalasia presents with gradual onset of dysphagia and characteristically has a tapered appearance on barium swallow. Esophageal cancer might present with gradual-onset dysphagia, but this would generally be accompanied by weight loss, and a tumor would be seen blocking the esophagus. Hiatal hernia and esophageal spasm would not present with gradual onset dysphagia, but with intermittent substernal pain.

126. The answer is B [Chapter 6 III D 2].
A 6-mm stone in the ureter may or may not pass spontaneously. Smaller stones could be managed on an outpatient basis, and stones larger than 10 mm should be managed on an inpatient basis. By carefully monitoring this patient and providing fluids and analgesia, management can be adjusted to treat any complications. This patient should probably be stabilized before referring to lithotripsy.

127. The answer is D [Chapter 8 II B 3].
In order to assess the viability of the pregnancy, both serial human chorionic gonadotropins (hCGs) and ultrasound may be necessary. In a normally developing pregnancy, hCG will increase by 66%–100% increments over 48 hours. This is used to assess viability of a pregnancy as well as to exclude ectopic gestation. Ultrasound findings in a nonviable pregnancy may include inappropriate development or interval growth, poorly formed or unformed fetal pole, and fetal demise. History and physical examination are unreliable in establishing the status of a pregnancy.

128. The answer is C [Chapter 9 IV G 4].
Volar wrist splinting at night and with activity during the day and vitamin B6 given daily is the best treatment. Endoscopic carpal tunnel release is a method of

treatment if the condition does not resolve after pregnancy or if profound nerve deficits are occurring. Nonsteroidal anti-inflammatory medications are not recommended in late pregnancy. Usually, carpal tunnel syndrome resolves after pregnancy. It is often amenable to steroid injections. Surgery should be avoided unless the condition persists.

129. **The answer is B** [Chapter 10 I C 1 c].
A patient with a history of either head or neck radiation therapy and a single thyroid nodule is at high risk for malignancy. "Hot" nodules are likely to be benign, while "cold" nodules are more likely to be malignant. Multinodular goiters are usually benign. Finally, recent or rapid enlargement of a nodule is more likely to be malignant. The diagnosis can be firmly established only by histologic or cytologic examination of the neoplastic tissue.

130. **The answer is D** [Chapter 11 V B 4 a, b].
The decision to administer prophylactic medication is generally based on the frequency of headache. When headaches occur only occasionally, abortive therapy is appropriate; frequent headaches warrant prevention with β-blockers, calcium channel blockers, tricyclic antidepressants, and others. In general, since specific antimigraine therapy in the form of serotonin receptor agonists and ergotamine products is available, the use of narcotic analgesics, in any form, should be avoided.

131. **The answer is C** [Chapter 12 III C; Table 12-1].
A patient who presents with inflated self-esteem, a decreased need for sleep, and pressured speech is exhibiting a manic episode. Individuals who present this way are not exhibiting the symptom picture expected for schizophrenic disorders, which would include disorders of perception, beliefs, or thought processes. A delusional patient would exhibit erroneous beliefs, a finding that we might also expect to see with schizophrenic disorders. Because patients experiencing a manic episode have an inflated self-esteem, they do not suffer from suicidal depression; however, they can pose a risk to themselves because they may engage in dangerous behaviors believing that they will not hurt themselves.

132. **The answer is D.** [Chapter 2 X A, B].
Infection, bronchospasm, or heart failure may precipitate acute respiratory failure in patients with kyphoscoliosis who already have compromised lung function. Lung compliance is decreased due to progressive atelectasis. Lung volume is also reduced because the chest wall is distorted, which causes stiffness of the chest wall, increasing the work of breathing.

133. **The answer is C** [Chapter 3 Figure 3-5].
In sinus tachycardia, nothing has changed about impulse generation or conduction other than the rate. Configuration of P waves, QRS complexes, and PR interval are all normal.

134. **The answer is A** [Chapter 4 III, B 2 a, 3 c].
Patients with Hodgkin's disease have varying presentations, but most present with cervical, supraclavicular, or mediastinal nodes. One third of patients will present with constitutional symptoms, including the classic Pel-Ebstein fever. This is one of the so-called B symptoms, associated with a poorer prognosis. Hodgkin's disease has a bimodal distribution, occurring most often in people between 15 and 45 years of age and those over 60 years of age. In the younger group, it occurs more often in women. Reed-Sternberg cells are diagnostic of Hodgkin's disease. Non-Hodgkin's lymphoma may present similarly, but fever is less common than in Hodgkin's. The classic feature of chronic myelogenous leukemia (CML) is the Philadelphia chromosome. Acute lymphocytic leukemia (ALL) occurs most often in children and young adults, typically presenting with abrupt onset of fever, lethargy, and headache. ALL has a fulminant course.

135. **The answer is A** [Chapter 5, II D 2 b (1), c (3)].
In a patient over 40, dyspepsia that does not respond to therapy should be considered to be gastric cancer until proved otherwise. Gastric cancer generally presents with anemia and occult gastrointestinal (GI) bleeding as well as weight loss and dyspepsia. Amylase and lipase detect pancreatitis, which presents with epigastric pain radiating to the back. A cardiac cause of the dyspepsia and weight loss is possible, depending on the history, but a Holter monitor would be inappropriate at this point. Barium swallow is not a particularly useful examination for gastric cancer.

136. **The answer is C** [Chapter 6 VII D 4 a].
Acute prostatitis should be treated for 30 days with trimethoprim–sulfamethoxazole or ciprofloxacin. Chronic prostatitis should be treated for up to 3 months. Shorter durations of treatment will result in recurrent infections and possible spread to other organs.

137. **The answer is B** [Chapter 8 II F 2].
Although generalized edema in pregnancy is common, swelling of the face or hands is of greater significance than swelling in the lower extremities in regard to preeclampsia. Neither nephrotic syndrome nor adrenal insufficiency is the most probable diagnosis in the pregnant woman.

138.   The answer is D [Chapter 9 III F 3].
Extension splinting of the distal joint should be done for approximately 6 weeks. This is the recommended treatment for mallet finger (avulsion of the terminal extensor tendon of the finger). Fractures of the finger are likely to be visible on radiographs, unlike fractures of the scaphoid bone. Continued movement of the hand is crucial but not compromised by the immobilization as recommended. Flexor tendon injuries are suspected when a patient is unable to actively flex the distal joint of the finger while the other joints are immobilized.

139.   The answer is B [Chapter 11 V A 4 a].
Simple analgesics such as aspirin, acetaminophen, or a nonsteroidal anti-inflammatory drug (NSAID) are indicated for mild, tension headaches. Products containing narcotics are not indicated in the setting of mild headache, and without evidence of muscular spasm or limited range of motion, splinting devices will not be of primary benefit. Although useful in chronic pain and in the setting of acute stress or depression, tricyclic antidepressants would not be indicated as initial therapy.

140.   The answer is A [Chapter 12 III C, D].
The major difference between hypomanic and manic episodes is not in the type of symptoms, but in their severity. A patient experiencing a manic episode is significantly impaired. In contrast, the hypomanic patient does not require hospitalization, and social and occupational functioning are not significantly impaired. The hypomanic patient may, however, engage in the same types of risky behaviors (e.g., inappropriate sexual behaviors) and be as easily distracted as an individual experiencing a manic episode.

141.   The answer is B [Chapter 13 IV B].
Psoriasis is a chronic, inflammatory, scaling condition of the skin. Psoriasis patches are usually raised, reddened areas with distinct margins and loosely adherent silvery scales. Psoriasis most commonly affects the elbows, knees, and scalp. Acne vulgaris is an inflammatory follicular, papular, and pustular eruption. Impetigo is characterized by superficial flaccid vesicles that erupt and form a thick, yellowish crust. Furuncles and carbuncles are infections of one or more hair follicles and are erythematous, hard, tender lesions in hair-bearing areas of the head, neck, or body.

142.   The answer is B [Chapter 1, III A 3 a].
Plain sinus radiographs are the most practical imaging modality for differentiating sinusitis from rhinitis. A radiograph is helpful in determining if there is an air–fluid level. It can also help determine if antibiotics are necessary or not. Computed tomography (CT)

scan has a high sensitivity but low specificity. Magnetic resonance imaging (MRI) and positron emission tomography (PET) have no place in the diagnosis of sinusitis.

143.   The answer is A [Chapter 2 XI C 4].
Normal scans virtually rule out clinically significant thromboembolism. Arterial blood gases will show a mild acute respiratory alkalosis, indicated by a low P_{CO_2} and slightly elevated pH. Results of chest radiographs are normal in most patients. A few show plate-like atelectasis, a unilaterally high diaphragm, and a small pleural effusion. Doppler ultrasonography can produce false-positive results, and it cannot be used to evaluate pelvic veins. Pulmonary angiography is the standard test for the diagnosis of pulmonary embolism. It is unequivocally diagnostic if emboli are visualized. Although invasive, this test should be performed when ventilation and perfusion scans are equivocal.

144.   The answer is C [Chapter 3 Figure 3-7].
In second-degree atrioventricular (AV) block, impulse generation still occurs in the atrium, but not all impulses are successfully conducted to the ventricles. An increased PR interval would indicate first-degree AV block. Uniform QRS complexes of ventricular origin and widened QRS complexes with irregular ventricular rate indicate dysrhythmias of ventricular origin.

145.   The answer is B [Chapter 5, III A 4 c].
Clostridium difficile is almost invariably the cause of antibiotic-related diarrhea. *Cryptosporidium* and *Vibrio* both cause watery diarrhea, but neither is a common cause of diarrhea in this country. *Giardia* may cause diarrhea, but is more likely associated with nausea and bloating.

146.   The answer is B [Chapter 8 II F 4 d].
Magnesium sulfate is used to arrest and prevent convulsions due to eclampsia. It does not produce central nervous system depression in the fetus or the mother. Hydralazine is the drug of choice for a hospitalized patient with marked hypertension. Neither diazepam nor carbamazepine has a role in the treatment of eclamptic seizures.

147.   The answer is B [Chapter 9 II A 1 c].
Trigger thumb (flexor stenosing tenosynovitis) is an inflammatory process of the tendon sheath. It can occur in the thumb or other digits when the pulley system, usually the A1 pulley, catches the tendon or a tendon nodule proximal to the pulley. The cause is unknown, but it is frequently seen in rheumatoid arthri-

tis and diabetic patients. Gamekeeper's thumb, also called skier's thumb, is a ligamentous injury to the ulnar collateral ligament of the thumb. Incomplete tears of the ligament are treated by immobilization and complete tears by surgical repair. Diabetic neuropathy has predominant sensory signs without associated stenosing tenosynovitis. Hypoplastic thumb is congenital absence or shortening of the thumb bones and is associated with other systemic abnormalities.

148. **The answer is A** [Chapter 10 I C 3 a].
Unless a thyroid cancer is associated with thyroiditis, thyroid function tests are likely to be normal. Patients most often present with painless neck swelling. The most common form (70%) of thyroid cancer is papillary carcinoma; this is also the most indolent. Follicular carcinoma is associated with distant metastasis, whereas medullary carcinoma tends to metastasize locally.

149. **The answer is B** [Chapter 12 I D].
Because the patient is not capable of providing the responses needed to determine a more specific diagnosis, and next of kin cannot be identified to provide additional important information, the appropriate diagnosis is psychotic disorder not otherwise specified. The patient should be hospitalized until competent authority deems that the patient is not a threat to self or others.

150. **The answer is A** [Chapter 13 III A 3].
Pyogenic granuloma is a misnomer because the lesion does not have an infectious origin. Therefore, antibiotics are not effective in the treatment of pyogenic granuloma. A pyogenic granuloma is actually a capillary hemangioma. Treatment consists of electrodesiccation and curettage or excision.

151. **The answer is A** [Chapter 1, III A 1 c].
Haemophilus influenzae, *Moraxella catarrhalis*, and *Staphylococcus aureus* are the most common causative agents in sinusitis. *S. aureus* is an unusual cause of acute sinusitis but may be present in chronic sinusitis. Anaerobes are usually present in chronic sinusitis.

152. **The answer is A** [Chapter 2 XII D 4 a].
Mycoplasma pneumonia is the most common cause of atypical community-acquired pneumonia. *Pseudomonas aeruginosa* is one of the organisms found in nosocomial infections. *Streptococcus pneumoniae* and *Haemophilus influenzae* are commonly found in classic typical community-acquired pneumonia. Atypical pneumonia is less severe than the classic kind and is characterized by lack of sputum production. Systemic symptoms (myalgia, arthralgia, and skin rash) are more prominent and chest pain and productive cough are less marked.

153. **The answer is D** [Chapter 3 Figure 3-6].
Monomorphic refers to the condition in which all QRS depolarizations are uniform (i.e., generated from the same site), which is ventricular in origin and operating at an excessive rate. In all of the other choices, QRS complexes will vary with the irregularity of generating sites or conduction variables.

154. **The answer is D** [Chapter 5, IV B 4 b].
Diverticulitis often requires that the patient be hospitalized for antibiotics, analgesics, and bowel rest. Dietary fiber is protective against diverticulosis, but treatment involves a low-residue diet. Barium enema should not be used during an acute episode because of the risk of perforation, and there is no association between diverticulosis and colon cancer.

155. **The answer is A** [Chapter 6 VII A 2 a].
Frequency, urgency, and dysuria are symptoms of bladder inflammation due to incomplete emptying and detrusor instability. The other symptoms are called obstructive symptoms reflecting decreased force and flow of stream due to mechanical obstruction and detrusor decompensation.

156. **The answer is A** [Chapter 7, III A 4 a].
The most common ovarian mass is an ovarian cyst. Of these, most are functional. In a premenopausal woman, a cyst smaller than 8 cm should be followed through 1–2 cycles. Cysts larger than 8 cm or those which persist should be evaluated laparoscopically. No study has validated the usefulness of oral contraceptives in the treatment of functional cysts. CA-125 tests have a high false-positive rate in premenopausal women and are most useful in following the progress of women with diagnosed ovarian cancer. This patient is best treated with reassurance, pain relief, and a follow-up pelvic examination in 6–8 weeks.

157. **The answer is C** [Chapter 8 II C 1 d].
Multiple pregnancy is the most frequent cause of preterm birth. Both pregnancy-induced hypertension (PIH) and cord accidents occur more frequently in multiple pregnancies than singleton pregnancies but are not the most common complication. There is no increased incidence of gestational diabetes in multiple gestation.

158. **The answer is D** [Chapter 9 II A 1 b].
Patellar tendinitis is most common in athletes participating in jumping sports such as basketball and volleyball. Pain is in the inferior patellar border, and is most marked in extension. Prepatellar bursitis is the most common form of knee bursitis and is usually associated with prolonged kneeling. Iliotibial band friction syn-

drome is a result of abrasion between the iliotibial band and the lateral femoral tendon. Tenderness is most prominent with the knee flexed approximately 30°. This syndrome most commonly occurs in cyclists or runners. Patellar tendon rupture is most likely to occur in younger adults as a result of direct trauma. A palpable defect and inability to extend the knee are diagnostic.

159. **The answer is A** [Chapter 10 III C 1 a, c, 2 b, 3 a].
In the United States type II diabetes mellitus is most common in African-Americans, Hispanics, and Pima Indians. In addition, the patient is significantly overweight, another risk factor for type II diabetes. Many patients have few symptoms; however, vaginal candidiasis may be a presenting complaint. Depending on her sexual history, HIV, gonorrhea, and syphilis screening may also be in order. Demonstration of hyphae and spores means fungal culture is not necessary at this time. Reinforcing appropriate vaginal hygiene is appropriate, but evaluating her for diabetes mellitus is more important.

160. **The answer is D** [Chapter 11 VI A 1 d, 4 a].
Benign essential tremor has the tendency to be accentuated in stressful settings and suppressed by small quantities of alcohol. Other movement disorders would not follow this pattern and would not benefit from low doses of β-blockers like propranolol. Amantadine and benztropine have anticholinergic effects and are useful for milder presentations of Parkinson's disease, but not essential tremor. Dopamine medications are the mainstay of therapy for Parkinson's, but would not be appropriate initial therapy to rule it out in this setting.

161. **The answer is A** [Chapter 12 III G 2].
Treatments for bipolar I and bipolar II disorders include the use of lithium, anticonvulsants, and, when psychopharmacological interventions are not effective, electroconvulsive therapy. The use of certain types of antidepressants is warranted but they do present certain risks with bipolar patients (e.g., rapid cycling between depressive and manic phases). Patients need to be monitored closely for this side effect because, among other problems, the patient becomes a suicide threat while in the depressive phase of the cycle.

162. **The answer is C** [Chapter 13 II D 5].
Acne vulgaris is an inflammatory, follicular, papular, and pustular eruption involving the sebaceous glands. Acne consists of open and closed comedones as well as fluid-filled cysts. Acne is most commonly found on the face, neck, back, and shoulders, but not the feet. Treatment for mild acne may include benzoyl perox-

ides, tretinoin, topical erythromycin, clindamycin, or sodium sulfacetamide. Erythromycin, doxycycline, tetracycline, and minocycline are frequently used. Tetracyclines are the drugs of choice.

163. **The answer is B** [Chapter 1, III D 1 b, 2].
Haemophilus influenzae type B typically presents in children aged 2–7 years. Group A β-hemolytic streptococcus, *Mycoplasma pneumoniae*, and *Chlamydia trachomatis* may cause a sore throat that presents without stridor, drooling, or dysphagia.

164. **The answer is B** [Chapter 2 XII D 4 c (4)].
Chest radiographs in atypical pneumonia show unilateral segmental lower lobe infiltrates. Classic community-acquired pneumonia is associated with dense consolidation confined to a single lobe with visible air bronchograms. Patchy or streaky opacities are seen with pneumonias caused by *Mycobacterium pneumoniae*, viruses, and mixed anaerobic and aerobic organisms. Radiographs of tuberculosis demonstrate a cavitary infiltrate in a posterior apical segment of an upper lobe or in a superior segment of a lower lobe.

165. **The answer is A** [Chapter 3 X A 4 b].
Class I antiarrhythmics include Na^+ channel blockers. β-Adrenergic antagonists are class II antiarrhythmics, slow K^+ channel blockers are class III, and calcium channel blockers are class IV.

166. **The answer is A** [Chapter 8 II D 1 b].
Large birth-weight infants with subsequent difficult deliveries are the primary complication of gestational diabetes. Pregnancy-induced hypertension (PIH), multiple pregnancies, and smoking are all associated with small birth weights.

167. **The answer is A** [Chapter 9 III E 2 a].
The radiograph shows anterior dislocation of the hip with no evidence of fracture. Anterior hip dislocations are noted by the hip position in *abduction*; posterior dislocations typically are noted to have hip *adduction*. Although posterior hip dislocations are more common, both types need to be reduced promptly to avoid impairment of the blood supply leading to osteonecrosis. Overlapping of the inferior margin of the acetabulum by the femoral head, seen on anteroposterior radiograph projections of the hip, indicate anterior dislocations. Posterior dislocations are marked by the femoral head posterior to the acetabular rim margin on radiograph. Acetabular margin fractures are most often associated with posterior dislocations.

168. **The answer is D** [Chapter 10 III B 1 a, 2 a].
Insulin-dependent diabetes mellitus (type I diabetes) is classically a disease of the young. Thought to be an au-

toimmune phenomenon, it does seem to have a higher incidence in people of Scandinavian descent. The classic symptoms include polyuria, polydipsia, and polyphagia. If the condition develops subacutely over a period of weeks, weight loss despite increased appetite is commonly found. Bulimia nervosa is characterized by serial binging and purging (by self-induced vomiting, cathartic or laxative use); however, the typical bulimic patient hides her food intake. Non–insulin-dependent diabetes mellitus (NIDDM) is more often a disease of older age and is most common in African-Americans, Hispanics, and Pima Indians. While NIDDM patients may present similarly to those with type I diabetes, they may be asymptomatic or have less obvious symptoms. Patients with Addison's disease may present with weight loss; however, other symptoms are more likely to include weakness, easy fatigability, nausea and vomiting, diarrhea, and abdominal pain.

169. The answer is B [Chapter 13 III B 2].
Squamous cell and basal cell carcinomas are the most common "nonmalignant" neoplasms of the skin. The lesions are usually located on sun-exposed areas of the body (e.g., the face, head, neck, and, in men, the trunk). The lesions can be asymptomatic but can itch or bleed; in addition, they may seem to never heal. Metastasis in basal and squamous cell carcinomas is rare.

170. The answer is C [Chapter 2 V B 4].
A small spontaneous pneumothorax often resolves by itself. A more severe or a secondary pneumothorax calls for reexpansion of the lung via placement of an intercostal chest tube and application of appropriate negative pressure. Spontaneous pneumothorax has a tendency to recur and surgical treatment should be considered, which involves an open thoracotomy. If a tension pneumothorax is suspected, a large-bore needle is inserted and prompt decompression of the involved pleural space is indicated.

171. The answer is A [Chapter 3 IX A 4 a; X A 4 a; XI D].
Permanent cardiac pacing is appropriate in most instances of supraventricular dysrhythmias and atrioventricular block. Ventricular ectopic events are treated with pharmacotherapy or surgical ablation only.

172. The answer is A [Chapter 5, II C 3 a].
Burning epigastric pain associated with eating or with an empty stomach is classic for ulcer disease. Pain radiating to the back is classic for pancreatitis, and pain lying flat is consistent with reflux disease.

173. The answer is A [Chapter 6 VIII D 3].
Transurethral resection of the prostate (TURP) is the treatment of choice for benign prostatic hyperplasia (BPH) although many patients may select medical management or watchful waiting while symptoms are tolerable. Prostate cancer is treated with radical retropubic prostatectomy, radiation therapy, or hormonal manipulation. Bladder cancer treatment is called transurethral resection of the bladder (TURB). TURB is not the treatment of choice for prostatitis but in long-standing, intractable cases it may be considered.

174. The answer is B [Chapter 8 II G 1 e].
Known as fetal hydrops, the antibodies to the Rh-positive infant's blood attack developing red blood cells leading to severe anemia and, eventually, death. Rh incompatibility does not adversely affect the mother. Fetal–maternal hemorrhage is an indication for the administration of immunoglobulin to prevent the development of antibodies to the Rh factor.

175. The answer is B [Chapter 9 I A 2, 3 b].
Osteoarthritis with joint space narrowing is the correct diagnosis. This condition is associated with flexion contractures of the hip because of the limited motion in the hip and inability to fully extend the joint. Lytic changes are characteristic of malignancy and are not present. Osteonecrosis of the hip, when present with this much joint space narrowing, would most likely be accompanied by collapse of the femoral head. Age-related changes in the hip would not be this severe.

176. The answer is C [Chapter 10 III C 4 a, b].
The centerpiece of treatment of patients with type II diabetes is diet, exercise, and weight loss. Even a 10-pound weight loss improves tissue sensitivity to insulin. Often diet, weight loss, and exercise are sufficient for control of non–insulin-dependent diabetes mellitus (NIDDM). An ophthalmologic referral once her glucose is under better control is appropriate. Sulfonylureas are often used when diet and exercise alone have failed to control glucose levels. Insulin is occasionally used in NIDDM when other measures have failed to control the disease.

177. The answer is C [Chapter 12 IV D 1 b].
The components of an obsessive-compulsive disorder are the mental acts, or intrusive thoughts, which are the hallmark of an obsession. The obsession drives the patient to the repetitive behaviors or compulsion. By engaging in ritualistic or repetitive behavior, the patient hopes to prevent or control the anxiety or distress brought on by the obsession. Treatment of the condition can be geared toward stopping the obsession or stopping the compulsion. The approach taken depends on the techniques felt appropriate by the therapist.

178 through 182.

The answers are: 178-C [Chapter 13 IV A 2 a], 179-D [Chapter 13 II A 1 b], 180-B [Chapter 13 IV A 1 a (1)], 181-A [Chapter 13 IV A 1 a (3)], 182-E [Chapter 13 IV A 1 a (2) (a)].

Scarlet fever is an exanthem caused by *Streptococcus* infection. It is characterized by a rash that spares the face, palms, and soles of the feet.

Pityriasis rosea is characterized by a herald patch (i.e., a solitary, round or oval, pink lesion with a raised border and fine, adherent scales in the margin) and a rash that begins on the trunk and is usually confined to the trunk.

Measles is an exanthem characterized by a confluent rash that progresses from the hairline toward the feet. Koplik's spots (i.e., tiny, punctate, whitish spots on the buccal mucosa) may precede the rash by a couple of days, and are pathognomonic for measles.

Varicella is characterized by contagious, umbilicated, vesicular lesions that may cover the entire body and later become crusted. The lesions begin as faint macules, progress to vesicles on an erythematous base within 24 hours, and then rapidly become pustular, umbilicated, and crusted. Many health care providers feel that seeing patients with lesions in all three stages at the same time is diagnostic.

The 5-year-old girl with the reddened cheeks most likely has fifth disease, which mainly affects children 3–12 years of age. Macular erythema of the cheeks (a "slapped cheek") appearance that can resemble sunburn is part of the prodrome.

183. The answer is D [Chapter 1, III E 1].
Kiesselbach's plexus is the most common site of all nosebleeds. Less common is the posterior nosebleed, which generally arises from the turbinates or the nasal wall.

184. The answer is A [Chapter 2 VII A, B, C].
Interstitial lung diseases comprise a heterogeneous group of disorders that have in common the features of inflammation and fibrosis of the interalveolar septum in response to lung injury. The chest radiograph demonstrates a diffuse ground-glass nodular, reticular, or reticulonodular infiltrate. Patchy, diffuse bilateral fluffy infiltrates are seen with adult respiratory distress syndrome (ARDS). A unilateral high diaphragm occurs with pulmonary emboli although the chest radiograph is normal in most patients. The earliest visible signs of effusion on plain-film radiographs are blurring of the posterior diaphragm in the lateral view.

185. The answer is D [Chapter 3 XII A 1].
Excessive alcohol consumption is a significant factor in the patient history that should alert the clinician to the potential of dilated cardiomyopathy. Hypertrophic obstructive cardiomyopathy is a genetic disorder. Fibrosis causes restrictive cardiomyopathy. Endocarditis is not associated with cardiomyopathy.

186. The answer is C [Chapter 5, III B 1 a].
Abdominal distention is associated with small-bowel obstruction. Vomiting is of partially digested food, bowel sounds are high-pitched, and gas is unable to reach the colon.

187. The answer is D [Chapter 6 IV C 1 c (2) (c)].
The changes in the electrocardiogram (ECG) reflect the potassium level. Early manifestation of hyperkalemia is peaking of the T waves. More severe hyperkalemia reveals changes to P wave, PR interval, and QRS complex. The sine wave pattern anticipates cardiac arrest.

188. The answer is A [Chapter 8 IV A 1].
The frequency of ovulation is markedly reduced during lactation, leading to amenorrhea. The patient's examination is consistent with both lactation and a hypoestrogenic state. Stress can also contribute to anovulation leading to amenorrhea. If the lack of menses persists after discontinuing lactation, it would require further evaluation. Scarring of the uterus leading to amenorrhea can occur after surgical procedures, but it is not the most likely diagnosis in this case.

189. The answer is C [Chapter 9 III B 1].
Fracture of the dome of the talus and lateral malleolus is the most likely diagnosis. Isolated fractures are common in the malleolus and may be treated with below-the-knee cast. Fractures of the talus are less common. Osteochondral fractures involving the lateral corner of the talus are usually a result of inversion injuries. Casting will lead to healing if nondisplaced. If a fragment is loose and causes pain or locking, surgery is indicated. Bimalleolar fractures are unstable and require reduction with rigid fixation to avoid talar shift. The calcaneus, the largest bone of the foot, lies inferior to the talus. The distal prominence of the fibula is referred to as the lateral malleolus, and the distal prominence of the tibia is the medial malleolus.

190. The answer is B [Chapter 10 IV A 2 a, g, 3 b].
The patient's symptoms are most consistent with adrenocortical insufficiency (Addison's disease). He might also complain of headache and abdominal pain. Physical examination might reveal cyanosis, dehydration, and skin pigmentation in exposed areas. Oral lesions of Kaposi's sarcoma are red, purple, or dark plaques or nodules that may occur on skin or mucous membranes; coexisting darker pigmentation of the skin, however, is more consistent with Addison's disease. Weight loss and dark mucosal pigmentation do

not fit with the clinical picture of hypothyroidism. The physical findings point to an endocrine cause of his lethargy and apathy, rather than a neurotransmitter-related depression.

191. The answer is D [Chapter 11 VI B 4 d].
Levodopa alone, or in some combination with carbidopa, is most likely necessary for the patient with severe, disabling Parkinson's symptoms. Dopamine depletion is the source of the problem, and replacement is required in advanced disease. In earlier, milder disease the anticholinergics like benztropine and amantadine may reduce symptoms but they are not helpful with later, disabling symptoms. Propranolol is useful in benign essential tremor, but would provide no benefit in this case.

192. The answer is B [Chapter 12 IV C 3 a].
Alprazolam (Xanax) has historically been the only FDA-approved medication for panic disorder, even though SSRI's, monoamine oxidase (MAO) inhibitors, and tricyclic antidepressants have been used successfully with some patients. (The importance of this information is in the fact that there is only one approved medication. If a practitioner has a patient who is litigious or who presents with a symptom picture that is not clear-cut, then the treatment of choice is to select the one medication approved for the condition.)

193. The answer is B [Chapter 2 IX C].
Sarcoidosis should be suspected in any patient with mediastinal or hilar adenopathy and interstitial lung disease. Diagnostic confirmation requires tissue biopsy demonstrating typical granulomas. Transbronchial biopsy is often diagnostic. A clinical diagnosis may be made in asymptomatic patients with typical chest radiograph findings, but the diagnosis must be considered in the presence of the most common symptoms and signs, even if (as in approximately 10% of patients) the chest radiograph is normal. If the transbronchial approach is not available or fails to show granulomas, other possible biopsy sites include the mediastinum. Bronchoalveolar lavage is a newer diagnostic method that may be helpful in special situations.

194. The answer is A [Chapter 3 XII A 2].
Hypertrophic obstructive cardiomyopathy (HCM) is an insidious and often silent killer of patients who are asymptomatic and therefore unaware of their risk. Sudden cardiac death occurs in HCM patients under the age of 30 years at a rate of 2%–3% annually.

195. The answer is A [Chapter 5 V B 3)].
Sonogram is the most accurate, noninvasive method of diagnosis, and will show evidence of inflammation as well as most stones. Hepato-iminodiacetic acid

(HIDA) scan is helpful for confirmation in cases where the diagnosis is unclear. Only 20% of stones will be visible on X-ray, and endoscopic retrograde cholangiopancreatography (ERCP) is generally used to evaluate pancreatic and biliary ducts.

196. The answer is A [Chapter 8 IV B 2 b, 3 a].
Infection is the most common cause of fever in the postpartum period. The patient's examination is consistent with subinvolution of the uterus, which often results from either infection or retained products. Lacerations of the cervix or vagina tend to present immediately after delivery. Thrombophlebitis is an important cause of fever in the postpartum patient although neither historical nor physical data are consistent with this diagnosis. Pelvic inflammatory disease is an unlikely differential 5 days after delivery.

197. The answer is D [Chapter 9 III B 2].
Stress fracture of the third metatarsal is the most likely diagnosis. If symptomatic, as in this case, the fracture can be treated with a short leg walking cast. There is an increased incidence of stress fracture related to disuse. Myositis ossificans is a late complication following injuries with large hematomas. It is common after elbow fracture and dislocation and soft tissue trauma to the thigh. Conservative treatment is best. Reflex sympathetic dystrophy can follow trauma or surgery and is characterized by a vicious cycle of pain, swelling, discoloration, and stiffness of the affected extremity.

198. The answer is A [Chapter 10 IV A 3 a].
Hyponatremia or hyperkalemia or both usually occur. Patients are also often hypercalcemic and hypoglycemic. Eosinophilia is another common finding.

199. The answer is B [Chapter 11 VI D 1–2].
Persistent motor and phonic tics characterize Tourette's syndrome. The diagnosis requires a variety of signs occurring over at least a year, without any other evidence of neurologic or metabolic disease. In Tourette's, the electroencephalogram is normal, making seizures an unlikely diagnosis. While familial tremor may occur at any age, it is consistent in its presentation and not accompanied by phonic signs. It would be unlikely for these presenting signs to be related to an emotional problem.

200. The answer is C [Chapter 12 VI B 6].
Substance intoxication is the appropriate diagnosis when a patient develops a reversible substance-induced syndrome soon after ingesting an illicit substance. The behavioral and/or psychological changes are caused by the effects of the substance on the central nervous system; the symptoms are not caused by a medical or psychiatric condition.

201. The answer is A [Chapter 1, I D 3 b].
Strabismus is the correct choice. Both the corneal light reflex test and the cover test will assess an imbalance in the muscles of the eye. If there is muscle weakness, the eye will drift with the cover test and show an uneven light reflex. Amblyopia must be tested with a visual acuity test. Occlusive disease is assessed with funduscopy.

202. The answer is A [Ch 2, X B].
Exertional dyspnea is the outstanding respiratory symptom in kyphoscoliosis. The onset and severity of dyspnea correlate with the degree of spinal angulation. Hypoventilation supervenes in those patients whose deformity is severe. Chest pain is more often associated with an acute process such as pulmonary embolism, and bronchitic symptoms such as productive cough are unusual unless the patient has chronic bronchitis or atelectasis.

203. The answer is B [Chapter 4 I F 3 b (2)].
The most important difference between folate and B_{12} deficiency is the irreversible neurologic changes associated with the latter. These changes may be masked, but are not cured by folate administration, making correct diagnosis vital to appropriate treatment. Folate and B_{12} deficiencies are the two most common causes of megaloblastic anemia; however, other disorders can cause identical pathological changes in the bone marrow. Macrocytosis (MCV more than 100) is often the earliest sign of vitamin B_{12} and folate deficiency and may precede anemia. Other findings with these deficiencies include oval shape and lack of central pallor of red cells, anisocytosis and poikilocytosis, teardrop cells, Howell-Jolly bodies, and hypersegmented neutrophils. Neither folate deficiency nor B_{12} deficiency is likely to have remarkable physical findings; however, both may cause patients to complain of a sore tongue.

204. The answer is D [Chapter 5, VII A 2 a (2)].
Hepatitis E can be transmitted by water or by the fecal–oral route. Hepatitis B, C, and D are all transmitted by parenteral or mucous membrane contact.

205. The answer is C [Chapter 7, IV C 2; Table 7-1].
Any woman with a diagnosis of low-grade squamous intraepithelial lesion (LSIL) should undergo colposcopic evaluation to determine the location and severity of the lesion. Conization is reserved for patients when the results of colposcopy are unsatisfactory or when cervical biopsies or endocervical curettage scrapings suggest more severe disease. Women with atypical squamous cells of uncertain significance (ASCUS) may be evaluated for presence of cervicitis. If found, it is appropriate to treat the cervicitis and repeat the Pap smear in

6–12 weeks. A young woman with LSIL and koilocytic changes only [associated with human papillomavirus (HPV) infection] may be followed with Pap smears and colposcopy every 6 months or more often.

206. The answer is C [Chapter 8 II C 3 b].
Ultrasound can detect multiple gestation early in the first trimester and is very accurate in detecting multiple gestation. Serum alpha-fetoprotein is elevated in multiple gestation but could not confirm the diagnosis of multiple pregnancy. Clinical confirmation by hearing 2 fetal heart tones is not accurate in verifying multiple gestation.

207. The answer is A [Chapter 9 III E 2 a].
Osteonecrosis of the femoral head is the correct diagnosis. In advanced stages, there may be collapse of the femoral head, joint space narrowing, and arthritis. Osteoarthritis is unlikely to be present in a young man unless it is post-traumatic arthritis from severe trauma in early childhood. Acute osteomyelitis may show only soft tissue changes. Chronic osteomyelitis usually has soft tissue involvement and periosteal involvement with radiographs showing new periosteal bone formation and indiscrete borders of bone lysis.

208. The answer is D [Chapter 10 IV B 1 a].
Hypercortisolism is most commonly caused by corticosteroid drugs used to treat other conditions. An adrenocorticotropic hormone (ACTH)-secreting pituitary tumor causes more than half of endogenous hypercortisolism and is the second most common cause of all hypercortisolism; adrenocortical tumors account for approximately a quarter of cases of endogenous disease; and ACTH-secreting neoplasms in organs other than the pituitary gland represent approximately 15% of cases of Cushing's syndrome.

209. The answer is C [Chapter 12 VII B].
The initial precursors of ADHD are apparent before the age of 7 years. These precursors include signs of impulsivity, inattentiveness, and/or hyperactivity. While the absence of these symptoms prior to the age of 7 years does not rule out the diagnosis, it does call it into question and suggests strongly that a situational factor precipitated the current behavior. This should be explored in depth prior to medicating the child.

210. The answer is C [Chapter 1, I A 4 b].
The history and physical findings point to a diagnosis of acute angle-closure glaucoma. Temporal arteritis would not affect the anterior chamber. Acute iritis causes headache and eye pain but, as with temporal arteritis, the anterior chamber would be normal. Acute keratitis includes pain with increased lacrimation but, again, the anterior chamber is spared.

211. **The answer is D** [Chapter 2 XII A 1, 2].
Upper respiratory tract infections (URIs) almost invariably are viral; rarely is a specific cause sought or found. However, some URIs are complicated by bacterial infections, many of which can be detected by Gram stain and cultures. Common causative agents are anerobic fusobacteria, *Bacteroides* species, and anaerobic and aerobic streptococci.

212. **The answer is C** [Chapter 3 XII D 1].
Positive inotropic therapy will strengthen ejection force and enhance cardiac output in the underactive heart in dilated cardiomyopathy, but would place increased strain on the already overworked heart in hypertrophic cardiomyopathy, restrictive cardiomyopathy, or infectious pericarditis.

213. **The answer is B** [Chapter 5, III D 3 a].
Crohn's disease classically presents with segmented areas of cobblestoning. Colon cancer will be seen as a mass, diverticulosis as outpouchings, and ulcerative colitis is continuous distal to proximal (see Table 5-2).

214. **The answer is D** [Chapter 6 VI B 1].
Because her laboratory findings are normal, the patient is unlikely to have renal failure. Pheochromocytoma (adrenal tumor) presents with the classic triad of headache, tachycardia, and diaphoresis. The distinction between essential hypertension and renal artery stenosis rests on the presence of a flank bruit, lack of family history, and early onset of hypertension.

215. **The answer is A** [Chapter 7, V A 1].
The definition of infertility is failure to conceive following 1 year of unprotected intercourse. (In a woman closer to the end of her reproductive years, it would be appropriate to begin an infertility evaluation sooner than 1 year, however.) If the patient does not become pregnant in the next 4 months, her husband should have a complete reproductive history taken. A complete physical examination for the husband could be performed at this time, or later, if semen analysis is abnormal. If his history and physical examination are normal, the first test in the couple's evaluation should be a semen analysis. If two analyses 2–3 months apart are abnormal, he should be evaluated further. The next step is determination of the presence or absence of ovulation by basal body temperature charting, ovulation prediction tests, or serum progesterone levels. Hysterosalpingogram and laparoscopy are appropriate as later steps in the evaluation of infertility.

216, 217, 218.
The answers are: 216-A [Chapter 8 III A 2 a], 217-A [Chapter 8 III B 1 a], and 218-A [Chapter 8 III B 4 b, C 1 b].

The first stage of labor is the stage of cervical dilatation to delivery. The second stage of labor ends with the delivery of the infant. The third stage of labor entails separation and expulsion of the placenta. The hour following delivery is sometimes called the fourth stage and is critical in assessing the mother's status after labor and delivery.

Abnormal labor, or dystocia, occurs when the cervix fails to dilate progressively over time and the fetus fails to descend. Dystocia is often associated with abnormal presentation or an inadequate pelvis. Maternal fatigue can be a factor in the progress of labor. Analgesia often helps relieve fatigue.

Not only is the patient experiencing dystocia, but the fetus is also showing signs of distress. Contractions usually decrease the blood flow to the placenta, which is poorly tolerated by the stressed or abnormal fetus, leading to hypoxia and concomitant relative bradycardia. Decelerations have been defined as a decline in fetal heart rate (FHR) of 15 beats per minute or lasting more than 15 seconds. The patient does not seem to be responding to labor augmentation with oxytocin. Forceps delivery or vacuum extraction is used only when the cervix is fully dilated and the head engaged. Because the fetus is showing signs of stress and labor is failing to progress, watchful waiting might further endanger the health of the fetus.

219. **The answer is C** [Chapter 10 IV B 2 a, b].
The triad of hypertension, diabetes, and obesity should alert the provider to the possibility of Cushing's syndrome. In this case, the wide (more than 1 cm) purple striae make the diagnosis more likely than a coincidence of the 3 conditions. To diagnose hypertension, 3 abnormal readings must be documented on separate occasions. Two fasting plasma glucose levels more than 140 or a random plasma glucose more than 200 mg/dl with the classic symptoms of polydipsia, polyuria, and polyphagia is required to diagnose non–insulin-dependent diabetes mellitus (NIDDM).

220. **The answer is B** [Chapter 12 III G].
A major depression, or major depressive disorder, must meet the criteria for a major depressive episode. The patient's bubbly personality, propensity to talk, and energy level are not consistent with that diagnosis and suggests the presence of a bipolar disorder. A diagnostic re-evaluation is called for because the health care provider making the initial diagnosis may not have been made aware of the manic content of the patient's problem. In fact, some patients with bipolar disorder prefer not to have their manic symptoms treated because they enjoy the productivity, energy level, and elation during the manic phase, fearing only the low that follows with the onset of the depressive phase.

221. **The answer is B** [Chapter 1, I A 1 d (3)].
Irrigation for a chemical burn is imperative to stop the action of the chemical on the tissues. Patching without irrigation could increase the damage to the eye. Fluorescein staining is used to evaluate for a corneal abrasion, and tonometry is used to measure the intraocular pressure.

222. **The answer is B** [Chapter 2 XIII B 1].
Complications of obstructive sleep apnea include cardiac abnormalities (e.g., sinus arrhythmias, extreme bradycardia, atrial flutter, ventricular tachycardia), excessive daytime sleepiness, morning headache, and slowed mentation. Arrhythmias occur during periods of marked desaturation, most commonly sinus arrest and other bradyarrhythmias, and sometimes atrial fibrillation. Pulmonary hypertension and cor pulmonale may be seen, and many patients also have systemic hypertension.

223. **The answer is C** [Chapter 3 XIII B 1].
Pericarditis is almost always a very painful condition in which the pain is relieved by sitting up and leaning forward. Pulmonary embolus would occur more quickly and probably not show signs of infection (fever and elevated white blood cell count). In pneumonia and restrictive cardiomyopathy, chest examination would reveal rales related to pulmonary congestion.

224. **The answer is A** [Chapter 5, V B 1 a].
Alcohol abuse is the most common cause of pancreatitis. Perforated ulcer and cholelithiasis are far less common causes, and diabetes mellitus may be a complication.

225. **The answer is C** [Chapter 6 VII C 3 b].
Pyelonephritis is due to an ascending infection of the urinary tract. It may present with any manifestations of lower urinary tract infection although urethral discharge is uncommon. Hematuria and pyuria may be present in any lower urinary tract infection as well as pyelonephritis. White blood cell casts will appear only as the result of inflammation in the parenchyma of the kidney due to pyelonephritis.

226. **The answer is B** [Chapter 7, VI B 3 a, 4 a].
The clinical suspicion of trichomoniasis would be confirmed by demonstration of unicellular flagellated organisms on saline wet prep. The recommended treatment is oral metronidazole for the patient and her sexual partner(s), with warnings about alcohol avoidance. Ketoconazole is indicated for vaginal yeast infection, clindamycin cream for bacterial vaginosis, and doxycycline for infection with *Chlamydia trachomatis*.

227. **The answer is B** [Chapter 8 III C 2].
The incidence of rupture with a classic or vertical incision is 12%. A low transverse uterine incision is usually used in a nonemergent cesarean section. It is attractive because of the decreased blood loss associated with its use and the ease of repair and has a relatively low incidence of rupture (1:200). Obviously it is also important to obtain obstetric and medical history on each patient as well.

228. **The answer is A** [Chapter 9 II E 1 b (1)].
Pathologic fracture is shown on the radiograph. Plain films show a lytic lesion with intralesional calcification typical of an enchondroma, the most common primary neoplasm of the hand skeleton. They are asymptomatic unless complicated by a pathologic fracture. Exostosis is a common lesion affecting any bone preformed in cartilage. It is a hard, immovable, smooth bone mass firmly fixed to the bone and is nontender unless traumatized. The callus associated with fractures occurs in the repair phase of healing, starting with granulation tissue and leading to a large quantity of woven bone. Chronic osteomyelitis is an infectious process present for longer than 3 months with radiographic evidence of a sclerotic fragment of dead bone (sequestrum) surrounded by periosteal new bone (involucrum).

229. **The answer is B** [Chapter 10 V A 2 a (4)].
Osteomalacia may be induced by phenytoin use. Phenytoin also decreases serum folate and increases the turnover of vitamin K. Sulfasalazine impairs folate absorption. The oral contraceptive may cause vitamin B_6 and folate deficiency and increase the need for other nutrients. Isoniazid is a vitamin B_6 antagonist.

230. **The answer is C** [Chapter 11 VII B 2 e (3)].
Compression of the posterior tibial nerve may cause these symptoms on the sole of the foot, whereas the lateral calf will be affected by pressure to the common peroneal nerve. On the thigh, a femoral neuropathy might account for symptoms anteromedially. In patients who are obese or in late pregnancy, it is common to directly compress the lateral femoral cutaneous nerve that innervates the lateral thigh.

231. **The answer is C** [Chapter 2 XII E 2 a].
Pulmonary tuberculosis in most adults is characterized by an increased cough (possibly with altered sputum), weight loss, hemoptysis, and fatigue. Night sweats and anorexia are also common. Cough, dyspnea, expiratory wheezing, and chest tightness are the hallmarks of obstructive lung disease. Congestive heart failure most often presents with dyspnea but also includes symptoms related to fluid overload (e.g., orthopnea, parox-

ysmal nocturnal dyspnea). Signs and symptoms of community-acquired pneumonia include cough, fever, chills, and rust-colored sputum.

232. The answer is A [Chapter 3 XIV A 1].
Streptococcus species, especially *S. viridans*, account for up to 60% of all cases of infective endocarditis although *Staphylococcus aureus* is the most common infectious agent seen in intravenous drug users. Enterococci account for 8%–10% of cases. *Mycoplasma* is not usually a cause of endocarditis.

233. The answer is D [Chapter 5, VII B 4 a].
The most crucial factor is removal of a causative agent, generally alcohol. Supportive therapy and treatment of resultant fluid overload are generally all that is indicated, with liver transplant used in selected cases. Salt and fluid are restricted, β-interferon has no role, and nodular regeneration is a part of the pathology rather than its resolution. Cirrhosis is irreversible.

234. The answer is C [Chapter 8 IV A 1 d].
Conferral of maternal antibodies is one of the many advantages of breastfeeding. Other advantages include convenience, decreased cost, enhanced maternal–infant bonding, and the easy digestibility of breast milk. Although both breast milk and formula contain sugar and fat, breast milk does not contain iron.

235. The answer is B [Chapter 9 II F 4 a].
At the present time, estrogen replacement therapy, adequate exercise, and adequate early calcium intake are the best preventative measures for osteoporosis. Alendronate 10 mg a day is an alternative treatment for women who are unable to use estrogen replacement therapy and is used in conjunction with calcium and vitamin D supplementation. Calcium 1500 mg a day, vitamin D supplementation, and calcitonin and etidronate 400 mg a day have also been used to treat osteoporosis.

236. The answer is B [Chapter 11 VIII A 3].
With evidence of elevated white blood cell (WBC) count, elevated protein, and decreased glucose, the diagnosis must be bacterial meningitis pending definitive studies. While the protein and glucose in all of these may be similar, only bacterial infection produces WBC counts with predominant polysegmented neutrophils. Viral and cryptococcal disease results in elevated lymphocytes, and the cerebrospinal fluid of Guillain-Barré syndrome patients is normal early in the disease.

237. The answer is C [Chapter 1 III E 3].
Localizing the site of bleeding is the most important step in managing epistaxis. Once the site is localized, measures to control the bleeding, such as insertion of

packing and compression of the mobile part of the nose, can be taken.

238. The answer is C [Chapter 2 III B 1, 2].
In bronchiectasis, patients often present with rales and digital clubbing. Emphysema may also present with rales but more likely during early inspiration and with decreased breath sounds. Chest tightness and wheezing is consistent with asthma and may also include intermittent occurrence of cough and breathlessness. A pleural effusion, when it is small, causes pleural pain (pleurisy) and a friction rub may be heard.

239. The answer is A [Chapter 3 XVI A 3].
While the male smoker with a lymphatic tumor and the 75-year-old man with chronic angina are at moderate risk, major surgery (especially abdominal or lower extremity) is the most significant risk factor for pulmonary embolus (PE). The sedentary woman with recent hip replacement is more at risk than the athletic woman who had knee surgery, because her case involves the predisposing factor of sedentary lifestyle. Active individuals are at minimum risk.

240. The answer is C [Chapter 5, V B 3 a].
Amylase is the most useful enzyme in making a diagnosis of early acute pancreatitis, although lipase may also be helpful. Other liver enzymes may be elevated but are not specific to pancreatitis.

241. The answer is D [Chapter 6 X A 4].
Stage D prostate cancer has distant metastases that can respond to hormonal interventions that decrease circulating testosterone. Chemotherapy has limited or no usefulness in prostate cancer. Tumor grading is relevant to prognosis, but staging is more important for treatment planning. Surgical treatment is effective in stage A and B disease and less effective in stage C disease.

242. The answer is C [Chapter 7, VI E 4 b].
This patient probably has pelvic inflammatory disease. Because she has an adnexal mass and is vomiting, she must be treated as an inpatient. Another appropriate antibiotic regimen is intravenous clindamycin 900 mg every 8 hours and intravenous or intramuscular gentamicin 2 mg/kg loading dose with 1.5 mg/kg every 8 hours. The history and physical findings are inconsistent with an ectopic pregnancy; however, a pregnancy test is advisable before starting treatment. Initiating treatment promptly may decrease her chances of requiring surgical treatment for tubo-ovarian abscess. Her boyfriend must also be evaluated and treated.

243. The answer is A [Chapter 8 IV B 4 b].
Pain and swelling are the classic signs and symptoms of deep venous thrombosis. The patient also gives a his-

tory of prolonged stasis. Thromboembolic events such as deep venous thrombosis are more than 5 times more common during pregnancy and in the postpartum period than in the general population. Deep venous thrombosis during pregnancy and in the postpartum period often involves the iliac veins and may present solely with fever. Superficial thrombophlebitis has palpable tender veins and the resulting thrombi are not likely to migrate. Dependent edema improves postpartum and would not be associated with pain. Hypertension is usually asymptomatic.

244. **The answer is D** [Chapter 9 III B 2].
Bone scans show increased rather than decreased uptake in the area of fracture. It is not uncommon for radiographic findings to be subtle initially and, because complications such as nonunion (10% or less) and osteonecrosis occur, close follow-up is required. Adults suspected of having a scaphoid fracture should be treated in a cast that includes the metacarpal phalanges joint of the thumb for 2 weeks, and then the radiographs should be repeated. A minimum of 12 weeks immobilization is required for healing.

245. **The answer is A** [Chapter 10 V A 3 b (4)].
Deafness is the most common neurologic finding in patients with Paget's disease of bone. In advanced disease, patients may progress to ataxia and paraplegia. A symmetrical peripheral neuropathy in a stocking-glove distribution is characteristic of diabetes and alcoholism.

246. **The answer is B** [Chapter 11 VIII B 4 a–b].
With a presumptive diagnosis of viral meningitis, only symptomatic therapy is required in most cases. Minor analgesics can be used for discomfort, but low-grade fevers may actually enhance the host response. If seizure activity is noted, anticonvulsants can be used to suppress, but are not necessary routinely. Careful analysis of the cerebrospinal fluid, coupled with other evidence of a viral disease, precludes the need for antibiotics.

247. **The answer is B** [Chapter 2 V A 3].
Pleural effusion is an abnormal accumulation of fluid in the pleural space. The mediastinum is usually shifted away from the side of the effusion. Blunting of the costophrenic angle may also be seen. A pneumothorax is an abnormal accumulation of air in the pleural space, and a radiograph of the chest demonstrates the presence of this pleural air. Flattened diaphragms and hyperinflation of the lungs are seen with advanced stages of emphysema. The chest radiograph in a patient with adult respiratory distress syndrome may be normal at first, but then tends to demonstrate peripheral infiltrates with air-filled bronchi, also called air bronchograms.

248. **The answer is A** [Chapter 3 XVII C 1].
Abdominal aneurysms are often painless, and only become apparent during routine abdominal examination. Ultrasound is a readily available, noninvasive technique to verify an abdominal aneurysm with minimal risk to the patient. While magnetic resonance imaging (MRI) or angiography may be subsequently employed for better visualization, for the initial examination they are more expensive and angiography poses increased risk. Electrocardiogram (ECG) is not useful in evaluating aortic aneurysms.

249. **The answer is A** [Chapter 5, III E 2 a].
A tender, palpable sigmoid colon might be found. Resonance is increased because of trapped air in the colon. Occult bleed is found in diseases causing inflammation or in cancers of the gut, whereas pain referred to the flanks might indicate obstruction.

250. **The answer is A** [Chapter 6 IV B 1 c].
Syndrome of inappropriate antidiuretic hormone (SIADH) presents with hyponatremia and increased urine osmolality and can be caused by exogenous production of ADH-secreting lung tumors. Nephrotic syndrome would present with proteinuria and edema. The lack of edema decreases the likelihood of congestive heart failure (CHF), and the increased or normal volume is not typical of hypothyroidism.

251. **The answer is B** [Chapter 8 II E 1 a, b].
Preterm delivery is a significant cause of fetal morbidity and mortality. Low birth weight infants born prematurely often have visual or hearing impairment, developmental delays, cerebral palsy, and lung disease. Multiple gestations account for 10% of all preterm births. Recurrence is common, occurring in 17%–37% of patients. Abruptio placentae has a high association with fetal death but is much less common than preterm delivery. Fetal complications related to gestational diabetes are related to large birth weights and subsequent difficult deliveries. Although pregnancy-induced hypertension (PIH) could eventually lead to fetal death, it is not the most common cause of neonatal death.

252. **The answer is C** [Chapter 9 III D 1].
In children, injuries to the ligamentous attachments of the bone are not likely to cause ligamentous tears. Injury to the ligamentous attachment of a bone is more likely to cause fracture of the physis, or growth plate, and, therefore, when injury occurs, suspect fracture.

253. **The answer is C** [Chapter 11 VIII C 1 a].
Previous otitis, sinusitis, or pharyngitis is commonly noted in brain abscess, with direct spread of the infection to the brain. Prior to surgery, closed head injury or distant soft tissue infection is rarely related.

254. **The answer is B** [Chapter 1, III C 3 c (2)].
Eighty to one hundred percent of patients with mononucleosis will develop a maculopapular rash when taking ampicillin. The true mechanism for this reaction is unknown.

255. **The answer is A** [Chapter 2 I A 1].
Chronic obstructive pulmonary disease (COPD) is a clinical pathophysiologic syndrome comprising three diseases: emphysema, chronic bronchitis, and asthma. The COPD disease state is characterized by the presence of airflow obstruction that is progressive. Bronchiectasis is a congenital or acquired disorder of the large bronchi, characterized by abnormal dilation and destruction of bronchial walls.

256. **The answer is D** [Chapter 3 XVII B 2].
Mitral stenosis causes enlargement of the pulmonary artery while thoracic aortic aneurysm causes enlargement of the aorta, either of which may put pressure on the nearby laryngeal nerve, causing impaired function of the larynx manifested as hoarseness. The other conditions listed do not cause enlargement of major vessels apposing the laryngeal nerve.

257. **The answer is A** [Chapter 5, V A 1 a, b, 2 e].
The patient should be checked for appendicitis, the most common surgical emergency causing abdominal pain in this age-group. The physician must check for the psoas sign by placing his hand on the patient's right knee and having him flex against pressure. The right lower quadrant should be examined last, not first. Murphy's sign indicates gallbladder or liver pathology. A musculoskeletal examination is not warranted.

258. **The answer is A** [Chapter 6 I B 1 b; Table 6-2].
Diabetes and hypertension are both very common causes of irreversible renal failure. Recent data suggest that diabetes is responsible for 30% of chronic renal failure and hypertension for 25%. Polycystic kidney disease is responsible for 4%–10%, benign prostatic hypertrophy (BPH) less than 5%, and glomerulonephritis less than 2%.

259. **The answer is C** [Chapter 8 III B 1 d].
Because prolonged ruptured membranes can lead to amnionitis, the patient will need to be delivered in a timely manner after this occurs. Braxton Hicks contractions are the weak, slow, and usually painless contractions that accompany the increasing uterine irritability of the last 6 weeks of pregnancy. "Bloody show," or loss of the mucous plug that protects the cervix to the end of pregnancy, does not necessitate delivery. Labor may or may not begin soon after this sign. Cervical dilatation is common late in pregnancy and does not require any action.

260. **The answer is B** [Chapter 2 II D 1, 2].
β-blockers may worsen bronchospasm and should be avoided in patients with asthma. Even ophthalmic β-blocker preparations may cause severe bronchospasm. For prophylaxis, inhaled corticosteroids are the most effective anti-inflammatory medication for asthma management. Cromolyn sodium may also be helpful in reducing inflammation. Theophylline and β_2-agonists are used during acute attacks of asthma.

261. **The answer is A** [Chapter 3 II A 3].
The most common cause of cardiogenic shock is myocardial infarction. Other causes include arrhythmias, heart failure, valvular or septal defects, hypertension, myocarditis, and myocardiopathies. Hypovolemic shock is associated with hemorrhage or with loss of plasma, fluids, or electrolytes. Tension pneumothorax, pericardial tamponade, obstructive valvular disease, and pulmonary problems are all potential causes of obstructive shock. Neurogenic shock causes changes in the distribution of blood volume.

262. **The answer is C** [Chapter 4, Table 4-4].
The Centers for Disease Control and Prevention and the Council of State and Territorial Epidemiologists have expanded AIDS surveillance case definition that is divided into 3 categories: (1) definitive AIDS diagnosis with or without laboratory evidence of HIV infection; (2) definitive AIDS diagnosis with laboratory evidence of HIV infection; and (3) presumptive AIDS diagnoses with laboratory evidence of HIV infection. *Pneumocystis carinii* pneumonia falls into the first category, Kaposi's sarcoma at any age and invasive cervical cancer into the second, and cytomegalovirus retinitis based on serial ophthalmic examinations in the third.

263. **The answer is B** [Chapter 5, III C 3 a].
A 72-hour fecal fat test is the "gold standard" for evaluation of malabsorption. The albumin test will detect protein deficiency, but it is nonspecific. The stool test for white blood cells (WBCs) will detect inflammation; and in malabsorption there will not likely be any cause visible on endoscopy.

264. **The answer is A** [Chapter 6 IV A 3].
Decreased ability to concentrate urine with increased sodium burden is evidence of nephrogenic or central diabetes insipidus. In hyperosmolar coma the glucose would be elevated. Hypertonic dehydration would result in an increased urine osmolality. Excess salt ingestion would result in increased urine sodium and urine osmolality.

265. **The answer is B** [Chapter 8 III B 2 d].
When the presenting part does not completely occupy the lower segment of the uterus, cord prolapse between

the maternal pelvis and the fetal presenting part can result. Manual elevation of the fetal presenting part should be maintained until delivery. Palpation of a fetal presenting part will be commensurate with corresponding fetal anatomy. Bimanual examination of the placenta would probably result in marked bleeding. Evidence of amniotic fluid is not consistent with intact membranes. The diagnosis of compound presentation, which occurs when a fetal extremity presents with the presenting part, is made by palpating the presenting parts. A cephalohematoma should also be palpable on examination. It would not extend into the vagina.

266. **The answer is D** [Chapter 9 I B].
Heel pain and Achilles tendinitis are not found in cases of rheumatoid arthritis, but may be found in Reiter's syndrome, psoriatic arthritis, and ankylosing spondylitis. Radiographs show osteopenia more commonly than the osteosclerosis, which is commonly found in osteoarthritis. When the diagnosis is confirmed, aggressive treatment with medications is required to stop or slow progression of destructive synovitis before permanent articular damage occurs.

267. **The answer is D** [Chapter 10 V B 4 b (3)].
Niacin is associated with reduced long-term mortality in patients with hyperlipidemias. The effect of probucol on total mortality is unknown. It reduces low-density lipoprotein (LDL) cholesterol by 10%–15%, but also reduces high-density lipoprotein (HDL) cholesterol. Gemfibrozil reduces coronary heart disease rates in middle-aged men with elevated total cholesterol, but in men with previous myocardial infarction, overall mortality increases. Cholestyramine reduces the incidence of coronary events, but does not affect total mortality significantly.

268. **The answer is A** [Chapter 11 IX A 4 a].
In a normally healthy person presenting with signs and symptoms of disc prolapse, initial management is conservative and includes bed rest and minor analgesics. The pain and signs, even if disc prolapse is seen on imaging studies, will usually resolve with sufficient rest. Aggressive physical therapy and referral are not necessary unless conservative measures fail.

269. **The answer is D** [Chapter 12 I B, C].
Any patient between 18 and 30 years of age, presenting with psychotic symptoms, should automatically have drug-induced psychosis ruled out. In the current case, track marks are found on the inside thigh, indicating that drugs are probably involved in the symptom picture presented. Whenever drugs or a medical condition is responsible for psychiatric symptomatology, the diagnosis of drug or medical condition–induced psychosis takes precedence over any other competing diagnosis.

270. **The answer is D** [Chapter 2 VIII A].
Sarcoidosis is a multiorgan disease of unknown cause characterized by granulomatous inflammation in affected organs. Pneumoconioses are chronic fibrotic lung diseases caused by the inhalation of coal dust; various inert, inorganic, or silicate dusts; or organic dusts. Three common forms of pneumoconioses include exposure to cotton dust (byssinosis), silica (sand, quartz), and asbestos fibers (construction materials).

271. **The answer is B** [Chapter 3 V A 2].
Risk factors for atherosclerotic cardiovascular disease include male sex, increasing age, cigarette smoking, and elevated (more than 200 mg/dl) cholesterol levels. Men are affected approximately 4 times as often as women until menopause. Women who do not receive hormone replacement approach the same risk as men by age 70.

272. **The answer is A** [Chapter 5, III C 4].
A gluten-free diet is prescribed for celiac disease. Tetracycline will treat malabsorption from bacterial overgrowth, and pancrease is used to treat pancreatic insufficiency. Corticosteroids are not used in treatment of malabsorption.

273. **The answer is C** [Chapter 6 XI A 2, 3].
Most cases of impotence have a psychological component but the etiology is organic. Particularly important in evaluating cases in which the etiology is uncertain is the examination for nocturnal penile tumescence. Absence of erections during sleep strongly suggests, but does not necessarily prove, an organic basis. Although critical to diagnosis and treatment, information about medical and sexual history cannot distinguish between an organic and psychogenic etiology. The same holds true for evaluation of the arterial and venous vasculature, as well as the results of direct injection of vasoactive substances into the penis.

274. **The answer is D** [Chapter 7, VII B 1 a, b].
Most women with breast cancer have no identifiable risk factors other than increasing age and female sex. About 5% seem to have a genetic susceptibility to the disease. In addition to delayed childbearing, factors associated with breast cancer include nulliparity, early menarche and late menopause, long-term estrogen exposure, and radiation exposure.

275. **The answer is D** [Chapter 8 II F 3].
The young age of this patient is a risk factor for pregnancy-induced hypertension (PIH). Swelling in the upper extremities is a significant symptom for this dis-

order. Random elevated urinary protein is of limited value, but a 24-hour urine measurement of urinary protein greater than 300 mg/24 hours may indicate the need for delivery. The complete blood cell count (CBC) and liver function studies would be necessary to exclude HELLP syndrome (hemolytic anemia, elevated liver enzymes, and low platelets). The urinary excretion of protein would probably not be from an infection in this case.

276 through 279.

The answers are: 276-D [Chapter 9 II E 1 b (1)]; **277-B, 278-A, 279-C** [Chapter 9 II E 1 b (2)].

Enchondroma is the most destructive benign lesion of the bone. It usually occurs in the proximal phalanx.

A mucous cyst refers to a tumor located on the dorsal, distal interphalangeal joint. These cysts are actually ganglions originating in the distal interphalangeal joint, frequently associated with Heberden's nodes and osteophytes.

A ganglion is a soft, nontender, transilluminant tumor, which most commonly occurs as a dorsal hand mass over the scapholunate ligament but may occur elsewhere.

A lipoma is a soft, nontender, mobile tumor. It is a common tumor and may occur at many locations in the body. It consists of mature fat.

280. The answer is C [Chapter 11 IX C 4].
Acyclovir, as well as corticosteroids, are helpful in reducing the duration and severity of episodes of zoster. Only steroids, however, can lessen the risk of postherpetic neuralgia if utilized during the acute phase. Neither steroids nor the antivirals will be useful in the setting of the chronic pain syndrome seen after the acute phase.

281. The answer is C [Chapter 12 II D 1 c].
In an almost identical situation to the case described in the question, a therapist was told by his patient at the University of California counseling center that he was going to kill his girlfriend. The therapist requested and was denied permission from his supervisor to warn the intended victim. The therapist's patient made good on his threat and killed his intended victim. The victim's parents sued the University for negligence and won. The Tarasoff ruling has, after surviving appeal, become the accepted practice for all health care practitioners and requires that patient–practitioner confidentiality be breached when a credible threat has been made against someone's life. The practitioner is obligated to report the threat to the intended victim, the authorities, or both.

282. The answer is A [Chapter 1, II C 1 c].
Fungal infections are rarely a cause of otitis externa. When present, the infections caused by fungi are less acute than those caused by other organisms.

283. The answer is D [Chapter 2 VIII D].
Treatment for pneumoconioses is primarily supportive and the patient should be removed from the offensive environment. Corticosteroid treatment may be helpful for acute attacks. Smoking cessation is important for all patients with occupational lung disease but especially with asbestosis because it interferes with short asbestos fiber clearance from the lung. As the disease does not have an infectious etiology, antibiotics would be used only with superimposed infection.

284. The answer is D [Chapter 3 VII B 1, 2].
Myocardial infarction usually causes prolonged, severe anterior chest pain. Patients may also present with diaphoresis, weakness, anxiety, restlessness, syncope, dyspnea, nausea, and vomiting. The pain of costochondritis is more of local tenderness. Patients may fear taking a deep breath. The pain of reflux esophagitis may mimic that of myocardial infarction; however, the restlessness and dyspnea are more typical of infarction. The pain of pulmonary embolism (PE) is likely to be pleuritic, rather than aching. However, a major embolism will cause dyspnea, with or without central chest pain. Electrocardiogram (ECG) changes help differentiate infarction and PE.

285. The answer is D [Chapter 5, IV B 2 a].
Diverticulosis, which classically presents with left-sided, sudden-onset abdominal pain. Appendicitis and Crohn's occur in a younger population, and colon cancer is generally painless.

286. The answer is D [Chapter 6 XI A 4].
Although sex therapy may have some benefit, it will not restore erectile function in diabetic men. Testosterone is effective in men with an androgen deficiency. Finasteride is effective in men with vascular disease. Diabetes, however, affects vascular, neurologic, and endocrine function and can be most effectively treated with penile prostheses.

287 through 290.

The answers are: 287-A, 288-D, 289-C, 290-C [Chapter 8 I B 3 b, c, d].

The triple marker serum screening test, alpha-fetoprotein 3 (AFP 3), is offered universally to pregnant women as a screen for both neural tube defects and Down syndrome. Amniocentesis and chorionic villus sampling (CVS) are reserved for either those at high risk for congenital birth defects or those willing to undergo a higher risk procedure for prenatal diagnosis. All three tests can be used to screen for Down syndrome. CVS cannot be used to check for neural tube defects, and it is associated with limb defects and a higher risk of miscarriage than amniocentesis. Results from CVS can be made available earlier in pregnancy.

291. **The answer is C** [Chapter 10 V B 4 a (4)].
Hypothyroidism is associated with increased total cholesterol, whereas cirrhosis is associated with decreased total cholesterol. Alcohol use is associated with increased high-density lipoprotein (HDL) cholesterol and increased triglycerides.

292. **The answer is D** [Chapter 11 X A 2 a–b].
Myasthenia is characterized by the history of fluctuating symptoms, with weakness and fatigability improving after rest. Amyotrophic lateral sclerosis runs a progressive course and is not characterized by remission and relapse. Intracranial lesions and vascular occlusion would not present such a variable picture either.

293. **The answer is A** [Chapter 12 VIII C].
While both physical and cognitive deterioration is to be expected with advancing age, the bruising and the conflicting accounts of how it occurred are characteristic of abuse. Also characteristic of abuse is the observation that Mr. Jones has become withdrawn and the caregivers have taken over the majority of the communication for him. It would be appropriate for the practitioner to meet with the caregivers to discuss treatment options while a member of the clinic staff engaged Mr. Jones in conversation to see if he opened up while not in the presence of his daughters.

294. **The answer is B** [Chapter 1, II B 1 c].
Pseudomonas aeruginosa is not commonly seen in otitis externa. *Streptococcus pneumoniae*, *Haemophilus influenzae*, and *Moraxella catarrhalis* are among the most common pathogens in otitis media.

295. **The answer is A** [Chapter 2 XIII D].
Hypnotics exacerbate and contribute to the central suppression of respiration and airway obstruction. Obstructive sleep apnea, also called pickwickian syndrome, is treated by relieving upper airway obstruction, using continuous positive airway pressure (CPAP), uvulopalatopharyngoplasty, or tracheostomy. Central sleep apnea is treated by reversing the cardiac or neurologic cause or by giving supportive therapy.

296. **The answer is A** [Chapter 3 VII C 1].
The ST segment is usually elevated in the classic electrocardiogram (ECG) tracing for a patient with myocardial infarction, although the segment may be depressed. A shortened QT interval is characteristic of hypercalcemia. U waves are associated with hypokalemia. Widened QRS complexes when not preceded by a P wave indicate a premature ventricular contraction.

297. **The answer is A** [Chapter 4, I D 3].
As an African-American, this child is at risk for sickle cell anemia (SS disease). People of Middle Eastern, North African, Mediterranean, and East Indian de-

scent are also at risk. Patients with sickle cell disease usually are identified in their childhood or teenage years. The preferred test for demonstration of hemoglobin S in red cells is hemoglobin electrophoresis. The pain associated with the vaso-occlusive crises in this disorder may develop at more than one site. Bone pain may be caused by ischemia of the marrow. Abdominal pain may be associated with splenic or hepatic infarction. Rapid diagnosis is essential because a "sequestration crisis" (pooling of red cells in the spleen or liver) may be life-threatening in childhood.

298. **The answer is C** [Chapter 5, IV F 3 a].
Approximately 65% of cancer of the colon and rectum is within reach of the flexible sigmoidoscope. Fiberoptic colonoscopy should be done whenever cancer is suspected in any portion of the bowel and in every patient with symptoms referable to the colon. Elevation of carcinoembryonic antigen (CEA) is not specifically associated with colorectal cancer, but levels are high in 70% of patients. If CEA is high preoperatively and low after removal of a colonic tumor, monitoring CEA may help to detect recurrence. Testing of the stool for occult blood is advised as part of screening and high-risk surveillance programs but is not specific. Barium should not be given orally when an obstructing colonic lesion is suspected, because resorption of water from the barium suspension by the colon may precipitate barium sulfate and produce complete large-bowel obstruction.

299. **The answer is B** [Chapter 6 XI E 2].
A "bag of worms" textured mass on the left side is classic for varicocele. A hydrocele is a painless transilluminable mass; although it typically is not reducible, it may wax and wane in size. An inguinal hernia is characterized by a nontender mass that occasionally goes away but will return, especially after a Valsalva maneuver. A strangulated hernia is characterized by a nonreducible mass, fever, and diffuse abdominal tenderness.

300. **The answer is D** [Chapter 7, IV A 1, 2].
Cervical dysplasia and neoplasia are linked to human papillomavirus infection, especially types 16 and 18. In addition to early age at first intercourse and cigarette smoking, other risk factors include multiple sexual partners or a sexual partner who has multiple partners, low socioeconomic status, and African-American race.

301. **The answer is B** [Chapter 10 VI B 2 b].
Glossitis, cheilosis, and sore mouth are associated with various vitamin B deficiencies. Vitamin A deficiency is associated with areflexia, gait problems, and decreased proprioception and vibratory sense. Vitamin K deficiency is associated with bleeding diatheses. Vita-

min C may also be associated with bleeding abnormalities in addition to poor wound healing and anemia. Vitamin E deficiency is fairly rare and is not associated with a distinct clinical syndrome.

302. The answer is B [Chapter 11 X A 4 a].
Cholinesterase inhibitors such as pyridostigmine produce an improvement in strength in affected muscles and are the mainstay of therapy. Edrophonium is limited to injectable use and, because it is very short-acting, is used for diagnostic purposes only. Corticosteroids and immunosuppressive agents are both limited to refractory cases where cholinesterase inhibitors are inadequate.

303. The answer is B [Chapter 12 III F 4].
A patient with a major depressive episode often lacks the psychic energy to make a suicide attempt. As they start to show improvement, they develop that energy and must be monitored for both suicide ideation as well as intent. The best course of action is to limit the amount of medication prescribed and use the visits for refills to monitor progress.

304. The answer is A [Chapter 1, I A 1 b (3)].
Because of the possibility of further damage to the orbit, a Schiøtz tonometer would not be utilized. A radiograph might be helpful to identify a foreign body that was not visible to the naked eye. It is almost always safe to give tetanus prophylaxis and antibiotics.

305, 306, 307, 308, 309.

The answers are: 305-E, 306-C, 307-A, 308-B, 309-D [Chapter 2 XII E 4; Table 2-1].

Treatment of pulmonary tuberculosis (TB) infection in children consists of isoniazid 10 mg/kg/d, not to exceed 300 mg every day and rifampin 15 mg/kg/d, not to exceed 600 mg for 12 months; for extrapulmonary infection in this age-group, streptomycin 20 mg/kg/d or ethambutol 15 mg/kg/d is added. Patients with latent infection, but who are not HIV infected, receive the same regimen of isoniazid 300 mg/d for 6–12 months; HIV-infected patients receive the therapy for one full year. A 4-drug regimen is needed during the initial phase (months 1 and 2) for active infection in adults; the continuation phase (months 3 through 6) includes isoniazid and rifampin. For meningeal or miliary (disseminated) tuberculosis, ethambutol hydrochloride 25 mg/kg/d (months 1 and 2) not to exceed 2.5 g should be added. This dosage should then be decreased to 15 mg/kg/d at 3 or more months. Treatment should be continued for a minimum of 9 months and at least 6 months after culture conversion is noted by 3 negative cultures. For suspected drug-resistant tuberculosis, a 4- or 5-drug regimen should be used and reflect known local drug resistance patterns. The 5th drug used should be streptomycin 15 mg/kg/d not to exceed 1 g/d. Final treatment regimen should be based on final sensitivity results. If isoniazid resistance is demonstrated, rifampin and ethambutol should be given for at least 12 months.

310. The answer is B [Chapter 3 VII B 8].
Dressler's syndrome is also known as postmyocardial infarction syndrome. Patients may also have a pericardial or pleural effusion. Wolff-Parkinson-White syndrome represents an anomalous electrical pathway in the heart, with electrocardiogram (ECG) changes showing a shortened PR interval, a prolonged QRS, and a delta wave. Adams-Stoke syndrome involves episodic cardiac arrest and syncope, the main clinical manifestation of severe heart block. Bradbury-Eggleston syndrome is one of postural hypotension without tachycardia, found primarily in older males, due to impaired peripheral vasoconstriction.

311. The answer is B [Chapter 5, VIII C 3 a, b].
Hypertrophic pyloric stenosis develops within the first 4–6 weeks of life. The presenting symptoms are projectile vomiting without bile and a movable "olive" mass. Hirschsprung's disease will present with constipation or obstipation, vomiting, and failure to thrive. Esophageal atresia and diaphragmatic hernia will be discovered at birth.

312. The answer is C [Chapter 6 XI H 3].
The analysis of the sperm for concentration and mobility should guide the remainder of the evaluation. Serum testosterone may provide other information about testicular function and endocrinologic disorders in the face of low sperm counts. Serum glucose helps evaluate for diabetes and scrotal ultrasound may detect a varicocele, but both are only useful after a sperm analysis has been completed.

313. The answer is B [Chapter 7, IV C 1].
The American Cancer Society with consensus of the American Medical Association, the National Cancer Institute, the American Nurses' Association, the American Academy of Family Physicians, the American Medical Women's Association, and the American College of Obstetricians and Gynecologists recommend that Pap smear screening should begin when a woman becomes sexually active or reaches the age of 18, whichever comes first. Thereafter, annual screenings should be continued; however, after 3 or more Paps have been normal, the study may be performed less often if recommended by the woman's physician. Older women should continue to have Pap smears at intervals determined in consultation with the physician.

314 through 317.

The answers are: 314-D, 315-D, 316-A, 317-A [Chapter 8 II H, I].

Both placenta previa and abruptio placentae are associated with the risk factors of advanced age, smoking, and high parity. Smoking is a significant risk factor for many problems in pregnancy, including low birth weight, mental retardation, and placental problems such as abruptio placentae and placenta previa. To preserve both maternal and fetal health, cesarean section is often the preferred route of delivery with placental problems. The painless bleeding that is the hallmark of placenta previa is in contrast to the frequently painful, irritable uterus associated with abruptio placentae. Ultrasound is very accurate in diagnosing the low lying placenta, whereas abruptio placentae is a clinical diagnosis.

318 through 321.

The answers are: 318-A, 319-B, 320-C, 321-D.

Osteoporosis has thin cortices and fine medullary trabecula. Osteoarthritis shows narrowing cartilage, reactive sclerosis of subchondral bone cortex, osteophytic spurring along joint margins, and intraosseous subchondral cysts. Metastatic bone lesions are usually lytic although adenocarcinoma of the breast, prostate, and lymphoma can show a blastic appearance. Osteosarcoma is a primary bone malignancy showing infiltration, permeation, and violation of the anatomic borders.

322. The answer is A [Chapter 10 VI B 1 b (1)].

Alcoholism is the most common cause of thiamine deficiency in the United States. Lack of intrinsic factor is a cause of pernicious anemia, associated with B_{12} deficiency. Biliary atresia causes vitamin E deficiency in children. Fat malabsorption syndromes cause deficiencies of the fat-soluble vitamins A, D, E, and K.

323. The answer is A [Chapter 11 XI B 2 c].

Brown-Séquard's syndrome results from a unilateral cord lesion with resulting ipsilateral motor and proprioceptive impairment, and contralateral impairment of pain and temperature. A complete transection of the cord produces flaccid paralysis and loss of all distal sensation, whereas a central cord lesion spares the posterior column functions below the lesion.

324. The answer is D [Chapter 12 X].

Uncomplicated bereavement is a normal response to a major loss. The shock, confusion, and symptoms that are characteristic of depression will not be resolved by medicating the patient. Instead, social contact and reassurance are indicated.

325. The answer is D [Chapter 3 VIII A 1 a (3)].

All cyanotic congenital heart anomalies involve right-to-left shunts. The so-called hypoplastic left heart syndrome is actually a group of defects with an abnormally small left ventricle and normally placed great vessels. All the other defects are classified as noncyanotic types.

326. The answer is A [Chapter 5, IV C 1; Table 5-2].

Toxic megacolon is a complication of ulcerative colitis. Fistulas are a complication of Crohn's. Malabsorption and hemorrhoids are unrelated to ulcerative colitis.

327. The answer is B [Chapter 6 XI F 4].

Seminomatous tumors are known to be radiosensitive, including those in the abdominal and mediastinal lymphatics as well as the left supraclavicular area, depending on staging. Orchiectomy is always performed in testicular cancer for diagnostic and therapeutic reasons, but further therapy is usually necessary. Chemotherapy with cisplatin, alone or in combination with other agents, may cause regression and control of metastatic, nonseminomatous tumors. Stage I disease limited to the testis in nonseminomatous tumors can be treated with retroperitoneal lymph node dissection or rigorous surveillance without surgery or chemotherapy.

328 through 331.

The answers are 328-A, 329-B, 330-A, 331-B [Chapter 8 II C 1 c].

Two thirds of twins are dizygotic or fraternal and have been formed by the fertilization of two ovum. The incidence of dizygotic twins is increased in those taking fertility drugs, with increased weight and height, and is greater among the black race. Monozygotic twins are those formed from the fertilization of one egg and occur randomly.

332. The answer is D [Chapter 1, III B 1 b (1)].

A complete blood cell count (CBC) will not be helpful in the diagnosis of allergic rhinitis. There is a low yield of abnormalities. Nasal smears will show more than 10% eosinophils. Skin testing would be indicated if the patient complained of seasonal problems. Radioallergosorbent testing (RAST) is expensive but gives a semiquantitative measurement of immunoglobulin E (IgE).

333. The answer is A [Chapter 3 VIII A 1 a (1)].

The description is that of the 4 problems found in the tetralogy of Fallot. In patent ductus arteriosus, the channel in the heart to the aorta that bypasses the lungs and allows placental gas exchange during fetal life remains open following birth. Transposition of the great arteries most commonly involves reversal of the aorta and pulmonary artery. Coarctation of the aorta usually involves narrowing in the proximal thoracic aorta.

334. **The answer is C** [Chapter 5, I D 2 c].
Patients demonstrate elevated basal-state gastrin levels that do not increase 1 hour after a meal. To confirm the diagnosis, patients are given 2 units/kg secretin intravenously, after which gastrin levels increase (rather than decline) by 200 units and increase markedly (rather than modestly) after intravenous calcium administration. Angiography may be helpful because gastrin-secreting tumors may be highly vascular. Endoscopy may be helpful in localizing the tumor after the diagnosis has been established.

335. **The answer is D** [Chapter 6 XI G 2 d].
The patient presents with the first sign of syphilitic chancre after exposure to risky, unprotected sexual intercourse. Confirmatory serologic testing, urethral cultures, and HIV testing should be done, but treatment should not be delayed because untreated syphilis and gonorrhea can be very serious. As long as the patient is penicillin-tolerant, therapy with benzathine penicillin, ceftriaxone, and azithromycin has few risks. The azithromycin covers the chlamydial infection that is usually concurrent. Acyclovir is appropriate therapy for genital herpes, and lesions frequently develop 4–7 days after contact. Primary lesions are more painful, prolonged, and widespread than recurrent outbreaks. The patient may also experience generalized malaise and fever and inguinal lymphadenopathy.

336 through 339.
The answers are: 336-D [Chapter 9 I C 2 b (2)]; **337-C** [Chapter 9 I C 3 a (1)], b (1)]; **338-A** [Chapter 9 I F 2 b]; **339-B** [Chapter 9 I D 2 a].
Irregularity and pitting of the nail is a clue to diagnosing psoriatic arthritis.
Reiter's syndrome has a triad of arthritis, urethritis, and conjunctivitis usually presenting initially with urethritis and symmetric arthritis, and possibly a "painful heel."
Systemic lupus erythematosus (SLE) is a nonerosive arthritis involving two or more peripheral joints. SLE primarily involves the small joints of the hands, wrists, and knees.
First metatarsal phalangeal joint involvement is a common initial presentation of gout. Gout will probably affect this joint either at initial presentation or at some time in the patient's lifetime.

340. **The answer is B** [Chapter 1, I D 1 b].
Chronic subdural hematoma does not cause papilledema. Only an acute subdural hematoma will

show papilledema. Malignant hypertension and hemorrhagic stroke will also have papilledema as a manifestation.

341. **The answer is D** [Chapter 3 XIV A 2].
Tricuspid valve involvement is classic in infective endocarditis in intravenous drug users. The presentation of endocarditis is similar for all sites, except that right-sided endocarditis rarely causes a murmur, whereas left-sided endocarditis usually does. The left-sided valves (i.e., the aortic and mitral valves) are more often infected than the right-sided valves. This occurs because the left-sided valves are more often abnormal or damaged, providing a nidus for bloodborne organisms. Intravenous drug users are most often infected with *Staphylococcus aureus*, spread from the skin, nose, or throat. They are also at risk for fungal and gram-negative infections.

342. **The answer is B** [Chapter 5, I A 1 c].
Reflux esophagitis causes erosion that may lead to Barrett's esophagitis, in which metaplastic columnar epithelium replaces the normal squamous epithelium, predisposing to esophageal cancer. Zenker's diverticulum is an outpouching of the posterior hypopharynx; achalasia is a motor disorder; and esophageal atresia is a congenital disorder diagnosed at birth.

343. **The answer is A** [Chapter 11 XII A 1].
Gliomas account for approximately 50%, or half, of all primary central nervous system tumors, and astrocytomas account for 65%–70% of those. Meningiomas are usually benign and account for approximately 13%–18% of intracranial tumors. Pituitary adenomas and neurofibromas are less common.

344. **The answer is A** [Chapter 3 XV A 2 a].
The first symptom of peripheral arterial disease (arterial insufficiency) is lower leg pain exacerbated by exercise and relieved by rest. Venous insufficiency is characterized by itching, dull pain with standing, skin changes, and ulceration medial or anterior to the ankle. Varicose veins may be asymptomatic or associated with aching and fatigue. Deep venous thrombosis presents with swelling, heat, redness, and a positive Homan's sign.

345. **The answer is C** [Chapter 5, III A 4 a].
Pancreatic insufficiency can cause a secretory diarrhea. *Clostridium difficile* and ulcerative colitis both cause inflammation in the colon, and *Salmonella* is an invasive organism causing inflammation (see Table 5-1).

346. **The answer is D** [Chapter 11 XII B 3 a–e].
The temporal lobe is usually associated with seizures and a number of emotional and behavioral changes

when affected. Sensory disturbances and impaired stereognosis are associated with parietal lobe lesions, whereas visual field defects are typically related to lesions of the occipital lobe. Brain stem and cerebellar lesions can be expected to produce problems with balance and coordination.

347. The answer is D [Chapter 10 II A 2 a, b, c].
Tetany is pathognomonic of hypocalcemia. Chvostek's sign, contraction of the facial muscles in response to tapping on the facial nerve anterior to the parotid gland, can also be found in 10% of people with normal serum calcium. Trousseau's sign, carpopedal spasm elicited by compressing the nerves in the upper arm with a blood pressure cuff inflated above the systolic pressure for 3 minutes, is an important finding in hypocalcemia. Depressed deep tendon reflexes are found in hypercalcemia.

348. The answer is C [Chapter 3 IV B 2, 4].
Paroxysmal nocturnal dyspnea is a hallmark of congestive heart failure. Patients may also have peripheral edema. This patient has a predisposing risk factor for congestive heart failure (CHF), poorly controlled hypertension. Asthma presents with wheezing, dyspnea, and a cough, but is unlikely to cause peripheral edema, whereas a pulmonary embolus is likely to present with pleuritic chest pain and dyspnea. Heart disease due to atherosclerosis is a leading cause of CHF.

349. The answer is B [Chapter 11 XIII D 2].
Sleep apnea episodes are the result of multiple breath-holding events with associated oxygen desaturation in the blood. By maintaining an open airway throughout the night, desaturation does not take place and sleep is more efficient. Hypnotics are used for sleep onset problems, while clonazepam is effective in patients whose nocturnal myoclonus prevents proper sleep staging and resultant daytime sleepiness. Stimulants may be helpful for narcolepsy, but have no role in the setting of sleep apnea.

350. The answer is B [Chapter 10 III B 3 a, b].
Glycosylated hemoglobin (hemoglobin A_{1C}) is high in people with chronic hyperglycemia. It is an appropriate test of metabolic control during the previous 2–3 months. It is only 85% sensitive in detecting diabetes. The other choices are all valid tests for detecting diabetes.

351. The answer is D [Chapter 3 III D 3 d].
Clonidine is a central sympatholytic (or sympathoplegic) agent. It reduces sympathetic tone and increases parasympathetic tone, resulting in lowered blood pressure and slowing of the heart rate. Examples of β-blockers include propranolol and atenolol.

352. The answer is D [Chapter 11 VII A 4 a–d].
Gaining better control of the diabetes may be helpful in reducing the symptoms. Additionally, symptomatic treatment for pain with a tricyclic is helpful in conjunction with detailed patient education regarding footwear, foot hygiene and nail care, and prevention of thermal injury. Corticosteroids are contraindicated and would complicate diabetes management. Propranolol lowers blood pressure by decreasing cardiac output, while other β-blockers may either decrease cardiac output or reduce peripheral resistance. Diltiazem, verapamil, and nifedipine are all calcium channel blockers. These agents dilate peripheral arterioles and reduce blood pressure, in addition to having antianginal and antiarrhythmic effects. The α-adrenergic antagonists (e.g., prazosin) reduce hypertension by blocking α_1 receptors in arterioles and venules.

353. The answer is D [Chapter 11 XI A 1 d].
The degree of amnesia seen following head injury as well as the time spent unconscious are directly related to the severity of injury. Prognosis also hinges on the site of the injury and the severity of the injury.

354. The answer is C [Chapter 3 XIII D 2].
Inflammatory pericarditis may be appropriately treated with steroidal or nonsteroidal anti-inflammatory agents. Pericardiocentesis is necessary to relieve fluid accumulation in pericardial tamponade with hemodynamic compromise. An infectious pericarditis must be treated with antibiotics; the choice of antibiotic agent is based on blood and pericardial fluid culture. Diuretics are the mainstay of treatment for congestive heart failure and some hypertension.

355. The answer is C [Chapter 11 XIII B 1].
Depression is typically tied to complaints of early morning awakening, whereas smoking in excess of 1 pack per day and alcohol abuse are frequently tied to complaints of multiple nighttime awakenings. A medical history of uremia, asthma, or hypothyroidism is often seen in insomnia, but diabetes has little or no relation.

356. The answer is B [Chapter 3 XV C 4 c].
The current recommended treatment for deep venous thrombosis (DVT) is anticoagulation for a total of approximately 3 months, beginning with 7–10 days of heparin, followed by coumadin, both in maximal doses. The coumadin and heparin treatments should overlap for 3–5 days. For recurrent episodes of DVT, coumadin is often continued for 6 months. None of the other regimens is accepted practice.

357. The answer is A [Chapter 11 VI B 2 a–f].
The classic early sign of Parkinson's is the resting tremor that typically disappears with voluntary activ-

ity. Accompanied by slow movements (bradykinesia), rigidity noted with passive range of motion testing, and postural instability, they constitute the essentials of diagnosis for the disease.

358. **The answer is C** [Chapter 3 VII D 1].
To be effective, thrombolytic therapy [whether with tissue plasminogen activator (TPA), streptokinase, or urokinase] must be initiated within 12 hours of onset of chest pain. All the other treatments are appropriate in caring for the patient with infarction.

359, 360, 361, 362, 363.
The answers are: 359-E, 360-C, 361-B, 362-A, 363-D [Chapter 1 III C 3, D 2; Chapter 2 XII C 2].
Mononucleosis is an acute infectious disease caused by the Epstein-Barr virus and characterized by fever, malaise, sore throat, and lymphadenopathy. Patients generally present with nonspecific complaints that also include anorexia and headache. Treatment is directed at providing symptomatic relief. Acute epiglottitis is a life-threatening infection in which early recognition is key to successful management. Epiglot-

titis usually affects young children, but more than 10% of patients are adults. The most common pathogen is *Haemophilus influenzae* type b. The sequelae of streptococcal pharyngitis include suppurative complications from local extension of infection, and nonsuppurative complications (e.g., scarlet fever, acute rheumatic fever, and acute glomerulonephritis). Probably more than 80% of cases of pharyngitis are caused by the same viruses that cause the common cold. The patient does not require antibiotics; supportive care is sufficient. Patients with tracheobronchitis characteristically have an incessant cough. Most cases of tracheobronchitis are caused by viruses. Again, treatment is based on symptomatic relief.

364. **The answer is A** [Chapter 5, I A 4 b (5)].
Nitrates decrease lower esophageal sphincter (LES) pressure and should be avoided, although they are used in the treatment of diffuse esophageal spasm. Cisapride increases the reflux barrier by increasing LES tone. Decreasing gastric acid effects may be accomplished by the administration of histamine$_2$-receptor antagonists (cimetidine) and a proton pump inhibitor such as omeprazole.

Index